Clinical Urology Illustrated

R.B. Brown
MB, BS(Melb.), FRACS, FRCS, FACS,
Head, Urology Unit, Alfred Hospital, Melbourne,
Consultant Urologist, Royal Australian Navy

with foreword by
Willard E. Goodwin, MD,
Professor Surgery/Urology,
University of California, Los Angeles

With 348 Illustrations —
including line drawings, x-rays
and clinical photographs

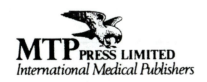
MTPPRESS LIMITED
International Medical Publishers

Falcon House, Cable Street,
Lancaster, Lancashire, LA1 1PE, UK

Clinical Urology Illustrated

Published in UK. Europe and Middle East
by MTP Press Limited
Falcon House
Lancaster
England

First printing
ISBN 978-94-009-8098-3   ISBN 978-94-009-8096-9 (eBook)
DOI 10.1007/978-94-009-8096-9

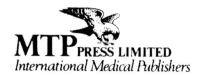

MTPPRESS LIMITED
International Medical Publishers

Falcon House, Cable Street,
Lancaster, Lancashire, LA1 1PE, UK

Dedication

This book is dedicated to my teachers and my colleagues: to Mr J.B. Somerset, Mr D.B. Duffy, Mr W.H. Graham, the late Mr J.D. Ferguson, Professor W.E. Goodwin and Professor J.J. Kaufman in particular; to my present and past associates at the Alfred Hospital, especially Mr David Kennedy, Mr Don MacDonald, Mr Douglas Druitt, Mr David Westmore, Mr Alex Wood and Mr David Yoffa — with whom many discussions have enabled me to express the views in this book while still appreciating that there are often two or more satisfactory ways of dealing with the same problem.

Foreword

In this precise and authoritative urological text Mr Ronald Brown and his associates have scored two firsts. In its emphasis throughout on the importance of clinical assessment, history taking and physical examination, together with its wealth of illustrations, it offers a unique view of genitourinary medicine; and it is the first clinical urology text to be written by an Australian.

The authors' approach to their subject is ideal for students and physicians confronted with patients with genitourinary problems. The text is concise, the references valuable and the index comprehensive. I was particularly interested in the chapter on Paediatric Urology with its admirably succinct discussion of hypospadias, but the outstanding feature of the whole book is the line drawings and illustrative x-rays, not only excellent in themselves but in their presentation: the clear uncrowded layout making it easy for the reader to consult the appropriate illustration nearby, and where helpful there has been no hesitation in using the same diagram in several different places. If my students know everything that's in this book they will know more than most urologists.

It is especially gratifying to me to see this fine book emanate from Australia and to know that four of the authors have had their stimulus to excellence in work here at UCLA.

Willard E. Goodwin, MD
Professor of Surgery/Urology
University of California, Los Angeles

Clinical Urology Illustrated

Preface

There are many outstanding textbooks of urology, yet there is a need for an approach which stresses basic clinical symptom presentation, diagnosis and treatment. For, although modern urological practice relies greatly on various specialised investigations — such as computerised tomography and fibre-optic visualisation — a careful history taking and a thorough general examination are still of paramount importance; together with a fundamental knowledge of embryology, anatomy, physiology and pathology, and, combined with cumulative clinical experience and simple investigations, these remain the basis for the diagnosis of most patients.

In writing the book we have been mindful of the important role illustrations can have in increasing understanding and retention of knowledge. By using not only line drawings, but wherever possible, x-rays, we have attempted to help the reader bridge the inevitable gap between the simple lecture room concept and the more complex reality of the clinic. Descriptions of operative techniques have only been included where it was thought to be essential to an understanding of a problem.

Urology is a major specialty. In Melbourne it accounts for a fifth of all elective surgical admissions and, on average, each general practitioner sees one genitourinary problem a day. Unfortunately this incidence is not always reflected in undergraduate student teaching programmes. Thus, whether as an introductory text or an opportunity for revision and updating, we hope medical students, urology residents and clinical practitioners will find something of value here.

Melbourne   R.B. Brown

Acknowledgements

I am very grateful for the speciality contributions from Mr Hussein Awang, Mr Peter T. Bruce, Professor Robert B. Smith, Mr E. Durham Smith, Mr J.C. Smith, Mr R.R.A. Syme, Mr D.D. Westmore and Mr R.H. Whitaker, whose expertise and experience in their respective areas indicates both the scope of the speciality and the continually changing approaches to both diagnosis and treatment.

I am particularly grateful to Mrs Maureen Farnsworth for her secretarial help and to Ms Kate Crowle for her excellent illustrations.

The following figures have been reproduced or adapted with the kind permission of the authors and publishers: figures 34, 40, 42, 252, 253 from Stephens: Congenital Malformations of Rectum, Anus and Genitourinary Tracts (Livingstone, Edinburgh) with the courtesy of Mr E. Durham Smith; figures 41, 248-251 from Holden and Ashcroft (Eds) Surgery of Infants and Children (Saunders, Philadelphia) with the courtesy of Mr E. Durham Smith; figures 145, 148 from Glen and Boyce (Eds) Urologic Surgery (Harper and Rowe, New York); figures 146, 147, 149 from Smith and Skinner (Eds) Urologic Surgery: Prevention and Management (Saunders, Philadelphia); figures 230, 231, 232, 235, 243, 244, 267, 268 from Jones (Ed) Clinical Paediatric Surgery (Blackwell Scientific Publications, Melbourne); and figures 255-257 from Jones and Campbell (Eds) Tumours of Infancy and Childhood (Blackwell Scientific Publications, Melbourne).

Contributing Authors

Mr Hussein Awang
MB, BS(Melb.), FRACS, Consultant Urologist Institute of Urology and Nephrology, General Hospital, Kuala Lumpur, Malaysia

Mr R.B. Brown
MB, BS(Melb.), FRACS, FRCS, FACS Head, Urology Unit, Alfred Hospital, Melbourne

Mr P.T. Bruce
MB, BS(Melb), CHM, FRCS, FRACS Senior Urologist, Queen Victoria Hospital, Melbourne

Professor Robert B. Smith
MD, FACS, Associate Professor of Urology, The University of California, Los Angeles, USA

Mr E. Durham Smith
MD, MS, FRACS, FACS, Paediatric Surgeon, Royal Children's Hospital, Melbourne

Mr J.C. Smith
MS, FRCS, Consultant Urological Surgeon, Oxford, England

Mr R.R.A. Syme
MB, BS(Melb.), FRCS, FRACS, Urologist, Austin Hospital Melbourne

Mr D.D. Westmore
MB, BS(Melb.), FRCS (Eng.), FRCS (Edin.), FRACS, Assistant Urologist, Alfred Hospital, Melbourne

Mr R.H. Whitaker
M Chir, FRCS, Consultant Urological Surgeon and Lecturer, University of Cambridge, England

Contents

Contents   xi

Chapter I

Embryology and Congenital Abnormalities

An understanding of the evolution of the genitourinary system is essential if the system's normal and abnormal anatomy is to be understood. Many of the congenital abnormalities in this chapter are further discussed elsewhere, especially in chapter XIV, Paediatric Urology.

Embryology

The evolution of man has seen the development of 3 distinct kidney systems — the pronephros, mesonephros and metanephros. Only the latter remains although the development of this system, and the retention of some of the earlier components, is responsible for occasional congenital abnormalities.

Figure 1 illustrates these changes diagrammatically. The pronephric and mesonephric renal elements have disappeared completely in man but the pronephric or Wolffian duct has persisted in both sexes as the bladder trigone, and in males as the posterior urethra, vas deferens and seminal vesicle, while forming almost all the urethra in the female. The mesonephric or Mullerian duct persists in the female as the fallopian tubes and as the prostatic utricle in the male. The ureter develops as a bud from the pronephric duct to rise and join the developing metanephrogenic renal tissue. Should two ureteric buds develop then a *bifid system* may result.

Renal system

1a The evolutionary replacement of the 3 renal systems.

1b The development of the ureter and vas deferens.

1c The development of the urogenital sinus and genital tubercle.

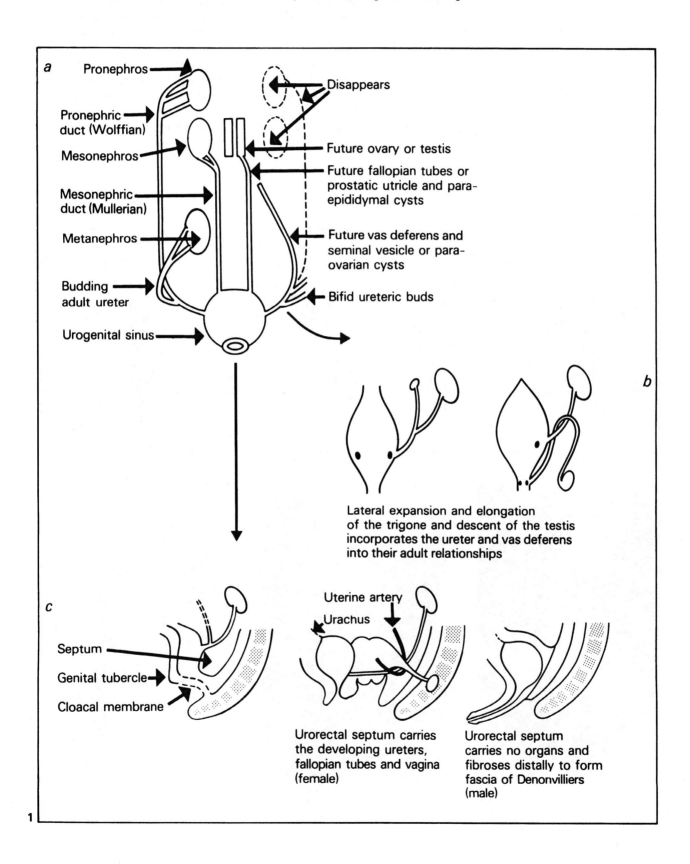

a

Pronephros

Pronephric duct (Wolffian)

Mesonephros

Mesonephric duct (Mullerian)

Metanephros

Budding adult ureter

Urogenital sinus

Disappears

Future ovary or testis

Future fallopian tubes or prostatic utricle and para-epididymal cysts

Future vas deferens and seminal vesicle or para-ovarian cysts

Bifid ureteric buds

b

Lateral expansion and elongation of the trigone and descent of the testis incorporates the ureter and vas deferens into their adult relationships

c

Septum

Genital tubercle

Cloacal membrane

Uterine artery

Urachus

Urorectal septum carries the developing ureters, fallopian tubes and vagina (female)

Urorectal septum carries no organs and fibroses distally to form fascia of Denonvilliers (male)

1

Figures 2-7 illustrate the development of completely bifid renal and ureteric systems while figures 8-9 illustrate the development of incomplete bifid systems.

The urogenital sinus elongates and widens, causing the future vas deferens to loop and to be crossed by the ureter. Further lateral expansion of the trigone incorporates the vas deferens and ureter into their adult relationships.

The urogenital sinus, with its thin cloacal membrane (fig. 1), is divided by the growth and descent of the uro-rectal septum of Rathke, which fuses in the mid-line to separate the future bladder and rectum. The development of the septum carries the mesonephric duct derived fallopian tubes, uterus and upper vagina into the pelvis, resulting in their adult relationships to both the ureter and the uterine artery.

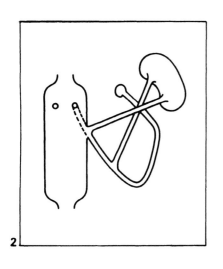

2

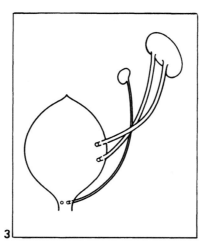

3

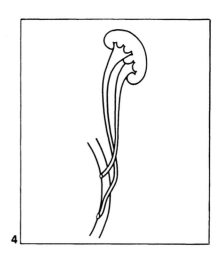

4

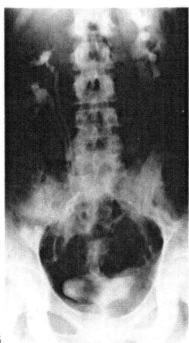

5

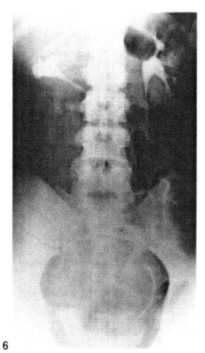

6

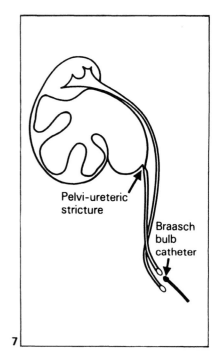

7

Pelvi-ureteric stricture

Braasch bulb catheter

The development of completely bifid renal and ureteric systems
2 Two ureteric buds develop from the pronephric duct in an 8-weeks-old embryo.

3 Elongation and widening of the urogenital sinus incorporates the 2 orifices with the upper segment ureter situated more caudally, irrespective of the number of times the ureters cross (Weigert-Meyer rule).

4 A completely bifid adult system. Note the shorter sub-mucosal length of the lower segment ureter which often results in vesico-ureteric reflux. Ectopic or ureterocele openings are also more common in bifid systems.

5 A completely bifid uncomplicated right system. Note the upper system ureter crossing the lower.

6 The apparent solitary presence of an upper calyceal system, with only 2 or 3 calyces, should always raise the suspicion of a bifid system.

7 Cystoscopy and Braasch bulb retrograde pyeloureterogram of patient in figure 6 reveals a bifid right system, with the lower half complicated by gross pelvi-ureteric obstruction which has destroyed its function. Note that the catheter must be inserted into the superior bladder ureteric orifice in order to outline the lower system.

An incompletely bifid ureteric system
8 Should 2 buds arise from the same ureteric mesonephric duct bud an incomplete bifid system may result.

9 A gross right-sided uretero-ureteric 'Yo-Yo' refluxing system; distension pain was reproduced and observed by cine studies after a heavy fluid load. Note the completely bifid but asymptomatic left system.

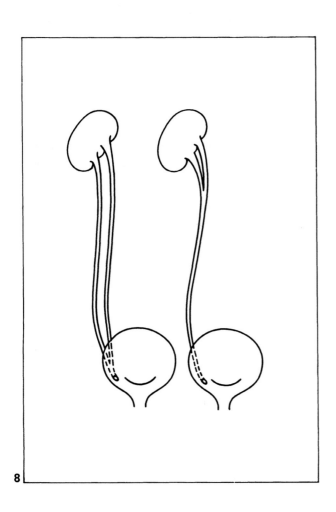

8

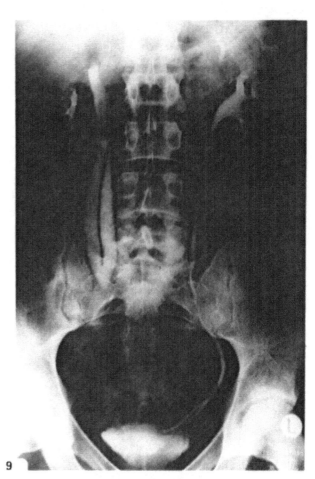

9

The bladder trigone, the posterior urethra in the male and almost all of the female urethra are derived from the expanded lower ends of the pronephric ducts, whilst the rest of the bladder is derived from the original urogenital sinus.

The gonadal ridge tissue develops medial to the disappearing mesonephric tissue and differentiates into ovarian or testicular tissue whilst associating with the respective mesonephric or pronephric duct and descending, in the uro-rectal septum, to the pelvis or scrotum, resulting in the anterior relationship of both of these ducts to the adult ureter.

The undifferentiated external sexual stage of the embryo is represented by the genital tubercle, which develops a groove on its under-surface together with two infro-lateral genital swellings. Future sexual differentiation results in:

Female: The genital tubercle persists as the clitoris whilst the under-surface groove disappears and the genital swellings enlarge to become the labia.

Male: The genital tubercle enlarges to form the penis whilst the under-surface groove joins together from behind forwards to form the urethra. The genital swellings become fused at the mid-line to form the scrotum. The testes have usually descended to the level of the internal inguinal ring just prior to birth and make their final descent and scrotal fixation at the time of birth.

Congenital Abnormalities

Renal and Ureteric Structural Abnormalites

It is not surprising that such a complex series of changes should occasionally result in errors of development.

Agenesis: There is no trigone, ureter or kidney (fig. 10).

Aplasia: There is a small trigonal and ureteric development but no renal tissue (fig. 11).

Fetal Lobulation: The normal fetal lobulation development persists (fig. 12). Congenital lobulation must be distinguished from pyelonephritic scarring.

Megacalycosis: This congenital but, usually non-obstructive dilatation of the calyces may be confused with obstructive hydrocalycosis (figs. 13-14) [see also p. 270].

10 Agenesis. There is no trigone.

11 Aplasia. There is a small trigonal and ureteric development but no renal tissue.

12 Fetal lobulation. The normal fetal lobulation development persists.

Megacalycosis
13 Schematic representation.

14 Left-sided megacalycosis.

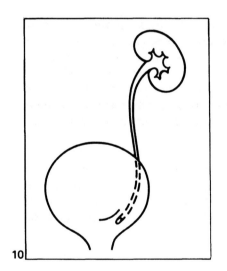

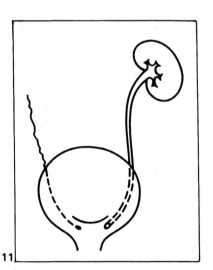

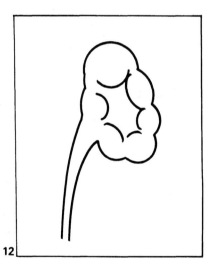

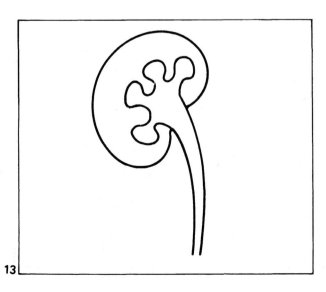

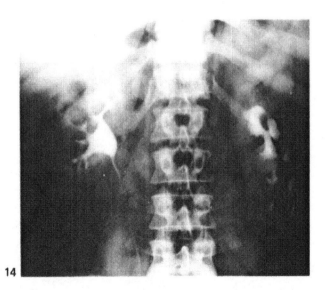

Dysplasia: A usually smaller than normal kidney with abnormal primitive duct development of renal tissue. In addition to renal elements other tissues such as small cysts, cartilage, bone or smooth muscle develop (fig. 15).

Hypoplasia: An otherwise normal but very small system (fig. 16).

Antero-medial Renal Rotation: The kidney does not completely flatten on to the posterior abdominal wall and the pelvis remains facing anteriorly and medially (fig. 17).

Horseshoe Kidney: A similar but bilateral antero-medial rotation of the kidneys occurs, in addition to a connective tissue or, uncommonly, renal tissue fusion of both lower poles in front of the aorta and inferior vena cava (figs. 18-19). The resultant close proximity of the pelvi-ureteric junction to this connection and the great vessels may account for the high incidence of pelvi-ureteric hydronephrosis in such patients. (See also chapter XII; p. 280)

Pelvic Kidney: A low development of the metanephrogenic tissue results in a pelvic kidney which, although flattened and receiving a multiple blood suppy from the adjacent iliac vessels, does not require any specific treatment unless it has an associated abnormality, such as a pelvi-ureteric hydronephrosis (fig. 20).

Ectopic Kidney: A pelvic kidney represents the most common form of renal ectopia but other abnormal loin to pelvis positions are occasionally found, together with the extremely rare condition of crossed renal ectopia, in which one kidney has developed in a normal manner but the other has crossed to fuse with it. The abnormal ureter crosses behind the great vessels to reach its own side and such a crossing may result in proximal dilatation, although this is rarely severe enough to require corrective surgery (figs. 21-22).

Retrocaval Ureter: This results from a normal ureteric development but an abnormal abdominal venous system development. The most common type involves the right ureter running behind the inferior vena cava, and severe proximal obstruction may result (see chapter XII; page 280) requiring surgical correction (fig. 23).

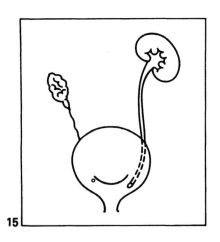

15

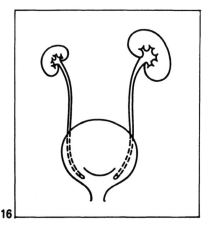

16

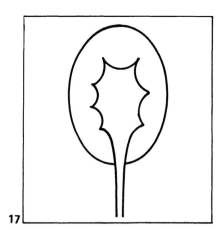

17

15 Dysplasia.

16 Hypoplasia.

17 Antero-medial rotation.

Horseshoe kidney.
18 Schematic illustration.

19 Horseshoe kidney with a left-sided pelvi-ureteric obstruction.

20 Ectopic pelvic kidney.

Crossed renal ectopia
21 With slight proximal dilatation.

22 Left-sided crossed renal ectopia without proximal dilatation.

23 Retrocaval ureter with gross proximal dilatation.

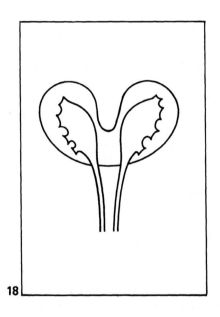

18

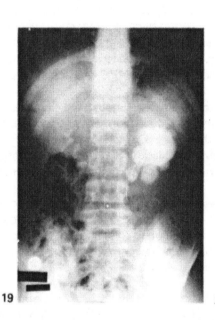

19

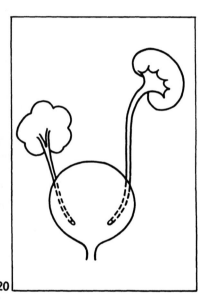

20

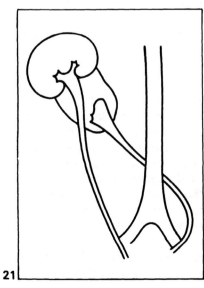

21

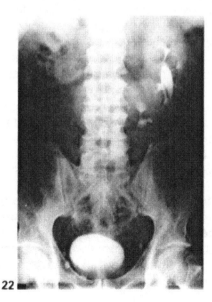

22

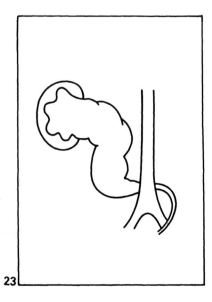

23

Pelvi-ureteric Obstruction and Aberrant Renal Vessels: See pages 36, 38, 274, 326.

Duplex System: Budding of the ureter may be partial or complete, leading to either two complete systems or an upper duplex system (see p. 4-5). The elongation and widening of the urogenital sinus, together with the looping of the lower aspect of the pronephric duct in a duplex system, results in the ureter which drains the upper renal segment always being situated below and medial to its fellow. This arrangement (see below) usually ensures that the more medial ureter, by virtue of its longer submucosal length, is non-refluxing whilst the more laterally situated ureter often refluxes (figs. 2-4). Uretero-ureteric reflux may also occur in some incomplete bifid systems (fig. 9).

Vesico-ureteric Reflux: (See also pages 52, 134, 336).

The length of the submucosal ureter determines whether or not congenital vesico-ureteric reflux occurs. The submucosal tunnel is surrounded by loose connective tissue, which ensures that if the tunnel is sufficiently long it is progressively flattened by increasing intra-vesical resting or voiding pressure, thus preventing reflux from occurring. Deficiencies in this submucosal length account for 95% of all cases of vesico-ureteric reflux, which is found in 30% of all children presenting with urinary tract infection.

Ectopic Ureter: Should the ureter arise from a very low position on the pronephric duct then it may open into the lower trigone, bladder, posterior urethra, vagina, vas deferens or seminal vesicle. Should the relationship be below the bladder and posterior urethral outlet sphincteric mechanism then day and night-time urinary incontinence may result (fig. 24).

Mega-ureter: The term *primary mega-ureter* refers to a congenital dilatation of a ureter, without the presence of bladder or urethral obstruction. The condition is distinguished from *secondary mega-ureter,* which may result from mechanical and/or function distal obstruction and/or vesico-ureteric reflux (see p. 328).

As illustrated in figures 25-28 a primary mega-ureter possesses a variable degree of dilatation, with or without hydronephrosis, due usually to a narrow distal ureteric segment which, for unexplained reasons, acts as a functional barrier to normal ureteric peristalsis. This narrowed area varies in length and the terms *supravesical* and *vesical mega-ureter* are sometimes used to describe these situations. The term *focal gigantism* is also used to describe a dilated primary vesical mega-ureter.

Dilatation of the ureter however does not necessarily mean significant obstruction (chapter XII). Radiological visualisation of an obstructed mega-ureter reveals vigorous, high pressure, muscle contractions of the proximal portion, resisted by a sustained contraction of the distal portion, resulting in a delay in emptying of the system. A grossly abnormal delay in emptying will result in urinary stasis, renal damage and eventual atonia of the hypertrophied proximal ureteric muscle bundles, leading to further proximal ureteric dilatation. Such severe cases require surgical re-implantation of the ureter into the bladder, above the level of the narrowed distal segment, or a nephrectomy in patients with gross renal damage. A long submucosal tunnel, reflux-preventing, implantation operation is employed, but may be difficult to achieve in the presence of gross ureteric dilatation (see p. 335).

24 Ectopic ureter.

Mega-ureter
25 Vesical mega-ureter without renal obstruction.

26 Vesical mega-ureter with renal obstruction.

27 Right supra-vesical mega-ureter without renal obstruction.

28 Left supra-vesical mega-ureter with renal obstruction.

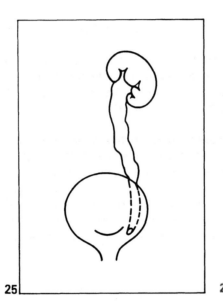

25

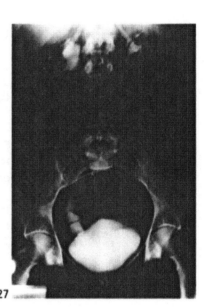

27

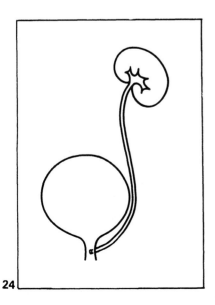

24

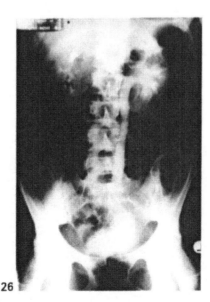

26

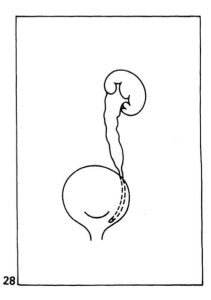

28

Fortunately, many cases of congenital mega-ureter do not result in such serious side effects, nor do they cause significant symptoms, other than infection, and therefore require only regular urological observation and intermittent chemotherapy rather than attempted surgical correction.

Ureteric Valves: Congenital obstructive flaps of tissue may, rarely, occur in the upper ureter.

Ureterocele: This term is used to describe an abnormally narrow and distended opening of the ureter into the bladder (see p. 330). There may be associated obstructive dilatation of the involved system which may require corrective surgery (figs. 29-30).

Renal Cellular Abnormalities

Renal Glycosuria: Glycosuria can result from diabetes mellitus or from failure of the proximal tubules to completely absorb all of the glomerular filtrated glucose. No specific treatment is available for this condition but it must be distinguished from diabetes mellitus.

Renal Tubular Acidosis: This is rare (see p. 210).

Cystinuria: This is extremely rare (see p. 209).

Diabetes Insipidus: This is a very rare male sex-linked Mendelian recessive gene disease which prevents the collecting tubules from responding to antidiuretic hormone. Severe dehydration, particularly in children, may result from this abnormality.

Phosphaturia: In this extremely rare abnormality phosphate is not reabsorbed in the tubules and very large doses of Vitamin D are necessary to prevent renal rickets occurring.

Fanconi Syndrome: Amino acids and phosphate are not reabsorbed by the tubules and, usually, an associated renal tubular acidosis is present. This condition also, is extremely rare.

Ureterocele

29 Left ureterocele with renal obstruction.

30 Left ureterocele without renal obstruction.

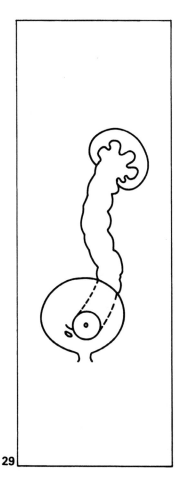

29

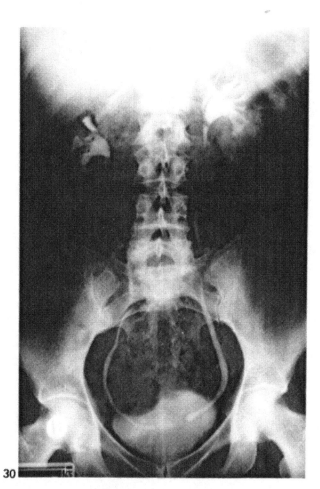

30

Bladder
Abnormalities

Agenesis: This is extremely rare.

Extrophy: As indicated in figures 31-32, if the cloacal membrane is larger than normal and extends onto the future lower abdominal wall before dissolving there may be a deficiency of anteriorly covered areas in this region, ranging from a minor epispadias to a complete extrophy of the bladder and urethra. Ectopia vesicae occurs once in every 50,000 births and is associated with ureteric and renal obstructive dilatation and damage, epispadias, a deficient pubic symphisis, umbilical hernia, undescended testes and inguinal hernia and an abnormally lax, prolapsed anal sphincter and rectum. The condition requires early expert reconstruction (p. 352) or urinary diversion (chapter VIII).

Ectopia vesicae
31 Extension of the cloacal membrane

32 The abnormalities which result from **31**

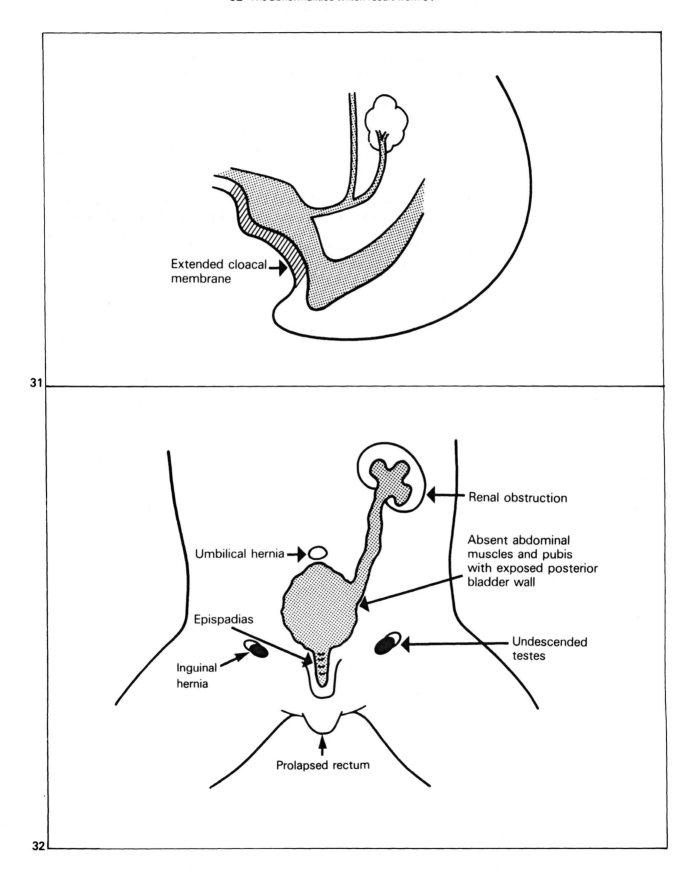

Recto-vesical, Recto-urethral and Recto-vaginal Fistulae: As indicated in figure 33 these congenital fistulae are associated with an imperforate anus and result from faulty development of the uro-rectal septum. Such cases require reconstruction of the anus together with removal and closure of the fistula track.

Patent Urachus: Very rarely the urachus remains patent and and urine escapes from the umbilical region. Encysted areas of the urachus may also, rarely, result from failure of complete obliteration and many become infected, requiring surgical excision (see p. 332).

Duplication: A second uro-rectal septum may, very rarely, partially or completely divide the bladder with a median wall, which may even require surgical excision in severe cases.

Triad or Prune-belly Syndrome: Failure of the abdominal muscles to develop is associated with intra-abdominal testes and gross hypodysplasia of several areas of the genito-urinary system. The abdominal skin is wrinkled early in life, hence the name, but later develops into a pot belly. Other congenital abnormalities are common and 50% of these children die within 2 years of birth (fig. 34).

33 Congenital cloacal fistulae.

34 Urinary abnormalities in the 'triad syndrome' — diffuse hypomuscularity causing bizzarre enlargement of the ureters.

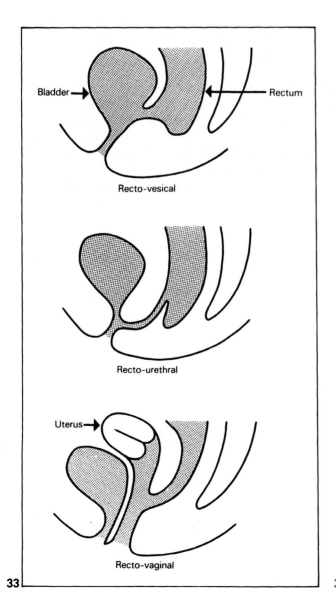

Bladder → ← Rectum

Recto-vesical

Recto-urethral

Uterus →

Recto-vaginal

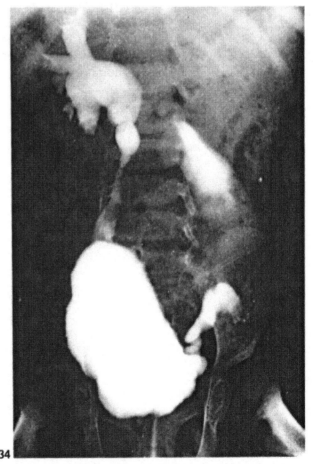

33   34

Megacystis-mega-ureter (Focal Gigantism of the Bladder and Ureter):
In this condition which, in its later stages, may be impossible to distinguish
from gross primary vesico-ureteric reflux, the congenital ureteric and pelvic
dilatation extends from the calyces to the ureteric orifice, producing a
vesico-ureteric refluxing system together with a large bladder, without evidence of any bladder outlet and/or urethral mechanical obstruction. In the
early stages of a megacystis-mega-ureter system there is vigorous
peristalsis of the muscle components of the bladder and ureter, but this excessive energy is not coordinated and fails to empty the system adequately. Urinary stasis, renal damage and eventual atonia of the muscle in
the walls of the ureter and bladder follow, leading to further dilatation. Such
serious side effects may require surgical, non-refluxing, ureteric re-implantation into a surgically reduced-capacity bladder. Unfortunately, some of
these children present with advanced renal failure and many require an initial cutaneous ureterostomy suprapubic urinary diversion, in order to
achieve optimal renal function, prior to reconstructive surgery. Cases of
minor megacystis-mega-ureter syndrome do not require surgical correction
of the abnormality but do require regular urological supervision for the rest
of their life.

Marion's Disease: This rare congenital bladder neck stenosis may require
transurethral or open resection, depending upon the degree of obstruction
and the age of the patient (p. 336).

Congenital Diverticulum: Most adult bladder diverticula are associated
with bladder outlet or urethral obstruction but a congenital diverticulum
does occasionally occur in the region of the ureteric orifices (see p. 336).
The diverticulum often contains bladder muscle fibres in its wall in contrast
to acquired or pulsion diverticula, which represent herniations of the bladder mucosa through hypertrophied muscle bundles (figs. 35-36). Surgical
excision of a congenital diverticulum is indicated if it is sufficiently large or
complicated.

Diverticula

35 Congenital and acquired bladder diverticula. Note the absence of muscle in the acquired or pulsion diverticulum.

36 A congenital bladder diverticulum. Note the narrow communicating neck.

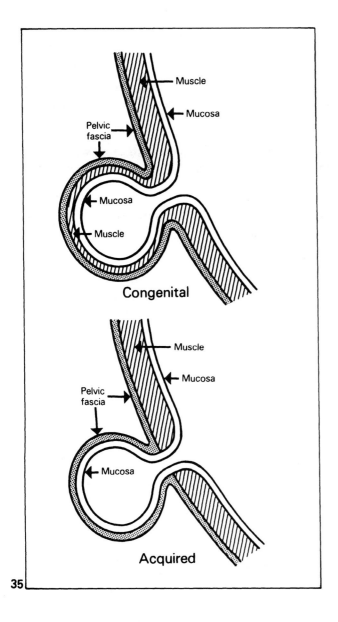

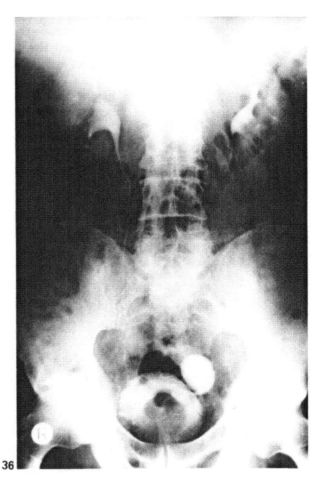

Urethral
Abnormalities

Hypospadias: Minor forms of hypospadias are not uncommon and a total incidence of 1 in 300 male births has been reported. The condition results from incomplete distal fusion of the genital tubercle under-surface groove and results in the urethra terminating proximal to the ventral surface of the penis (fig. 37).

Hypospadias may also result in:

1) A usually narrow, external urethral meatus
2) A shortening and associated fibrosis of the proximally developed and distally undeveloped urethra and related tissues, which produces a ventral deviation of this part of the penis, particularly evident on erection, and termed a *chordee* deformity
3) An incomplete ventral prepuce
4) A small blind pit on the tip of the glans penis.

Hypospadias is anatomically classified according to the site of the external meatus as:

Glandular   ⎫
Coronal   ⎬ 80%
Penile   ⎭
Peno-scrotal ⎫
Perineal   ⎬ 20%

Circumcision should never be performed in severe cases as the dorsal prepucial skin may be required for future reconstruction of the deficient urethra (p. 346).

Peno-scrotal and perineal hypospadias are usually associated with a small penis, and the question of intersex (see p. 354) must be settled before surgical and sociological advice is given.

Epispadias: A shortened dorsal opening of the urethra (fig. 37) is far less common than hypospadias (p. 352).

Hypospadias and epispadias

37a Subglandular (coronal groove) hypospadius

37b Peno-scrotal hypospadius

37c Perineal hypospadius

37d Epispadius

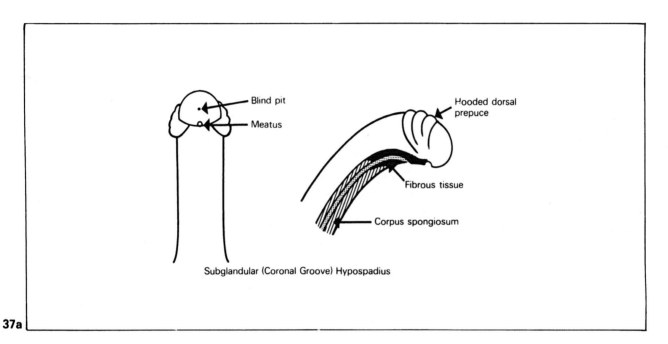

Subglandular (Coronal Groove) Hypospadius

37a

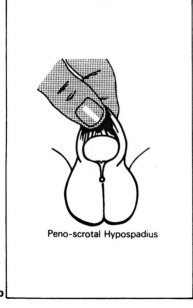

Peno-scrotal Hypospadius

37b

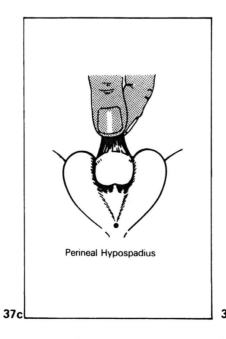

Perineal Hypospadius

37c

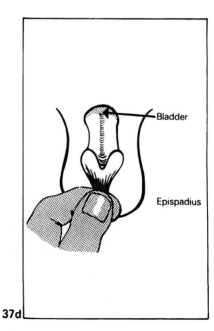

Epispadius

37d

Posterior Urethral Valves: This condition (fig. 38) occurs in males where persistence of the distal ends of the Wolffian ducts leads to faulty development of the posterior urethra, where valve-like flaps of tissue run from the verumontanum to the lateral urethral walls resulting in mechanical posterior urethral outlet obstruction (Young et al., 1919). Provided that the condition is diagnosed (see p. 338) before severe secondary obstructive or infective complications have occurred then the results of transurethral resection of the valves are excellent.

Distal External Meatal Stenosis: An excess of obstructive fibrous tissue at the external meatus is a rare occurrence (see p. 349) but may require surgical correction.

38 Young's classification of posterior urethral valves.

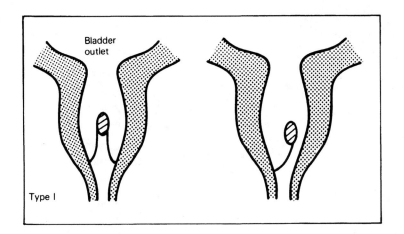

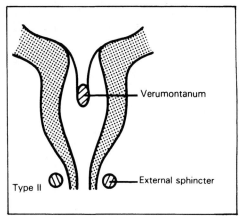

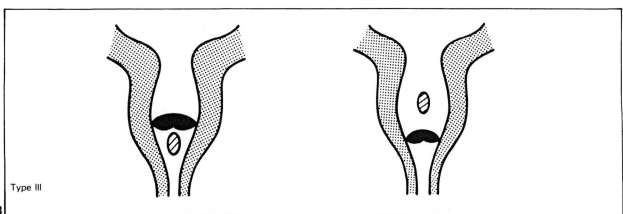

Urethral Diverticula: Congenital urethral diverticula are extremely rare and occasionally completely separated from the true urethra in a manner which suggests that their development may be due to faulty genital tubercle under-surface groove duplication as indicated in figure 39-41. More commonly such diverticula open into the lumen of the true urethra and many become secondarily infected because of their small opening.

Depending upon their size and symptoms, such as ballooning of the area during voiding, subsequent slow emptying and occasional abscess formation, they may require surgical excision.

Duplication of the Urethra and Agenesis: These abnormalities are extremely rare.

Anterior Urethral Strictures: Failure of the normal genital tubercle under-surface groove fusion may result in congenital anterior urethral stricturing or valves (fig. 39).

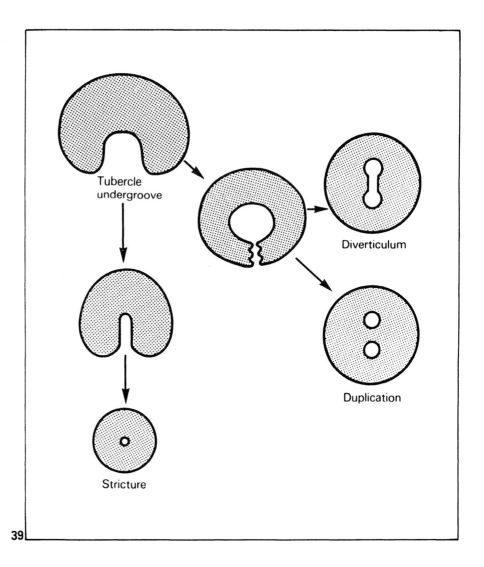

Urethral diverticula

39 Examples of abnormal genital tubercle under-surface groove fusion.

40 A saccular wide-necked urethral diverticulum. The orifice opens proximally (arrow) and, as the diverticulum fills, it may obstruct the urethra.

41 A spherical narrow-necked urethral diverticulum in the distal urethra, causing haematuria.

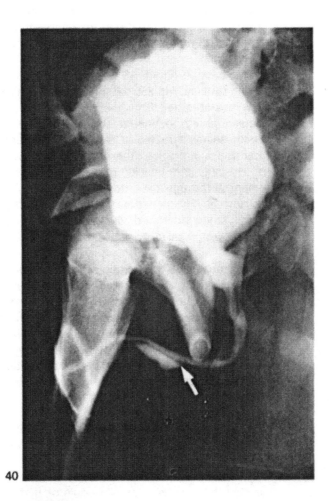

40

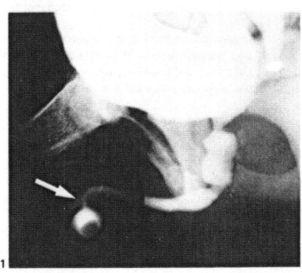

41

Megalo-urethra: An extremely rare condition where the anterior urethra expands widely, in association with a very large penis and often other tissue-related abnormalities (fig. 42). The defect is due to a loss of formation of the corpus spongiosa and a poor development of the corpora cavernosa.

Abnormalities of the Male External Genitalia

Testes. *Undescended testis:* The testis is arrested in the line of normal descent or descends to an ectopic position in 0.2% of males. An undescended testis is often associated with an indirect inguinal hernia and/or a hydrocele (see below). Such testes must be distinguished from a retractile testis which can always be manipulated into the bottom of the scrotum.

As indicated in figure 43 a testis arrested in the line of descent may be intra-abdominal, inguinal or high scrotal whilst an ectopic testis, by definition, has emerged from the inguinal canal to be situated in the superficial inguinal pouch, perineum, thigh or penile base. The clinical distinction between testes arrested in the line of descent or ectopically placed has no practical significance other than the fact that testes arrested high in the line of descent are usually grossly hypoplastic, whilst testes which have emerged through the external inguinal ring are often minimally hypoplastic or normal. Failure surgically, spontaneously or hormonally to bring the testes to the bottom of the scrotum by the age of 6 years will result in acquired, progressive, testicular atrophy.

Undescended testes are subject to a higher than normal incidence of infertility, trauma, possibly torsion and malignancy and therefore require either surgical or, rarely, hormonal repositioning in the scrotum or removal. Retractile testes do not usually require treatment.

Surgically fixing undescended testes in the scrotum does not imply normal fertility as the testis may be hypoplastic and/or may have suffered ischaemic damage during the operation (Retief, 1978).

Hypoplasia: Although hypoplastic testes have diminished hormonal and fertility function they are best left *in situ,* particularly in view of the modern doubt as to the incidence of possible future malignancy.

Agenesis: This is an extremely rare condition and many cases diagnosed as such have either a small nodule of testicular tissue at the distal end of the vas deferens or an intra-abdominal testis.

Inversion: Instead of a posterior attachment to the scrotal wall the testis and epididymis may be attached to the anterior or lateral wall. Torsion of the spermatic cord may occur when there is a lack of normal fixation of the testis to the posterior scrotal wall.

Polyorchidism: This is extremely rare.

42 A diffuse megalo-urethra, due to gross deficiency in the corpora.

43 A classification of undescended testes.

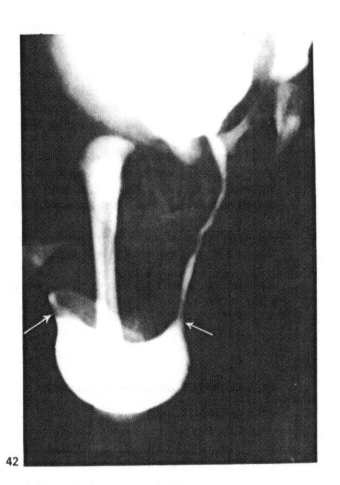

42

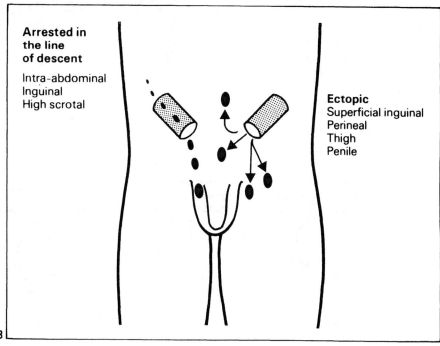

Arrested in the line of descent

Intra-abdominal
Inguinal
High scrotal

Ectopic
Superficial inguinal
Perineal
Thigh
Penile

43

Other Conditions Commonly Associated with Testicular Abnormalities. *Indirect inguinal hernia:* If the processus vaginalis fails to obliterate then abdominal contents may pass into the scrotum. Congenital, encysted, funicular and infantile types of indirect inguinal hernia may occur, depending upon whether the hernia descends to the base of the scrotum and whether or not an additional process of perineum covers the anterior surface of the original processus vaginalis (fig. 44).

Hydrocele: An excessive amount of fluid in the tunica vaginalis is termed a hydrocele and idiopathic, encysted, congenital and infantile types may occur, depending upon a continuing peritoneal cavity communication and the type of processus vaginalis obliteration occurring (fig. 45).

Epididymis: As described earlier congenital cysts derived from vestigial structures may form in relationship to the epididymis and testis. They are common but rarely reach a size sufficient to concern the patient and therefore only require surgical excision should they become torted.

Abnormalities of the Female External Genitalia

Agenesis of the vagina is extremely rare but labial adhesions are common (see p. 350) and are occasionally confused with agenesis.

An imperforate hymen is also extremely rare and is treated by surgical excision.

44 A classification of indirect inguinal hernias.

45 A classification of hydroceles.

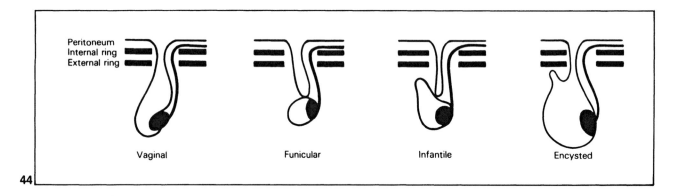

Peritoneum
Internal ring
External ring

Vaginal   Funicular   Infantile   Encysted

44

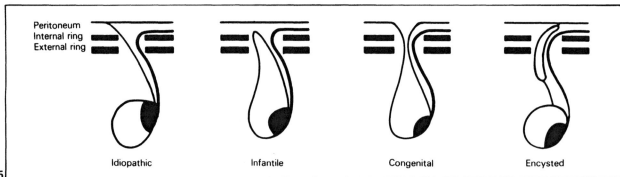

Peritoneum
Internal ring
External ring

Idiopathic   Infantile   Congenital   Encysted

45

Renal Cysts

Not all renal cysts are congenital in origin but they are included in this section for the purpose of classification and differential diagnosis and are further discussed in their appropriate chapters.

Dysplasia: See figure 15 and p. 363.

Congenital Bilateral Polycystic Kidneys: This uncommon condition presents either between 30 and 50 years of age or, far less commonly, at birth, where it may result in a stillborn uraemic child. The congenital polycystic disease developing in middle-age is due to a Mendelian dominant gene transmission but the aetiology of the condition occurring at birth is unknown. The kidneys are large, containing numerous similar-sized cysts, with varying amounts of normal functioning renal tissue sandwiched between them (figs. 46-47). There is an inevitable progression in the size of

Polycystic kidneys
46 Schematic illustration

47 One of 2 non-functioning polycystic kidneys being removed prior to renal homotransplant surgery.

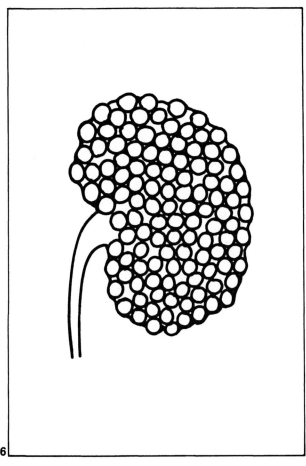

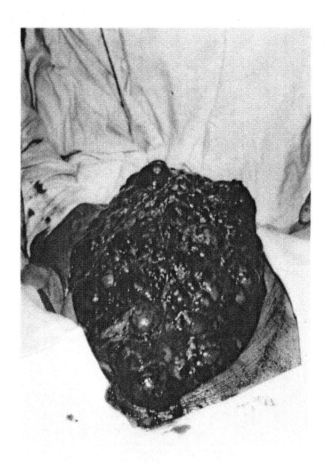

46

47

the cysts, leading to a further reduction in the amount of functioning renal tissue and eventually uraemia, but it is often not possible in the cases which develop later in life to give an accurate prognosis and many patients live, without support therapy, for 10 to 15 years after the initial diagnosis. Dialysis or renal homotransplantation however usually become necessary (see chapter XVI).

Unilateral Multicystic Congenita: This is a large unilateral multicystic kidney without functioning renal tissue. In view of its size and the development of complications, such as haemorrhage and infection, such kidneys are removed surgically on diagnosis (fig. 48).

Congenital Medullary Sponge Kidney: This congenital cystic dilatation of the collecting tubules, within the renal medulla, is uncommon. Because of urinary stasis and resultant infection, calculi may develop within the cysts. The condition rarely requires treatment unless calculi (see chapter IX) form. A localised meduallary sponge area can occasionally be excised with a partial nephrectomy operation if recurrent pain and calculus formation justify the procedure (fig. 49).

Congenital and Acquired Hydrocalycosis: Smooth congenital dilatations of the calyx are not uncommon. Acquired hydrocalycosis may result from fibrous inflammation (see p. 133) or neoplasia in the region of the calyceal neck and, very rarely, from an arterial aneurysm (figs. 50-51). Calculi may develop within the hydrocalycosis and may cause sufficient pain to justify surgical excision, together with an associated hydrocalycosis cavernostomy. Hydrocalycosis must be distinguished from (usually small) congenital or acquired protrusions of the calyx into the renal parenchyma, termed calyceal diverticula (p. 109).

48 Unilateral multicystic congenita.

49 Localised medullary sponge kidney.

Congenital hydrocalycosis
50 Schematic illustration

51 Urinary stasis is common in congenital hydrocalycosis and may result in the formation of calculi, which are usually easily removed through the thin overlying renal cortex. The cavity is then marsupialised.

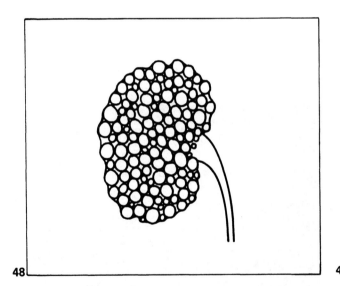

48

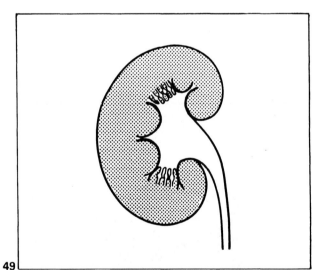

49

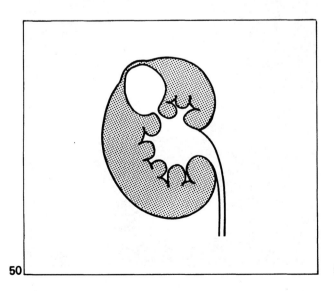

50

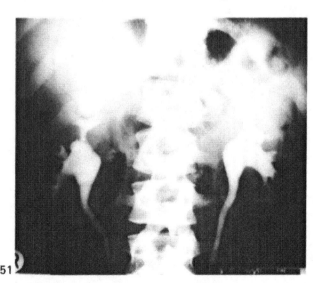

51

Solitary Cyst: This is a not uncommon large single cyst (figs. 52-54); differential diagnosis from other renal space occupying lesions is discussed in chapter III p. 94. Cyst needle aspiration is performed for both diagnostic and, often, therapeutic reasons. In very large cysts, or where there is some doubt concerning neoplasia, after selective renal angiography and computerised tomography, the kidney is surgically explored, the cyst unroofed and its cavity carefully visualised to exclude the presence of an intracystic carcinoma before its protruding walls are excised.

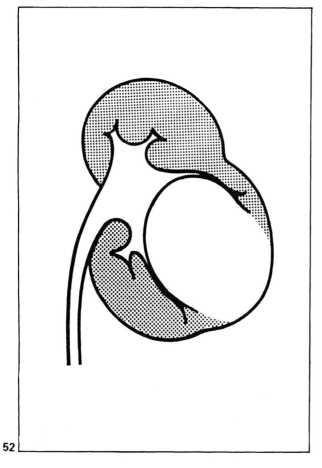

52

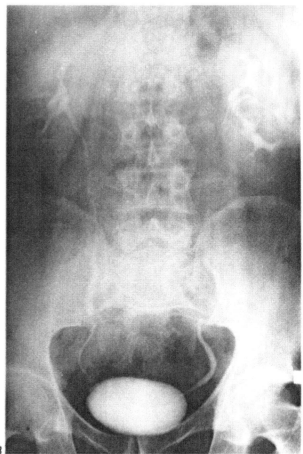

53

Renal cysts

52 Solitary renal cyst.

53 A smooth left renal space occupying lesion, consistent with a solitary renal cyst.

54 Solitary renal cyst at operation.

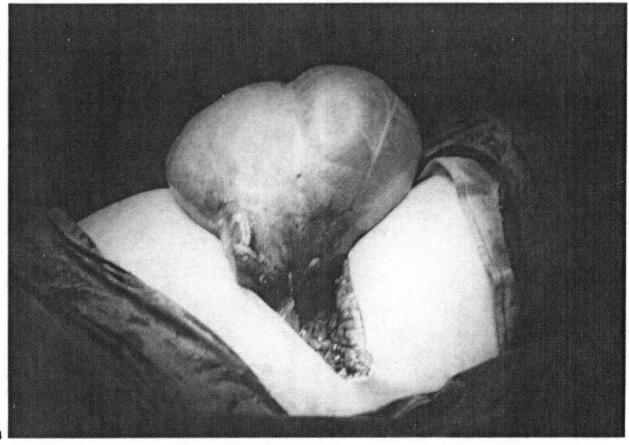

54

55 Multicystic kidney.

56 Bilateral multicystic kidneys. Note the smooth appearance of the space occupying lesions.

Peri-renal cyst
57 Schematic illustration.

58 A left-sided peri-renal (para-pelvic) cyst resulting from renal trauma and a subsequent encysted urinary extravasation. The renal obstructing mass was surgically drained.

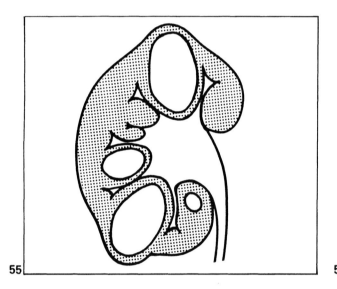

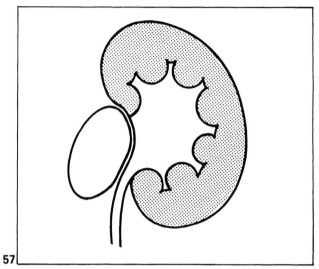

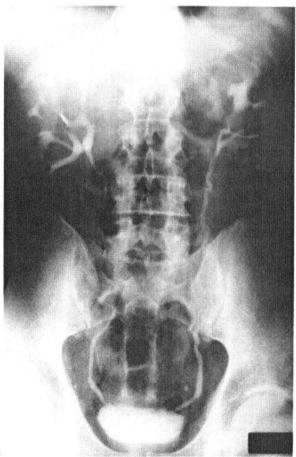

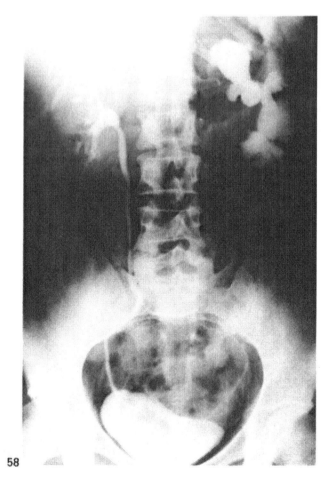

55

57

56

58

Multicystic Kidney: In this not uncommon finding the kidney contains 2 or more cysts but still retains ample functioning renal tissue (figs. 55-56). The condition must be distinguished from renal carcinoma (see p. 288).

Peri-renal (Para-pelvic) Cyst: These 'cysts' usually develop from urinary and blood extravasation following renal trauma (p. 288) or surgery and represent an encapsulated collection of fluid (figs. 57-58). They often require surgical drainage. Very rarely non-traumatic collections of presumed lymphatic cysts are found in this area.

As illustrated in figure 6 a grossly obstructed partial or complete kidney may present as a possible renal cyst.

References

Retief, P.J.: Fertility in undescended testes. South African Medical Journal 52: 610 (1978).
Young, H.H.; Frontz, W.A. and Baldwin, J.C.: Congenital obstruction of the posterior urethra. Journal of Urology 3: 289 (1919).

Further Reading

Arey, L.B.: Developmental Anatomy, 7th ed. (Saunders, Philadelphia 1974).
Segal, A.J.; Spataro, R.F. and Barbaric, Z.L.: Adult polycystic disease: Review of 100 cases. Journal of Urology 118: 711 (1978).
Stephens, F.D.: Congenital Malformation of the Rectum, Anus and Genito-Urinary Tracts (Livingstone, Edinburgh 1963).

Chapter II

Anatomy, Physiology and Related Pathology

A knowledge of basic genitourinary anatomy and physiology is essential in order to localise and appreciate the pathological changes occurring within the system.

The Kidney

The kidneys are paired, solid organs, which lie in the retroperitoneal upper part of the posterior abdominal wall. They are well protected by the rib-cage, vertebrae and related muscles and possess a high degree of mobility, an envelope of shock absorbing peri-renal fat and strong Gerota's fascia.

Anatomy

A pathological kidney, because of its abnormal and less solid architecture, is more easily damaged (p. 286). The kidney's medial surface contains a slit, the renal hilum, through which the renal arteries, veins and pelvis enter or leave the kidney. Enlargement of the renal pelvis, due to pelvi-ureteric or more distal obstruction (chap. XII) may obstruct the vessels within the hilum leading, together with increased renal tubule back pressure damage, and occasionally associated infection, to varying degrees of parenchymal ischaemia and atrophy.

The renal pelvis is termed extra-renal if it extends beyond the confines of the kidney or intra-renal if it is within these confines. The effects of urinary tract obstruction on the less distensible intra-renal pelvis are more rapidly damaging to the renal parenchyma than those occurring where there is an extra-renal pelvis.

The kidney is divided into a functioning cortex and medulla and a conducting calyceal-pelvi-ureteric system. As indicated in figure 59 the functioning and conducting systems join at the renal papillae. Urinary tract obstruction,

59 Renal anatomy. Macroscopic and microscopic renal anatomy. Note the foot processes on Bowman's cells.

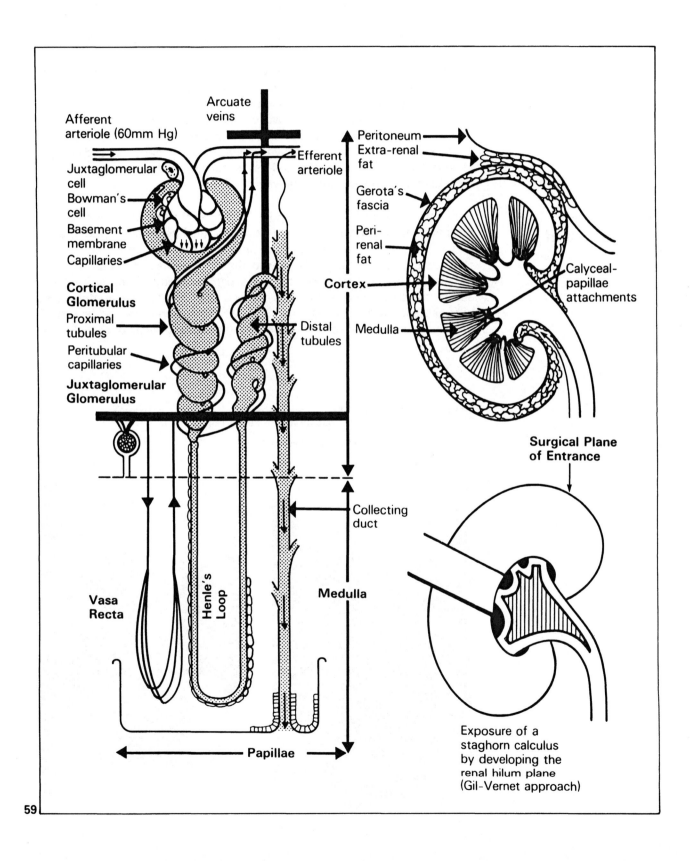

59

arterial disease, diabetes mellitus, excessive analgesic intake in susceptible people, tuberculosis, and other infections, can destroy the renal papillae (figs. 60-61 and see also p. 360). This intermittent anatomical attachment provides an important surgical entrance plane into the hilum of the kidney (fig. 59), which is of considerable help when removing large staghorn calculi or performing other intra-renal operations.

The left renal vein receives tributaries from the testis, ovary and the left adrenal gland, but the right renal vein receives no tributaries (fig. 62). Obstruction to the left renal vein, which may occur from a neoplastic or other vein thrombus (p. 372) may result in engorgement of the left testicular vein and a resultant varicocele which may be the first indication of such a neoplasm. Most varicoceles, however, result from incompetence of the vein valves and are not due to a renal vein thrombosis. Varicoceles are rare on the right side. Within the kidney the veins drain the nephrons and enlarge to form an arcade system (fig. 59) before running with the major renal arterial branches to form the renal vein.

Renal Vessels, Lymphatics and Nerves

Renal Veins: As illustrated in figure 62 the renal veins lie anterior to the renal arteries whilst both are anterior to the renal pelvis and upper ureter, with the exception that the posterior branch of the renal artery, and its accompanying vein, cross posteriorly to the renal pelvis and ureter to enter the hilum. This posterior branch, or a separate 'aberrant' vessel from the aorta, may cross close to the pelvi-ureteric junction and may contribute to pelvi-ureteric hydronephrosis (p. 274). Multiple 'abnormal' or 'aberrant' branching of the renal vessels is common (fig. 63) and rarely of pathological

Renal papillary necrosis
60 Resulting from grade III, bilateral vesico-ureteric reflux.

61 Resulting from analgesic abuse nephropathy.

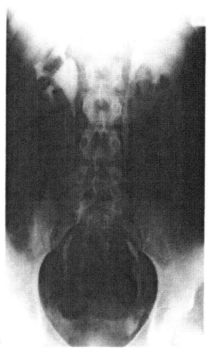

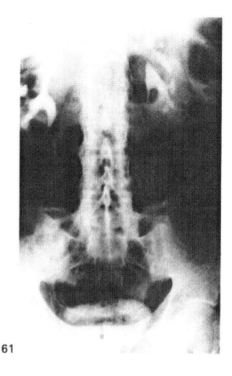

60   61

62 The renal and adrenal blood supply and lymphatic drainage.

63 Renal vessel abnormality. An aberrant right renal artery crossing the pelvi-ureteric junction of the right kidney but not resulting in pelvi-ureteric hydronephrosis.

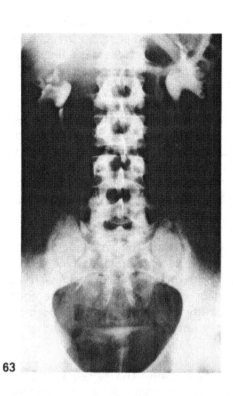

63

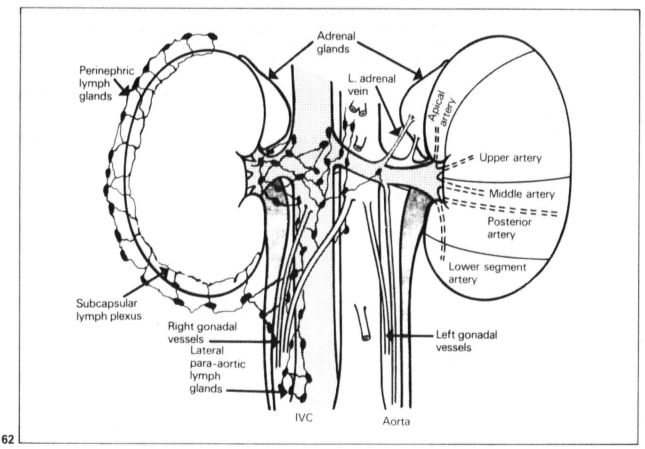

62

significance, although an accurate knowledge of such branching is essential for many renal operations, particularly renal homotransplantation, where a multiplicity of branching may be a contraindication to the procedure because of the resultant technical anastomotic difficulties (p. 366).

Renal Arteries: The main renal artery usually divides into major apical, upper, middle, lower and posterior branches (fig. 62) which supply these areas of the kidney. Although there is a fine anastomosis with small renal capsular vessels, which may increase under pathological conditions, these major branches are normally end-arteries and surgical ligation or severe trauma will result in death of the wedge shaped renal segment supplied. Advantage is taken of this arrangement during the performance of a partial nephrectomy operation, where the involved segment vessel is ligated early in the procedure, thereby demarcating the area to be removed and reducing the degree of operative bleeding. The renal arteries continue to divide into smaller branches until they supply the cortical glomeruli with an afferent arteriole (fig. 59). Despite the view expressed in some text books, the arteries do not form arcades.

Renal Lymphatics: The lymphatic circulation is divided into a sub-capsular plexus and a second system which accompanies the renal blood vessels (fig. 62). Both groups unite at the renal hilum and drain into the lateral aortic and inferior vena cava nodes. These nodes are removed when a radical nephrectomy for neoplasm is performed, both in order to determine whether or not metastases are present and to remove them if at all possible (p. 169).

Renal Innervation: The kidney is supplied by the tenth, eleventh and twelfth autonomic and sensory thoracic nerve roots which also supply the gut. This nerve sharing often results in patients with pelvi-ureteric hydronephrosis presenting with dyspepsia rather than loin symptoms and also plays a part in the development of the partial ileus which often accompanies renal surgery.

Macroscopic Renal Relationships and Their Surgical Significance

Macroscopic renal relationships and their surgical significance are shown schematically in figure 64.

Postero-lateral Relationships: The kidney is related to the diaphragm, pleura, twelfth rib, quadratus lumborum and psoas muscle.

64 **Macroscopic renal relationships and their surgical significance.**

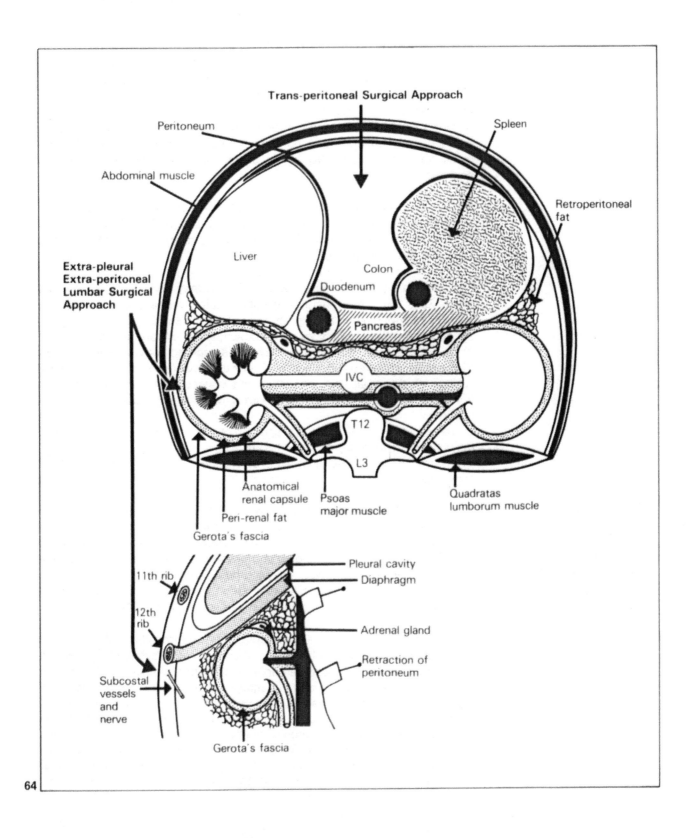

64

Renal operations are commonly performed through an extra-peritoneal postero-lateral or loin incision, incising the bed of the partially or completely removed twelfth rib, with the patient in a lateral operating position. Prolonged operations performed with the patient in this position may result in atelectasis and/or pneumonia, due to congestion and inhibition of movement of the contralateral lung during the operation and similar inhibition of the ipsilateral lung due to postoperative pain. Regular, early, postoperation deep breathing and coughing are mandatory exercises following renal surgery. This loin approach enables both an extra-peritoneal and an extra-pleural operation to be performed, so avoiding contamination of these compartments with urine, blood and/or pus. Opening the pleura may result in a pneumothorax, haemopneumothorax and/or a pyopneumothorax (fig. 64). Care must be taken to prevent damage to the subcostal nerve during the operation as trauma may result in persistent postoperative pain. Urinary or blood postoperative retroperitoneal extravasation may contribute to a partial postoperative ileus. A postoperative urinary fistula may result from distal obstruction, poor healing or a specific unrecognised infection or neoplasm.

Antero-medial Relationships: As indicated the kidney is related anteriorly to the peritoneum, spleen, pancreatic tail, colon, second and fourth parts of the duodenum and jejunum whilst medially it is related to the inferior vena cava and the aorta (fig. 64).

Extremely rarely fistulae occur between the kidney and the colon or small bowel (fig. 65). These fistulae usually result from a primary staghorn calculus or tuberculous renal pathology (Brown, 1966).
Anterior trans-peritoneal surgical approaches (fig. 64) are chosen:
1) To remove large neoplastic kidneys. This approach enables early ligation of the renal artery, so reducing the size of the renal mass, followed by early ligation of the renal vein, so preventing unnecessary metastatic cellular spread (which will occur if the neoplasm is excessively handled prior to such ligation).
2) To perform renal homotransplantation operations and to correct renovascular abnormalities (see chapter XVII).
3) To provide a fresh surgical plane of approach for secondary or tertiary renal operations.

Anatomy and Function of the Renal Parenchyma, Adrenal Gland and Calyceal-pelvi-ureteric System

As indicated in figure 59 the kidney consists of cortical and medullary zones and a pelvi-calyceal collecting system, enclosed by a strong, fibrous capsule. The cortex is composed of glomeruli, tubules and vessels, whilst the medulla consists of the ascending and descending loops of Henle, the vasa rectum vessels and the major collecting ducts which are known as the columns of Bellini. Renal plasma flow, filtration fraction and filtration rate are best estimated by gamma scintillation camera studies (p. 105).

A Nephron

Each nephron consists of a glomerulus, juxta-glomerular cells, proximal convoluted tubule, loop of Henle, distal convoluted tubule and a collecting duct. The number and quality of nephrons determines renal function. Figure 59 indicates the anatomy and function of a nephron system. The small afferent vessel enters the glomerulus, surrounded by granular juxta-glomerular cells, which are also connected to the distal convoluted tubules and are thought to be the source of the hypertensive enzyme *renin* (p. 369). The glomerulus is formed by division of the vessel into a ball of capillaries adherent to the basement membrane of Bowman's capsule. The cells of Bowman's capsule are attached to the basement membrane by many

65 Nephro-colic fistula. A 50-year-old woman, with a known right staghorn calculus, presented with acute right renal pain and fever. This resolved within 24 hours and subsequent intravenous pyelography and retrograde pyelo-ureterogram studies (a) revealed a nephro-colic fistula (b,c).

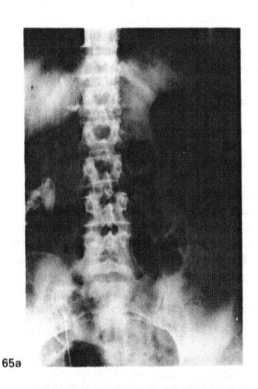

65a

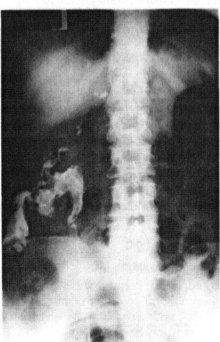

65b

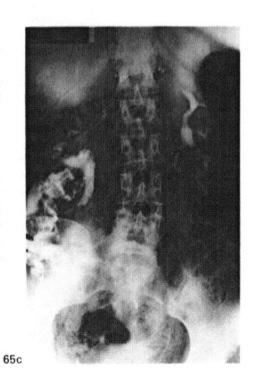

65c

separate 'foot processes', which fuse early in the development of *glomerulonephritis* (p. 364). Both these structures contain fine pores through which serum protein molecules above 150,000 molecular weight normally cannot enter.

The blood in the afferent vessel has a pressure of 60mm Hg, whilst the plasma resisting osmotic pressure is 20mm Hg, and the pressure inside Bowman's capsule is about 10mm Hg. This results in a filtration pressure of 30mm Hg and a *total glomerular filtrate* of 180 litres each 24 hours. Blood pressure alterations, glomerular disease and obstruction of the collecting system will all influence the amount and quality of the filtrate. *Glomerular filtration* is measured by estimating the excretion in the urine of a substance, of known plasma concentration, which, having passed through the filter, is neither further excreted nor absorbed by the system. The glomerular filtration rate (GFR) is then determined as follows:

$$GFR = UV/P$$
where,
U = urine concentration
V = volume of urine per minute
P = plasma concentration.

Inulin fulfills these criteria but *creatinine* rather than inulin clearance is usually used as it is far easier to measure, even though a slight amount of creatinine is added to the filtrate by the proximal tubules.
The efferent vessel conveys blood away from the glomerulus and divides again, either into capillaries which surround the proximal and distal convoluted tubules, or, in the case of the juxta-medullary glomeruli, long branches, termed the vasa rectum, which run down to the papillae, branch again into multiple capillaries in this area, and then return to the juxta-glomerular efferent venule (fig. 59).

Tubules. *Sodium and fluid balance:* The proximal convoluted tubules actively and passively reabsorb 80% of the glomerular filtrate. The active reabsorption of sodium produces a hypotonic urine, which then results in passive water and urea movement from the tubules to the peritubular capillaries.

The isotonic urine then enters the loops of Henle. The thin cells of the descending limb of the loop are permeable to water but the thicker ascending loop cells are not. These ascending cells actively remove further sodium from the filtrate resulting in a hypotonic urine entering the distal convoluted tubules. The removed sodium raises the osmolarity in the ascending cells and is thereby osmotically removed by the vasa rectae vessels. Because of this sodium osmolarity gradient, which is maximal at the papillae, water is passively lost from the descending limbs of Henle and the collecting ducts. The passive loss of water results in hypotonic urine entering the distal convoluted tubules where further active sodium and passive water absorption may occur, resulting in isotonic urine entering the collecting ducts. Passage of this urine down the ducts of Bellini, through the progressively increasing hyperosmolarity areas, again results in further water loss, influenced by the hypothalamic antidiuretic hormone, with the resultant final production of a hypertonic and, in our community, slightly acidic urine. This mechanism of active sodium absorption and the creation of differing areas of medullary hyperosmolarity, with a resultant passive distribution of water, is known as a counter-current multiplier system.

As indicated earlier, renal papillary necrosis (fig. 60-61) will grossly interfere with these vital kidney functions.

In addition to the tubular cells' capacity for active and passive reabsorption they are also able to selectively excrete hydrogen, potassium, ammonia and uric acid. Most of this active secretion occurs in the distal tubule. The tubular cells and the lungs are the major sites for preservation of the *normal body pH*. The tubular cells assist in this vital function by excreting hydrogen and/or bicarbonate ions. The former process occurs during the reabsorption of sodium, when either hydrogen or potassium ions are excreted into the tubular lumen, whilst the latter process occurs as the result of the action of the enzyme carbonic anhydrase, which forms carbonic acid within the cells which then disassociates into hydrogen and bicarbonate ions. The hydrogen ion passively moves into the lumen of the tubule, where it combines with bicarbonate to form carbonic acid, which then breaks down to water and carbon dioxide; these then diffuse back into the cell where the process continues whilst the bicarbonate component of the original breakdown passively passes into the peri-tubular capillaries. The end result being the body reabsorption of one bicarbonate ion and the secretion of one hydrogen ion. The tubules' inability to exchange hydrogen ions may result in renal tubular acidosis (p. 210) and resultant renal calculus formation.

At least 2 hormones act on the distal tubules to influence sodium and water retention. They are particularly active at times of body stress:

a) *Aldosterone* controls the active reabsorption of sodium and the subsequent passive reabsorption of water, based probably on blood pressure changes which are detected in the afferent glomeruli juxta-glomeruli granular cells. Renin, released from these cells, converts the liver produced protein, angiotensinogen, into *angiotensin* which, in addition to its vaso-constrictor action, also stimulates the adrenal gland to release aldosterone (p. 372).

b) *Antidiuretic hormone* is released by the hypothalamus in response to osmotic blood pressure changes. Antidiuretic hormone acts on the distal tubule and collecting ducts enabling passive water reabsorption to occur in these areas.

Renal Hormone Production

The kidney produces 3 essential hormones:

1) *Renin*
2) *Erythropoietin:* This is essential for red cell production (p. 365)
3) *Prostaglandins:* These are produced by the renal medulla and are known to influence metabolism, smooth muscle and nerve activity.

Adrenal Glands

The adrenal glands are attached to the upper poles of both kidneys but are usually separated by compartments of Gerota's fascia. The left adrenal is often related to the renal pedicle whilst the right is usually situated at a higher level. Both glands are supplied with branches from the inferior phrenic, aorta and renal arteries but the right adrenal vein drains into the inferior vena cava and the left into the left renal vein (fig. 62).

The adrenals consist of an outer cortex and an inner medulla. The adrenal cortex produces more than 30 steroid hormones which influence such vital body functions as carbohydrate metabolism, electrolyte and fluid balance and sexual characteristics. Excessive hormone production in children is characterised by premature sexual development in the male and virilisation in the female. In the adult, *Cushing's syndrome* results from an excess of cortical hormone production producing hyperglycaemia and glycosuria, obesity and male sex characteristics.

Addison's disease results from infective, traumatic or neoplastic replacement of the adrenal cortex and is characterised by a hypersensitivity to insulin, weakness, hypotension and excessive pigmentation of the exposed skin. Under conditions of body stress an acute adrenal crisis may occur in patients suffering from Addison's disease, requiring urgent and expert intravenous cortisone replacement therapy. Aldosterone is produced by the adrenal cortex and *Conn's tumour* (p. 372) results in an excessive production of the hormone, with resultant hypertension and muscle weakness due to the loss of potassium at the expense of sodium retention.

Adrenal cortical hyperplasia is treated by giving cortisone, which reduces the pituitary stimulus to further hormone production, and Addison's disease is also treated with replacement cortisone therapy. Primary adrenal neoplasms are treated by surgical excision (p. 374).

The adrenal medulla produces adrenaline and noradrenaline. A *phaeochromocytoma* produces excessive amounts of these hormones resulting in hypertension (p. 374).

The adrenal gland should always be carefully identified and left *in situ* during a nephrectomy operation as it may be the only functioning adrenal tissue in the body.

Calyceal-pelvi-ureteric Collecting System

The calyces and pelvis are lined with transitional epithelium and surrounded by smooth muscle. Urine passes from the renal papillae to the ureter by a combination of gravity and filtration pressure assisted by varying degrees of active peristalsis of the muscle.

The Ureter

The ureter is a thick walled, three layered, muscular tube, lined with transitional epithelium, with an internal adult diameter of only 6mm (fig. 66). The ureteric muscle consists of long interlacing bundles, called nexuses, and their contraction results in the easily observed peristaltic movements which carry urine from the kidney to the bladder. The ureter is enclosed in a thin sheath of loose connective tissue which greatly aids such movements. Sympathetic and parasympathetic nerve fibres from the aortic and hypogastric plexus freely supply the ureter but their role, apart from transmitting pain sensation (p. 210), is unknown as the denervated ureter continues to function normally.

Dilatation of the ureter may occur when there is either extra-ureteric (pelvic or retroperitoneal neoplasia, large benign masses, deep x-ray therapy oedema or fibrosis, inflammation or benign retroperitoneal fibrosis) or intra-ureteric mechanical (calculi or neoplasm) or functional (mega-ureter) obstruction (chap. XII).

66 The ureter. The ureteric 3-layered wall, blood supply, lymphatic drainage and normal sites of narrowing. Note the method of minimal-stricture oblique end-to-end interrupted suture repair of the ureter and the importance of preservation of the longitudinal adventitial vessel anastomoses during mobilisation and suturing.
A dilated ureter is not necessarily an obstructed ureter.

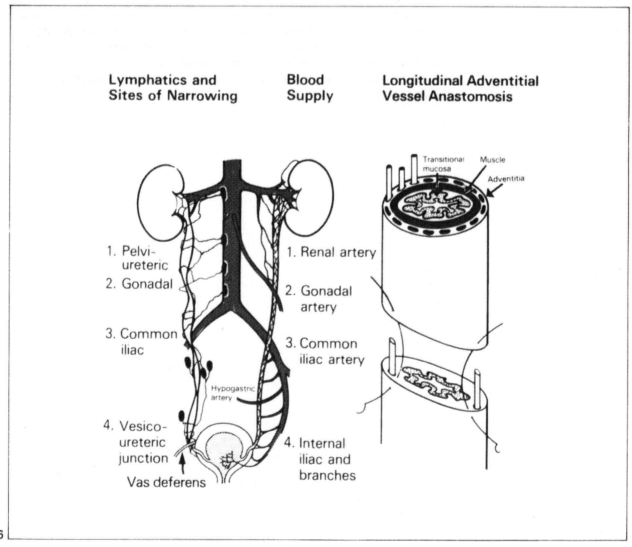

Dilatation of the ureter and kidney does not necessarily mean signficant obstruction, which is defined as an abnormally delayed emptying of the system together with progressive renal damage (see chapters X and XII).

Non-significant ureteric narrowing, with associated pre- and post-narrowing dilatation, often occurs at the pelvi-ureteric and vesico-ureteric junctions and where the ureter crosses the common iliac vessels, or is crossed by the gonadal vessels (figs. 67-68). Dilatation also occurs during pregnancy due to both the mass of the uterus and possible hormonal associated smooth muscle action.

Ureteric Vessels, Lymphatics and Nerve Supply

Arterial branches from the renal, gonadal, internal and common iliacs, and the superior and inferior vesical arteries supply the ureter and freely anastomose to form longitudinal vessels which run the length of the ureter in the outer adventitial layer (fig. 66). This arrangement means that division of the separate branches will not devitalise the ureter provided that the surgical dissection remains outside the longitudinal anastomosis. This enables extensive mobilisation of the ureter to be performed during ureteric anastomotic and other operations (see chapter VIII). The ureteric veins correspond to these arteries.

The lymphatic drainage of the ureter is to the nearest medial node group. The upper ureter drains to the renal glands whilst the middle ureter drains to the lateral aortic glands and the lower ureter drains to the internal iliac glands. The ureteric nerves arise from the renal, inferior mesenteric, gonadal and pelvic plexus and follow the course of the blood vessels to the ureteric adventitia which contains many small ganglia from which afferent fibres run to the ureteric muscle. Numerous sensory fibres are found in the muscle layer.

Ureteric narrowing
67 Illustrates the 3 most common sites of normal ureteric narrowing.

68 Post-micturition film reveals that the right pelvi-ureteric narrowing (fig. 67) is abnormal. A right pyeloplasty operation was performed.

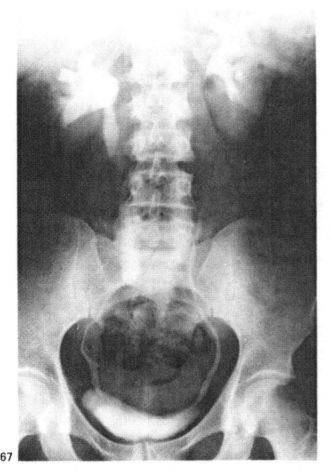

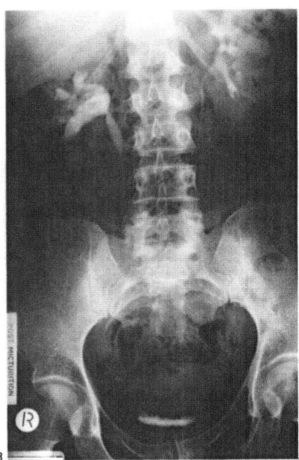

67 68

Ureteric Relationships and their Surgical Implications

Anterior Relationships: The main renal vein and artery cross anteriorly to the renal pelvis with the posterior branch of the renal artery crossing posteriorly as previously indicated. The testicular or ovarian vessels cross the mid-portion (fig. 66) and may, rarely, cause significant obstruction, requiring surgical correction; in the pelvis the superior vesical vessels proximally and the vas deferens distally also cross anteriorly (fig. 69). The vas deferens is a useful surgical guide to dissection of the lower ureter. The peritoneum must be kept intact and retracted during most surgical approaches to the ureter (fig. 70).

Posterior Relationships: The ureter crosses the psoas muscle and the bifurcation of the common iliac vessels before running through the pelvic connective tissue to the bladder. Intravenous pyelography indicates that this course is shown to cross the tips of the anterior lateral transverse processes and the sacro-iliac joint before running to the bladder in a slightly medial concave line, drawn from the inferior sacro-iliac joint to the superior pubic symphysis, with the vesico-ureteric junction situated at a point joining the middle and distal thirds of this line. Ureteric calculi should be situated along this course in plain x-rays or should be shown to be in the lumen of the ureter in an intravenous pyelogram or retrograde study (p. 114).

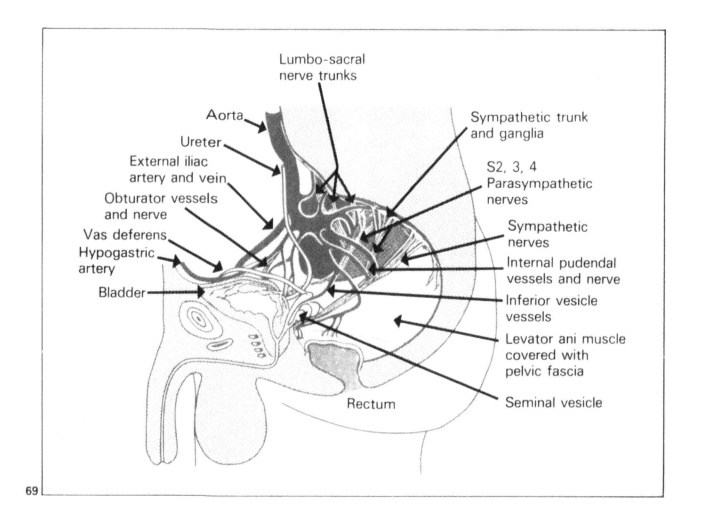

69 The male ureteric pelvic relationships. Note both the pudendal nerve leaving the pelvis to enter the ischio-rectal fossa and the intra-pelvic parasympathetic and sympathetic nerves (see fig. 73).

70 Ureteric surgery. Upper and lower extra-peritoneal surgical approaches to the ureter. Note the retraction of the peritoneum in both situations and the lateral mobilisation of the bladder in the lower approach.

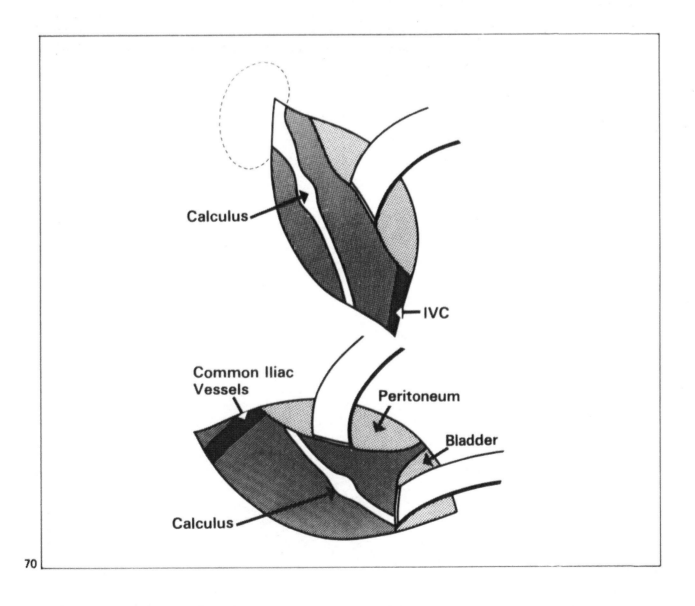

70

Medial Relationships: In both sexes the right ureter is related respectively to the inferior vena cava, the duodenum, colon, appendix, rectum, and bladder (figs 64 and 70) whilst the left ureter is related to the aorta, duodeno-jejunal junction, colon, rectum and bladder. These close relationships may result in damage to the ureter during abdominal or pelvic surgery.

In females the pelvic ureter is closely related to the lateral border of the ovary, the cervix and upper vagina and is crossed by the uterine artery (fig. 71). Ureteric trauma may occur during hysterectomy or vaginal prolapse repair operations where, in the latter, it may descend with the cervix and upper vagina and assume a position well below its normal site.

Ureteric Function

The ureter acts as a unidirectional conducting tube and does not require a nerve supply to achieve this function. Peristaltic contraction of the ureter often means that only portions of it are seen during a single intravenous pyelogram or retrograde ureterogram x-ray study and several films may be necessary.

The Uretero-vesical Junction

The ureter enters the bladder through a long sub-mucosal tunnel to be firmly attached to the lateral trigone (fig. 72). The length of this sub-mucosal tunnel and the shape of the associated ureteric orifice determines whether or not vesico-ureteric reflux will occur (p. 10, 134, 334). The normal sub-mucosal tunnel measures 2mm at birth, 10mm at 5 years and 20mm at the age of 20.

71 Female ureter. The relationship of the female ureter to the vaginal fornices and the uterine artery.

Uretero-vesical reflux surgery
72a A congenitally short grossly refluxing ureter.

72b,c Surgical correction by the distal creation of a minimum 2.5cm submucosal bladder tunnel.

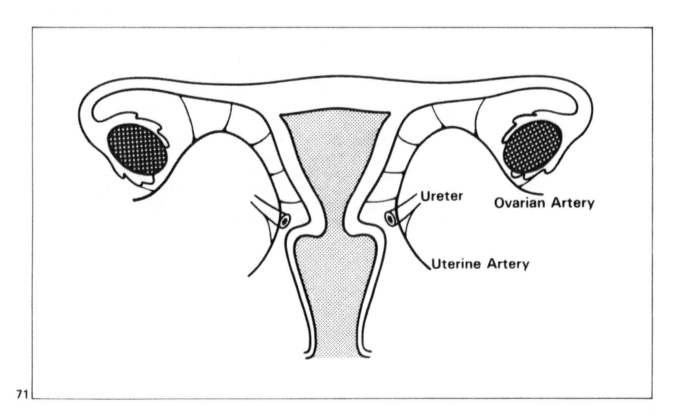

Ureter

Ovarian Artery

Uterine Artery

71

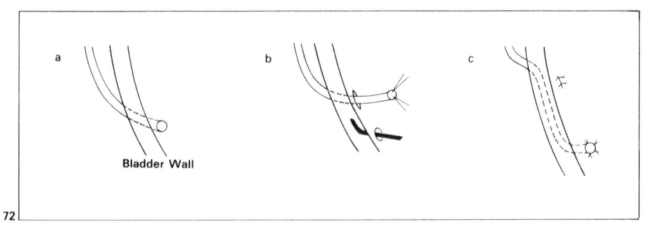

a

Bladder Wall

b

c

72

Bladder and
Posterior Urethra

Structure

Bladder and prostatic pathology cause the most commonly encountered genitourinary problems. The bladder is the urinary reservoir and, in children, it is situated principally in the abdomen with its upper two thirds covered with peritoneum, whilst in adults it descends with the growth of the pelvis to become a pelvic organ with only the superior surface covered with peritoneum. In order to prevent contamination of the intra-peritoneal cavity with urine, blood and/or pus most open conservative bladder and all prostate gland operations are carried out extra-peritoneally. The bladder wall contains an inner layer of thickened transitional mucosa and a vascular sub-mucosal layer, except over the trigone, where both the transitional layer and the sub-mucosal space is much thinner. The thickened mucosal layer and the loose sub-mucosal layer in the remainder of the bladder enable it to distend to its full adult capacity of 400 to 450ml. The middle wall of the bladder consists of thick smooth muscle fibres arranged in long intertwining helical groups whose circular arrangement predominates at the bladder neck (Tanagho and Smith, 1966, Yalla et al., 1977a), producing the autonomic internal sphincter (fig. 73). Further smooth bladder muscle fibres continue beyond the internal sphincter to attach both to the prostatic urethra and to the external sphincter, which is formed by the medial portion of the peri-urethral levator ani muscle (Hutch, 1972). The external sphincter is under voluntary control through the pudendal nerve (fig. 73) and actively contracts during abdominal straining to resist increased abdominal pressure.

In view of its mechanical, and possibly functional, obstructive elements the internal sphincter is always incised or damaged during a prostatectomy operation, but every care is taken to ensure that the external sphincter remains intact so that continence will be preserved. Deliberate division of the external sphincter to relieve neurogenic urinary retention (Yalla et al., 1977b) is occasionally necessary (see chapter XI).

73 Bladder muscles and nerves. Bladder and posterior urethral continuous smooth and striated muscle arrangements and their nerve supply (see fig. 69).

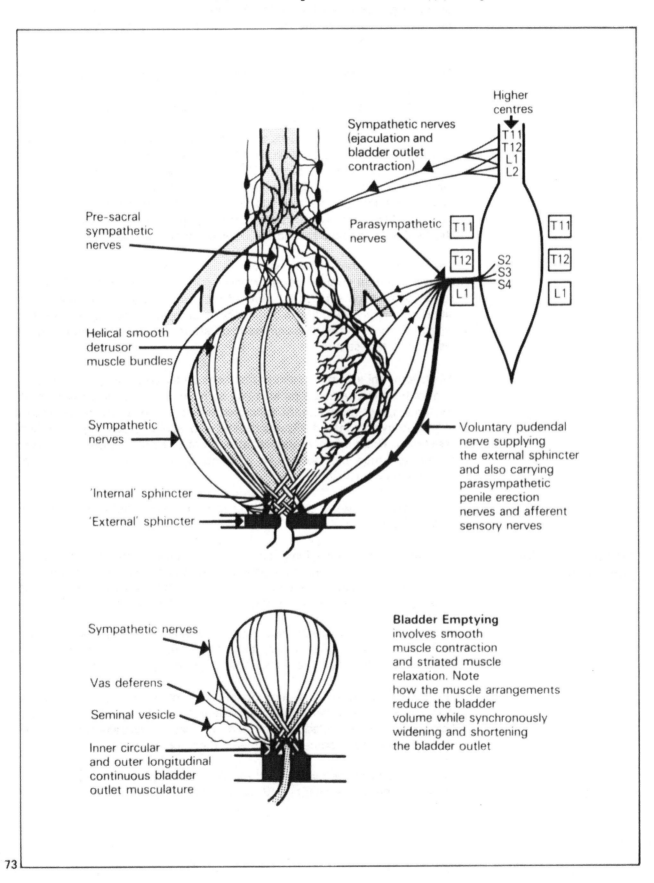

Higher centres

Sympathetic nerves (ejaculation and bladder outlet contraction)

T11
T12
L1
L2

Pre-sacral sympathetic nerves

Parasympathetic nerves

T11

T11

T12

T12

T12

L1

L1

S2
S3
S4

Helical smooth detrusor muscle bundles

Sympathetic nerves

Voluntary pudendal nerve supplying the external sphincter and also carrying parasympathetic penile erection nerves and afferent sensory nerves

'Internal' sphincter

'External' sphincter

Sympathetic nerves

Vas deferens

Seminal vesicle

Inner circular and outer longitudinal continuous bladder outlet musculature

Bladder Emptying involves smooth muscle contraction and striated muscle relaxation. Note how the muscle arrangements reduce the bladder volume while synchronously widening and shortening the bladder outlet

The female bladder outlet (fig. 74) musculature is weaker than the male and this factor, together with the shorter urethra and the occasional widening of the angle between the outlet and the urethra due to anterior vaginal prolapse, accounts for the high incidence of female stress incontinence of urine (p. 77, 358).

Nerve Supply

The bladder is supplied by sympathetic and parasympathetic nerve fibres. The efferent sympathetic fibres originate from the eleventh and twelfth thoracic and the first and second lumbar cord segments and run (figs. 69 and 73) in the superior hypogastric plexus and the pre-sacral nerve, crossing the bifurcation of the aorta, to innervate smooth muscle at the bladder neck and external sphincter region (Awad and Downie, 1976). Stimulation causes closure of the bladder outlet and occurs during ejaculation. Excessive efferent sympathetic activity may produce the rare condition of sympathetic dyssynergia resulting in lower urinary tract outlet obstruction (Krahe and Olsson, 1973). The afferent sympathetic nerve fibres arise from the fundus of the bladder and are believed to convey pain fibres.

The parasympathetic nerve supply is of far greater significance. The parasympathetic efferent detrusor fibres arise from the second, third and fourth sacral segments, at the level of the twelfth thoracic vertebra. This site is commonly traumatised during severe paraplegic back injuries, resulting in urinary retention. Parasympathetic afferent distension stimuli fibres also run to this centre.

The levator ani external sphincter muscle is under voluntary pudendal fibre control from the same sacral area and stimulation of this nerve will inhibit micturition, by contracting the sphincter, whilst division of the nerve results in an inability to contract this muscle and a consequent lowering of urethral resistance. This traditional surgical attempt at relieving neurogenic bladder urinary retention has now been replaced by the operation of external sphincterotomy (p. 266).

These nerve pathways are influenced and, normally, controlled by higher nerve centres (fig. 73).

Neurotransmitter Substances

Sympathetic post-ganglionic nerve fibres release noradrenaline whilst parasympathetic pre- and post-ganglion nerve fibres release acetylcholine. Ephedrine administration liberates noradrenaline from its storage sites and may be used to increase the resistance at the bladder outlet (p. 357).

Adrenergic blocking agents, such as phenoxybenzamine can occasionally be used to relieve lower urinary tract obstruction of urine in those rare patients suffering from the 'sympathetic dyssynergia' syndrome.

Anticholinergic drugs, such as propantheline, inhibit detrusor contraction and are used to combat detrusor over-action. Cholinergic drugs, such as bethanecol, increase bladder tone and are used to increase the detrusor muscle efficiency in some patients with detrusor inactivity.

These aspects of the bladder and posterior urethral nerve supply are discussed further in the chapters IV, XI and XV.

Normal Micturition

During normal micturition parasympathetic-induced contraction of the smooth bladder muscle, in the absence of excessive sympathetic activity and higher centre inhibition, results in a raised intra-vesical pressure and simultaneous opening of the bladder neck, due to shortening of the fibres attached to the posterior urethra (fig. 73). Synchronous voluntary relaxation of the external sphincter permits urine to leave the bladder and enter the urethra. The bladder normally empties completely and the inability to achieve this, or to void at will, indicates a mechanical, neurological or functional bladder, bladder outlet and/or urethral abnormality.

74 The female bladder outlet and urethra. Note that the posterior pubo-urethral ligaments attach to both the pubis and the superior levator ani fascia.

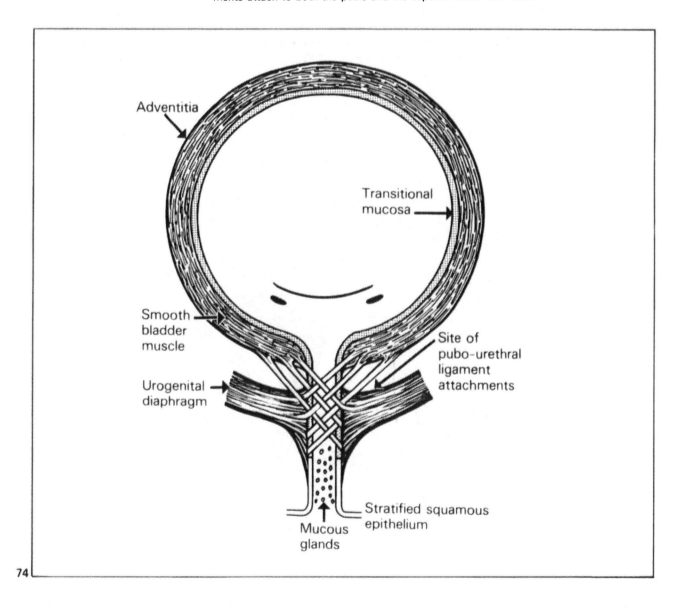

74

*Macroscopic
Relationships*

Superior Relationships: The bladder is covered with peritoneum, the uterus and small bowel in the female and the pelvic colon and small intestine in the male (figs. 75-76). The median umbilical ligament, or urachus, joins the superior aspect of the bladder to the umbilicus. These relationships are illustrated by the rare development of a vesicocolic fistula following malignancy or longstanding chronic inflammatory large bowel pathology.

External traumatic intra-peritoneal bladder rupture occurs in the fundal area while extra-peritoneal bladder rupture, which is almost always associated with a pelvic bone fracture, occurs low down on the anterior bladder wall (see chapter XIII).

Anterior Relationships: The bladder is related to the pubic symphysis, abdominal rectus muscles and the conjoint tendon. This relationship can result in bladder damage during inguinal herniorrhaphy operations in the uncommon event of a bladder diverticulum entering the hernial opening (fig. 83).

Posterior Relationships: The bladder is related to the lower uterus, cervix and vagina in the female and to the vas deferens, seminal vesicles and the fascia of Denonvilliers and rectum in the male. A vesico-vaginal or a vesico-cervical fistula can result from surgical, neoplastic, obstetric or radiotherapy damage in this area (p. 310).

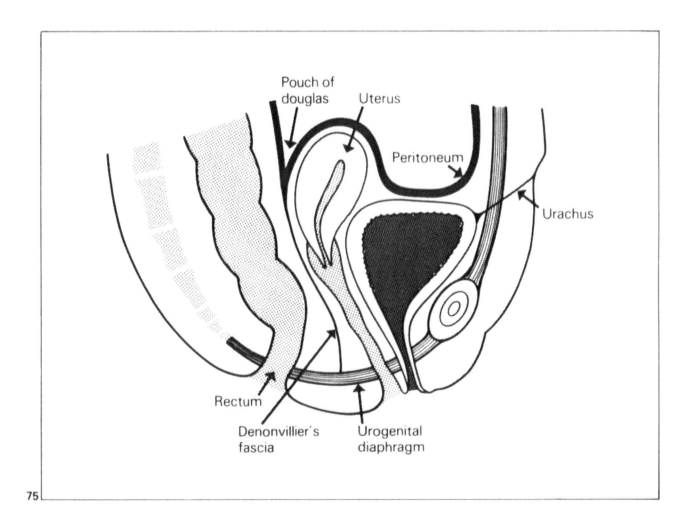

75

75 Female bladder relationships.

76 Male bladder relationships. The prostate gland, urethra, urogenital diaphragm and the fascial layers of the lower abdomen, penis, scrotum and perineum.

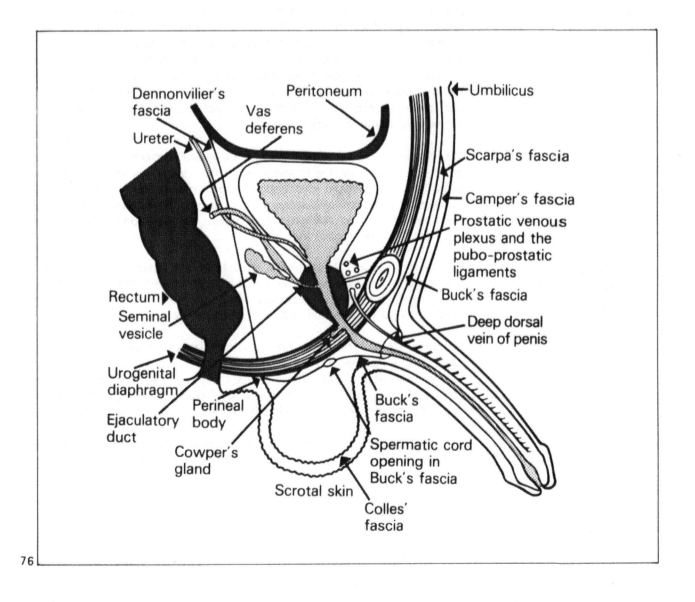

76

Infero-lateral Relationships: The infero-lateral surfaces of the bladder are related to the vesico-prostatic venous plexus, levator ani muscles, the internal obturator vessels and the pelvic girdle.

Inferior Relationships: In the male the prostate gland encircles the urethra below the bladder.

The Prostate Gland and the Urogenital Diaphragm

The prostate gland contains the prostatic urethra and has the shape of an inverted cone, surrounding the urethra from the bladder outlet to the urogenital diaphragm. The superior surface of the gland is intimately associated with the bladder outlet and internal sphincter, whilst inferiorly the prostate is related to the urogenital diaphragm which, as indicated in figure 76, is formed by strong layers of pelvic and perineal fascia enveloping the thick levator ani muscle. The diaphragm is weaker in the female as there is less muscle, thinner fascia and it is pierced by the urethra, vagina and rectum (fig. 75).

The prostate is surrounded by fatty pelvic connective tissue, containing the vesico-prostatic venous plexus, and is firmly attached to the pubic symphysis by the pubo-prostatic ligaments, which must be torn before a prostato-membranous traumatic urethral separation can occur. Open retropubic prostatectomy (p. 248) necessitates incising the anterior capsule of the prostate, after careful dissection and mobilisation of the related vesico- prostatic venous plexus. Posteriorly the prostate is related to the seminal vesicles, vas deferens, fascia of Denonvilliers and the rectum. The fascia of Denonvilliers results from fusion of the original peritoneal pouch in this area and forms a firm fascial plane which usually resists prostatic neoplastic invasion until a late stage.

The ejaculatory ducts enter the postero-lateral surface of the prostate gland and emerge on the lateral sides of the verumontanum, which contains the small vestigial mesonephric duct remnant, the prostatic utricle, situated between the ejaculatory duct openings. The prostate gland duct openings emerge on the groove between the verumontanum and the posterior urethral mucosa (fig. 77).

Blood Vessels, Lymphatics and Nerves

Prostatic Arteries: The arteries arise from the inferior vesical, middle haemorrhoidal and external pudendal. The major vessels enter the gland infero-laterally, just below the bladder neck, and must be ligated or diathermied at an early stage during a prostatectomy operation.

Prostatic Veins: The veins drain to the peri-prostatic venous plexus into which the dorsal vein of the penis also enters. The peri-prostatic plexus drains to the internal iliac veins, but also communicates with the pre-sacral venous plexus, and this accounts for the common findings of prostatic neoplasm metastases in the pelvic bones and the lumbar vertebrae.

Lymphatic and Nerve Supply: The lymphatic drainage and nerve supply of the prostate gland is similar to the inferior aspect of the bladder.

77 The urethra and prostate gland. A prostatectomy operation damages the internal sphincter, leading to retrograde ejaculation, provided that the ejaculatory ducts do not stenose. The external sphincter is responsible for postoperative continence of urine.

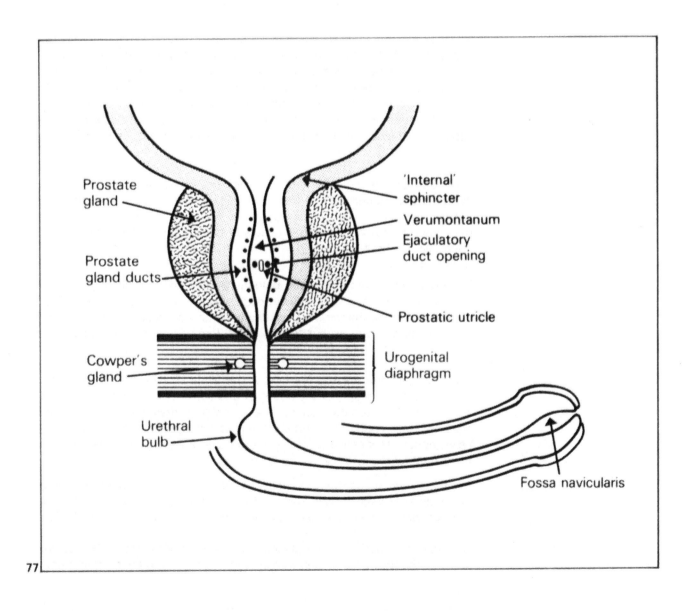

Prostate gland

'Internal' sphincter

Verumontanum

Ejaculatory duct opening

Prostate gland ducts

Prostatic utricle

Cowper's gland

Urogenital diaphragm

Urethral bulb

Fossa navicularis

Prostatic Histology, Function and Major Pathology

The prostate consists of numerous glands enclosed in a fibro-muscular stroma and surrounded by a fibrous capsule. Benign adenomatous prostatomegaly develops from the superficial and middle gland groups, creating the surgical plane of open prostatic enucleation indicated in figure 78b. Neoplastic changes develop in the peripheral glands and can be detected at an early stage by a rectal examination. The majority of the smooth muscle stroma fibres originate from the previously discussed bladder muscle fibres which insert into the posterior urethra.

The prostate glands are individually surrounded by smooth muscle which contracts during ejaculation, liberating about 0.5ml of prostatic fluid, the precise function of which is unknown, although it at least offers a fluid medium for the sperm.

The Urethra

The Male Urethra

The urethral urinary and semen conduit is divided into prostatic, membranous, bulbous and penile portions, with the prostatic and bulbous portions having the widest diameter and either the external urinary meatus, or an area just inside the meatus, having the smallest (fig. 77). The bulbous and penile urethra is surrounded by the extremely vascular erectile tissue of the corpus spongiosum.

Provided that the prostate gland is not enlarged the prostatic urethra is the widest part of the tube. The posterior mid-line of the prostatic urethra contains a raised area, termed the verumontanum, which contains the prostatic utricle, prostatic gland duct openings and the ejaculatory ducts (fig. 77). The inferior aspect of the verumontanum is an important land-mark in transurethral prostatic surgery, as resection beyond this area could damage the external sphincteric mechanism and produce permanent incontinence (p. 355).

The bend of the bulbous urethra must be appreciated when passing catheters and instruments as trauma in this region can result in death from septicaemia or a life-long stricture (p. 240). A traumatic prostato-membranous urethral separation occurs at the junction of the prostatic and membranous urethra, due to the tough nature of the male urogenital diaphragm.

The prostatic, membranous and bulbous portions of the urethra, together with a variable portion of the anterior urethra, are lined by transitional epithelium, whilst the remainder of the anterior urethra is lined by modified columnar epithelium, except for the distal 2cm where stratified squamous epithelium is found (p. 179).

Vessels, Lymphatics and Nerves of the Male Urethra: The blood, lymphatic and nerve supply of the posterior and some of the anterior urethra is similar to the prostate gland. The lymphatic drainage of the distal squamous cell epithelium lined urethra is to the inguinal and not the intra-pelvic nodes. This drainage influences the radical treatment of the rare anterior urethral malignancy.

The Female Urethra

The female urinary conduit urethra is a small tube, running from the bladder to the anterior vaginal wall, and lined by transitional cell epithelium in the proximal portion and by squamous cell epithelium in the distal (figs. 74-75).

Numerous mucous secreting glands are found in the mucosa. Their secretion aids the flow of urine and also acts as a deterrent to bacterial invasion.

The prostate
78a The normal prostate gland.

78b The sites of development of prostatic pathology and the surgeon's benign adenoma enucleation plane. Note the consequent distortion and obstruction of the prostatic urethra.

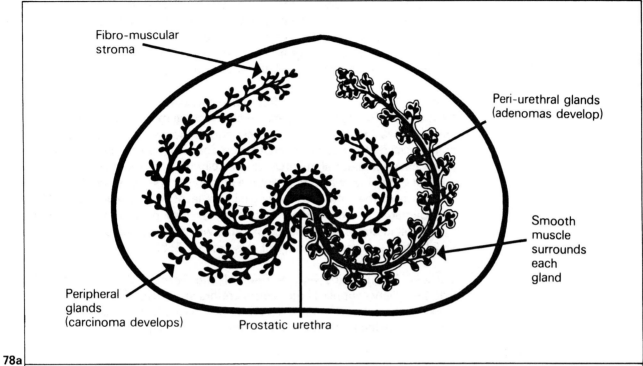

Fibro-muscular stroma

Peri-urethral glands (adenomas develop)

Smooth muscle surrounds each gland

Peripheral glands (carcinoma develops)

Prostatic urethra

78a

Surgeon's enucleation plane after incising the 'surgical capsule'

Enlarging adenoma and pseudo-capsule

Non-adenomatous compressed peripheral prostatic tissue

Fibrous prostatitis

Anatomical capsule

Stage III prostatic carcinoma

78b

Infected or non-infected urethro-trigonitis is very common and may result from interference with the secretion of these glands (p. 143).

The female urethra is surrounded by spongy erectile tissue, which is enclosed by the smooth and striated muscle derived from the bladder and levator ani respectively, and which forms the female outlet sphincteric mechanism. The arrangements of the muscle fibres in this area and raised intra-abdominal pressure, tends to both widen and lower the bladder outlet during voiding, as indicated previously. Anteriorly the female urethra is related to the pubic symphysis and pubo-vesical ligaments whilst posteriorly it is part of the anterior wall of the vagina and opens into it.

Krantz (1951) and Zacharin (1968) have stressed the importance of the female posterior urethral suspensory ligaments in maintaining urinary continence. These ligaments, which correspond to the male pubo-prostatic ligaments, include the anterior pubo-urethral ligament, which connects the anterior external urethral meatus to the clitoris and the posterior pubo-urethral ligaments, which connect the junction of the upper third and distal two thirds of the urethra to the pubic bone, levator ani fascia and the bladder. Damage to the posterior ligaments, as may occur during childbirth, may result in stress incontinence of urine, which may be cured by operative stabilisation and strengthening of this area (p. 358).

Vessels, Lymphatics and Nerves of the Female Urethra: Both the blood and nerve supply of the female urethra are derived from the pelvic inferior vesical internal pudendal vessels but, as with the male urethra, the lymphatic drainage of the distal portion is to the inguinal nodes.

The Fascial Coverings of the Lower Abdomen and Perineum

The fascial coverings of the lower abdomen, perineum, penis, scrotum and urethra are known as Scarpa's, Camper's, Colles' and Buck's fascia (fig. 79).

Midway between the pubis and the umbilicus the fatty superficial fascia of the abdomen forms a deep membranous layer termed Scarpa's fascia. The remaining, continuing, subcutaneous tissue becomes fibrous and is termed Camper's fascia.

Beyond the superficial inguinal ring Scarpa's fascia is termed Colles' fascia and continues to become the dartos muscle of the scrotum, which is responsible for the corrugations of the scrotal skin. Neither the scrotum nor the penis contains subcutaneous fat.

Colles' fascia encloses the scrotum and penis and is attached laterally to the ischial rami and pubis and, inferiorly, to the posterior border of the perineal membrane. Two openings in Colles' fascia permit the passage of the penis, covered with a layer of deep fascia termed Buck's fascia, and the spermatic cords.

Rupture of the urethra below the urogenital diaphragm (p. 298) may lead to blood and urinary extravasation below Colles' fascia and this extravasation is limited to the above attachments of the fascia. Superiorly the extravasation may extend to the abdomen and chest wall, although such delayed presentations are now extremely rare. External surgical drainage of such extravasated collections may be necessary and incisions must always pierce Colles' fascia to be effective.

79 Fascial coverings. The fascia covering the lower abdomen, penis, scrotum and perineum. Note the firm attachment areas of the superficial and deep fascia which limit the extravasation of blood and urine following rupture of the corpora and the anterior urethra.

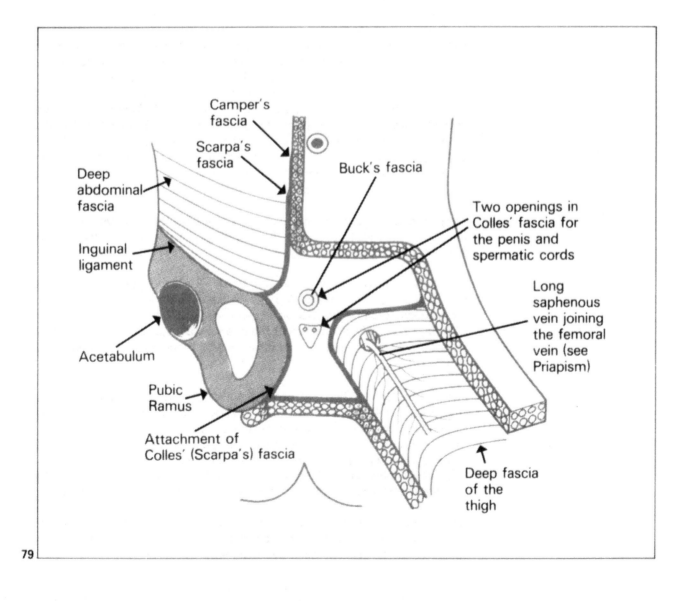

The Penis and Prepuce

The Prepuce

The Penis

Complications of the prepuce are discussed in chapters X and XIV.

The inability to replace the prepuce, after retraction, may result in considerable swelling of the involved skin, due to venous occlusion, and this condition is termed *paraphimosis*. Circumcision is required if manual reduction is unsuccessful.

The penis is the intromittent, copulatory, male organ and consists of 3 vascular compartments, surrounded by Buck's and Colles' fascia as previously described. Buck's fasica provides the septal vascular compartments and also encloses the deep dorsal vein, arteries and nerves.

In 1743 Francois de la Peyronie described a fibrotic change of unknown aetiology, occurring in Buck's fascia (fig. 80), and often infiltrating the cavernosum. The fibrosis can be painful in the early stages and, because of tethering, often results in lateral deviation of the penis during erection, making sexual intercourse difficult or impossible. β-adrenoceptor blocking drugs may cause *Peyronie's* disease (Osborne, 1977). Such patients occasionally have associated *Dupuytren's contracture* of the palms and soles and, rarely, other areas of the body. Early treatment, with cortisone and hyaluronidase injections, directly into the fibrotic area, may be of benefit in resolving the fibrosis (Chesney, 1963).

The 3 vascular compartments contain the twin corpora cavernosa and the corpus spongiosum enclosing the urethra. The corpus spongiosum expands at its distal end to form the glans penis and is surrounded on its lower aspect by the bulbo-spongiosis muscle. The corpora are each supplied by different arteries as illustrated in figure 80. These arteries are derived from the internal pudendal and divide into 3 branches for the spongiosum and cavernosum and 2 other branches, which run with the deep dorsal vein and nerves as illustrated. Venous drainage of the penis is divided into a superficial dorsal vein which drains into the saphenous vein, and a deep dorsal vein which drains into the prostatic venous plexus.

Lymphatic drainage of the body of the penis is to the external iliac group whilst the superficial lymphatics drain to the inguinal nodes and then to the external iliac group.

The shaft of the penis is covered with highly elastic, non-fatty skin and this stretch characteristic enables flap urethroplasty operations to be performed for both stricture and hypospadias operations (p. 256 and p. 346), as well as allowing for wide local excision of the rare scrotal carcinoma (p. 188). Penile sensation occurs through the terminal sensory branches of the internal pudendal nerve.

Penile Erection: When the penis is flaccid blood is shunted from the cavernosa and spongiosum channels by arterio-venous anastomoses (Conti, 1952), which may be activated by sympathetic nerve stimulation, as indicated in figure 80, whilst erection of the penis, resulting from pudendal nerve second, third and fourth parasympathetic sacral segment fibres (Hinman, 1960), initiated by higher centre and other stimuli allows blood to fill and intercommunicate with all three channels. (See also chapter XX.)

Semen Ejaculation and Emission: This requires a simultaneous contraction of the internal bladder neck sphincter and a relaxation of the external sphincter, whilst the vas deferens, seminal vesicles, prostatic and bulbo-

80 The penis and its blood supply.

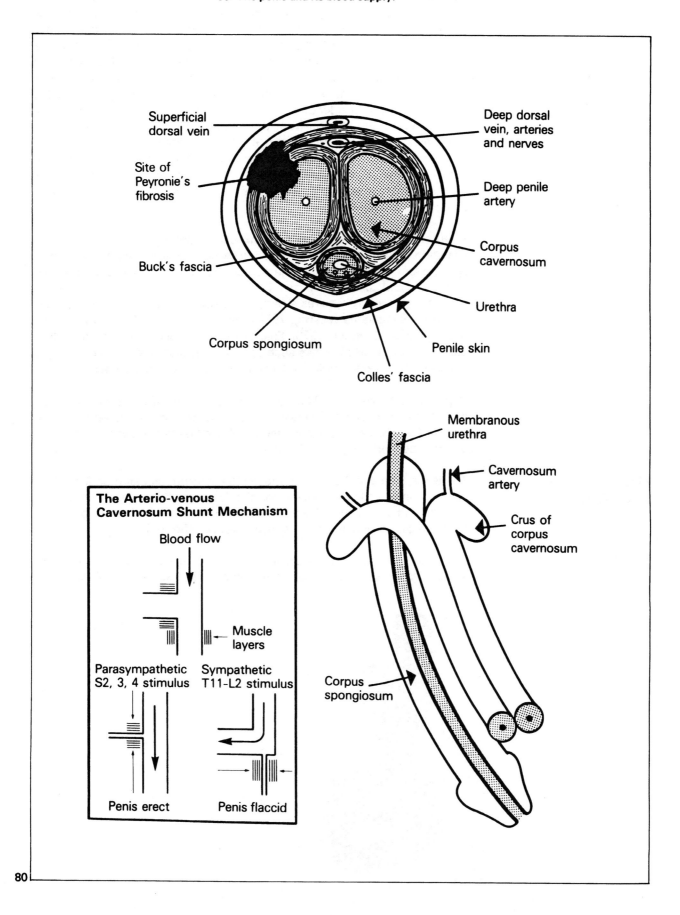

spongiosis muscles contract synchronously, propelling the ejaculate along the urethra. This mechanism is dependent upon an intact and normally functioning lumbar sympathetic nervous system, normal non-obstructive anatomy and a lack of higher nerve centre inhibition (fig. 73). Premature ejaculation (p. 392) is a common and distressing problem, which responds well to treatment directed at moderating this mechanism. The normal ejaculate has a volume of 4ml, with the sperm component occupying the first 0.5ml. The remainder of the fluid is secreted from the seminal vesicles, with a smaller contribution from the prostate gland and Cowper's gland. The ejaculate contains water and electrolytes, lipids, proteins, minerals, acid and alkaline phosphatase, coagulase and fibrinolysin enzymes, prostaglandins, bicarbonate, prostate citric acid, spermine and seminal vesicle fructose (see chapter XVIII). The role of most of these ejaculate constituents is unknown.

Priapism: In priapism, which is of unknown aetiology, there is a sustained dilatation of the vessels of the corpora cavernosum whilst the corpus spongiosum remains flaccid. The corpora cavernosa is painfully distended with blood and cannot return to a flaccid condition until the blood is drained from it. This usually requires a temporary, open, surgical anastomosis between the saphenous vein (fig. 79) and the related side of a corpora cavernosum (Eadie and Brock, 1970). Priapism is said to occur more commonly in patients with blood disorders such as leukaemia and sickle cell disease and occasionally follows prolonged sexual excitement in older patients.

Penile Shaft Fracture: This rare condition results from a direct severe blow to the erect penis. The resultant damage to the corpora leads to rupture of the delicate vascular channels, followed by fibrosis and, usually, impotence beyond the point of injury.

The Testis and Associated Structures

The Testis

The testis is an ovoid organ situated in the scrotum and surrounded by the visceral tunica vaginalis, except posteriorly, where it is fixed to the scrotal wall (fig. 82). A congenital lack of such fixation and a high insertion of the tunica vaginalis may result in testicular torsion (fig. 81).

The testis is surrounded by a small amount of fluid, sufficient to allow intra-scrotal movement and some protection against trauma, contained within

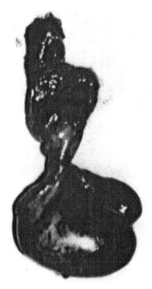

81

The testis and associated structures
81 Torsion of the spermatic cord resulting in death of the testis.

82 The testis, epidiymis, vas deferens, seminal vesicles, ejaculatory ducts and spermatic cord. Note the mesonephric paraepididymal and testicular remnanats which may tort if pedunculated (p. 80).

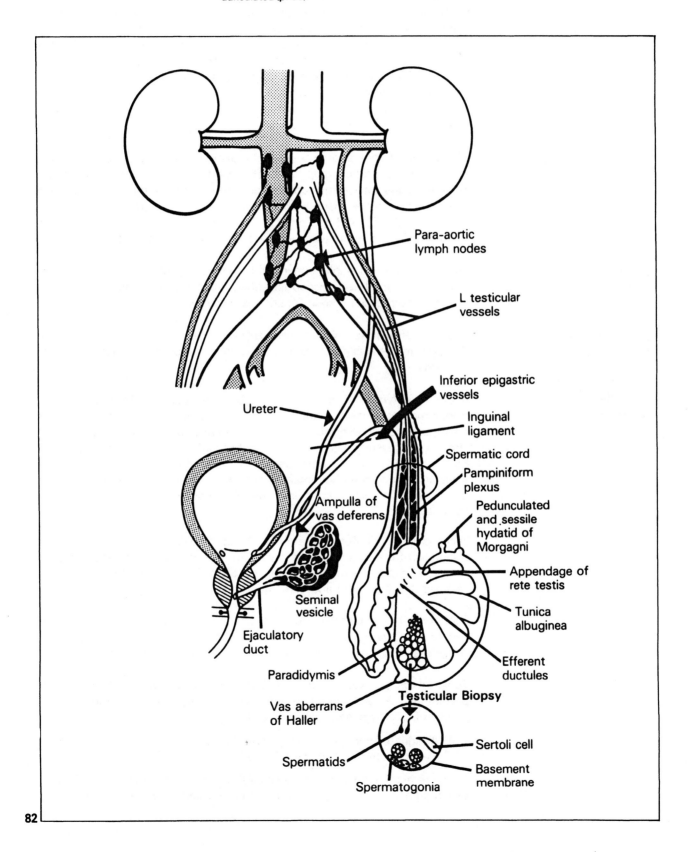

Para-aortic lymph nodes

L testicular vessels

Inferior epigastric vessels

Inguinal ligament

Spermatic cord

Pampiniform plexus

Pedunculated and sessile hydatid of Morgagni

Appendage of rete testis

Tunica albuginea

Efferent ductules

Ureter

Ampulla of vas deferens

Seminal vesicle

Ejaculatory duct

Paradidymis

Vas aberrans of Haller

Spermatids

Spermatogonia

Testicular Biopsy

Sertoli cell

Basement membrane

82

the tunica vaginalis. An excessive amount of fluid in this space results in a *hydrocele* (p. 28 and 81). The testis consists of tubules, extra-tubular connective tissue and Leydig cells, surrounded by a fibrous tunica albuginia, whose septa divide the testis into compartments providing added mechanical strength. The tubules contain a basement membrane from which both germinal and Sertoli cells grow. The germinal cells divide by meiosis and mitosis, eventually producing many millions of spermatozoa, but the role of the Sertoli cells is unknown. The extra-tubular Leydig cells produce testosterone (see chapters XVIII and XX). Testosterone secretion is essential for both libido and potency and is controlled by the serum levels of luteinising hormone, prolactin and gonadotrophic hormone, which are secreted by the anterior pituitary gland, in response to low serum testosterone levels (Wright, 1952).

All testicular lumps should be urgently explored, through a groin incision, after a non-traumatic clamp has been placed on the spermatic cord at the internal inguinal ring, as this enables both the diagnosis and initial treatment of a neoplasm to be made without disseminating the growth through the skin lymphatics (p. 186 and p. 187). The tubules of the testes join to form 10 to 20 efferent ducts (vasa efferentia) which join the epididymis.

Epididymis

The epididmyis is a single, convoluted, conducting tube, with a head, body and tail and lined with pseudostratified columnar epithelium possessing microvilli (stereocilia) whose function is unknown.

Epididymal and Testicular Inflammations, Infections and Torsion

Acute Conditions. *Acute epididymo-orchitis:* This traditional term, although anatomically accurate, is best considered as two distinct clinical problems.

Acute epididymitis: This is rare before the age of 21 years. Acute epididymitis is usually thought to result from a urinary tract infection, with the organisms travelling to the epididymis along the vas deferens following straining or severe physical exercise, but the infection may be blood-borne. Post-instrumentation or postoperative epididymitis is not uncommon. The epididymis gradually becomes inflamed, with or without a secondary hydrocele developing, and there is usually an associated mild testicular inflammation.

When occurring before the age of 21 years epididymitis is impossible to distinguish from *torsion of the testis* (fig. 81) and an immediate open exploration of the area is therefore necessary (Allan and Brown, 1966) to establish the diagnosis and instigate appropriate therapy (p. 80).

Recurrent epididymitis requires further special investigations, including an intravenous pyelogram and a cysto-urethroscopy, in order to exclude a congenital or acquired genitourinary tract primary abnormality.

Tuberculosis (p. 146) or, rarely, *inflammatory neoplasms of the testis,* can present acutely, and should be suspected if the inflammation does not respond to initial treatment consisting of:

1) Adequate broad spectrum chemotherapy
2) Elevation and rest of the inflamed area.

A severe epididymitis may take several months to resolve although most patients have adequate pain relief within the first week of treatment.

Gonorrhoea (chapter XIX), because of public education and adequate treatment, is now a very rare cause of acute epididymitis.

Acute orchitis: This uncommon condition is caused by blood-borne viruses including post-pubertal mumps, Coxsackie and infectious mononucleosis. In most patients only one testis is involved but the inflammation is usually severe and up to 50% of testes undergo subsequent atrophy (Werner, 1950).

Chronic Conditions. *Chronic epididymitis:* Most chronic epididymal infections in developed communities are non-tuberculous and result from persistent or recurrent infections which, as indicated earlier, require further investigation. In less affluent countries tuberculosis is by far the commonest cause.

The epididymis becomes irregularly thickened and, rarely, a scrotal sinus forms. The tuberculous epididymis, and any related involved skin, should be excised and the patient given a 2-year course of modern triple antituberculous drug therapy (p. 149).

Chronic orchitis: Sperm granuloma and granulomatous orchitis are rare lesions which cannot be distinguished from a possible testicular neoplasm and the diagnosis is therefore only made at exploratory operation (p. 186). Histologically, sperm granulomas exhibit the features of a foreign body reaction, whilst granulomatous orchitis exhibits the features of a granuloma (Morgan, 1964).

Vas Deferens

The tail of the epididymis becomes the tubular conducting vas deferens, which ascends the testis on its postero-medial side to join the spermatic cord and enter the retroperitoneal tissue by passing lateral to the inferior epigastric vessels, before descending the lateral wall of the pelvis to cross the external iliac vessels, obturator nerve and vessels and ureter, joining the duct of the seminal vesicle to form the ejaculatory duct, which pierces the prostate gland to emerge on the verumontanum (figs. 69, 77, 82). The course and relationships of the vas deferens in the pelvis are of considerable assistance to the surgeon dissecting in this area (e.g. as a guide to the lower ureter when performing a low ureterolithotomy operation).

Immediately prior to its junction with the seminal vesicle the vas deferens dilates and this region is termed the ampulla of the vas (fig. 81). The vas deferens is also lined with stereocilia and has a thick muscular wall, except for the ampulla, where, consistent with its reservoir role, the wall is thinner. The operation of scrotal bilateral vasectomy is performed on those males who desire permanent sterility.

Seminal Vesicle

The seminal vesicle is a sacculated, convoluted tube, lying in the recto-vesical connective tissue and, together with the ampulla of the vas deferens, acts as a sperm reservoir.

Testicular Vessels, Lymphatics and Nerves

The testicular artery runs from the aorta to join the spermatic cord. Multiple veins drain the testis and ascend in the spermatic cord as the pampiniform plexus joining, usually, as a single vein above the internal inguinal ring (fig. 81). The right testicular vein joins the inferior vena cava, whilst the left testicular vein joins the left renal vein and as discussed previously, this accounts for the occasional appearance of a left-sided *varicocele* in patients with an obstructed left renal vein due to a renal neoplasm. Most varicoceles however result from the absence or failure of venous valves and not from left renal neoplasms (Brown et al., 1967). Varicoceles are found in 8% of men (Clarke, 1966) and may cause poor sperm motility and morphology infertility (Tulloch, 1952) by raising the temperature of the testis (p. 375). Should ligation therapy be necessary it is best performed retroperitoneally, through a small abdominal incision, where the one or two vessels are easily identified (Palomo, 1949), rather than attempting a difficult ligation of the pampiniform plexus.

The lymphatic drainage of the testis ascends in the spermatic cord to the para-aortic lymph nodes, which are situated between the renal vessels and the bifurcation of the aorta. Testicular neoplasms may metastasise to these nodes (p. 185), which may require surgical excision if the neoplasm is a teratoma.

Spermatic Cord

The spermatic cord runs from the internal inguinal ring to the upper posterior part of the testis and contains the testicular artery, pampiniform plexus, vas deferens, sympathetic nerve fibres of the aortic plexus and the testicular lymphatics (fig. 82). These structures are covered by 3 coats: the external spermatic fascia, derived from the external oblique muscle; cremasteric muscle, derived from the internal oblique muscle, and the internal spermatic fascia, derived from the fascia transversalis.

Cremasteric muscle contraction is responsible for intermittent testicular retraction, which is often incorrectly diagnosed as an undescended testis (p. 26, 349).

Inguinal and Femoral Hernias

Indirect inguinal hernias traverse the inguinal canal, following the original pathway of the processus vaginalis (p. 28), while direct inguinal hernias emerge medial to the inferior epigastric vessels (fig. 83). Rarely the spermatic cord may be damaged during surgical repair of these hernias and this may lead to testicular infarction or hydrocele formation. Rarely, enlarged bladder protrusions or diverticula enter the hernial pouch and may be inadvertently traumatised during a repair operation.

Fournier's Gangrene

A rare, mixed infection of the scrotal skin, occurring in all age groups and leading to massive necrosis, is termed Fournier's gangrene (1884), although Pott (1779) originally described it. High dose broad spectrum chemotherapy, adequate wound debridement and drainage is usually curative, with or without secondary delayed skin suture and grafting, dependent upon the amount of tissue necrosis.

83 Hernias. An intra-abdominal view of inguinal and femoral hernias emerging above and below the inguinal ligament respectively.

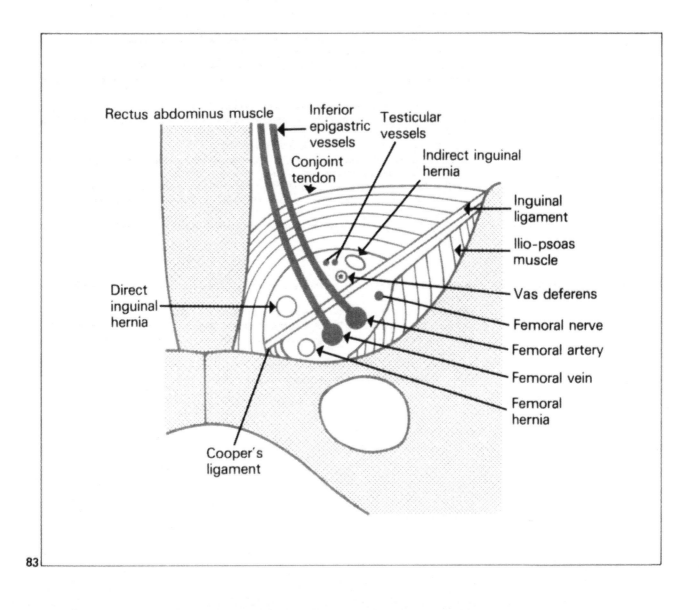

Rectus abdominus muscle

Inferior epigastric vessels

Testicular vessels

Conjoint tendon

Indirect inguinal hernia

Inguinal ligament

Ilio-psoas muscle

Direct inguinal hernia

Vas deferens

Femoral nerve

Femoral artery

Femoral vein

Femoral hernia

Cooper's ligament

References

Allan, W.R. and Brown, R.B.: Torsion of the testis: A review of 58 cases. British Medical Journal 1: 1396 (1966).

Awad, S.A. and Downie, W.G.: Relative contributions of smooth and striated muscle to the canine urethral pressure profile. British Journal of Urology 48: 347 (1976).

Brown, J.S.; Dubin, L. and Hotchkus, R.S.: The varicocele as related to fertility. Fertility and Sterility 18: 46 (1967).

Brown, R.B.: Spontaneous nephrocolic fistula. British Journal of Urology 5: 488 (1966).

Chesney, J.: Plastic induration of the penis: Peyronie's disease. British Journal of Urology 35: 61 (1963).

Clarke, B.G.: Incidence of varicocele in normal men and among men of different ages. Journal of the American Medical Association 198: 1121 (1966).

Conti, G.: L'erection du penis humain et ses bases morphologico-vasculaires. Acta Anatomica 14: 217 (1952).

Eadie, D.C.A. and Brock, T.P.: Corpus-saphenous by-pass in the treatment of priapism. British Journal of Surgery 57: 172 (1970).

Fournier, J.A.; in Semaine Medicale 4: 69 (1884).

Hinman, F. Jr.: Priapism: reasons for failure of therapy. Journal of Urology 83: 420 (1960).

Kaufman, J.J. and Bruce, P.T.: Testicular atrophy following mumps: a cause of testicular tumour? British Journal of Urology 35: 67 (1963).

Krane, R.J. and Olsson, C.A.: Phenoxybenzamine in neurogenic bladder dysfunction. II. Clinical considerations. Journal of Urology 110: 653 (1973).

Krantz, K.E.: Anatomy of the urethra and anterior vaginal wall. American Journal of Obstetrics and Gynecology 62: 374 (1951).

Morgan, A.D.: Inflammatory lesions stimulating malignancy. British Journal of Urology 36 (Suppl.): 95 (1964).

Osborne, D.R.: Propranolol and Peyronie's disease. Lancet 1: 1111 (1977).

Palomo, A.: Radical cure of varicocele by a new technique: preliminary report. Journal of Urology 61: 604 (1949).

Peyronie, F. de la: Sur quelques obstacles qui s'opposent a l'ejaculation naturelle de la semence. Memoires de l'Academie Royale de Chirurgie 1: 318 (1743).

Pott, P.: The chirurgical works of Percival Pott, Vol. 2 (Lowndes, London 1779).

Tanagho, E.A. and Smith, D.R.: The anatomy and function of the bladder neck. British Journal of Urology 38: 54 (1966).

Tulloch, W.A.: Varicocele in subfertility: results of treatment. British Medical Journal 2: 356 (1952).

Werner, C.A.: Mumps orchitis and testicular atrophy: occurrence. Annals of Internal Medicine 32: 1066 (1950).

Wright, S.: Applied Physiology, 9th Ed. (Oxford, London 1952).

Yalla, S.V.; Gabilondo, F.B.; Blunt, K.J.; Fam, B.A.; Castello, A. and Kaufman, J.M.: Functional striated sphincter component at bladder neck. Journal of Urology 118: 408 (1977a).

Yalla, S.V.; Fam, B.A.; Gabilondo, F.B.; Jacobs, S.; Di Benedetto, M.; Rossier, A.B. and Gittes, R.F.: Anteromedian external urethral sphincterotomy technique, rationale and complications. Journal of Urology 117: 489 (1977b).

Zacharin, R.F.: The anatomic supports of the female urethra. Obstetrics and Gynaecology 32: 754 (1968).

Further Reading

de Wardener, H.E.: The Kidney: An Outline of Normal and Abnormal Structure and Function (Churchill Livingstone, London 1973).

Gilmore, J.P.: Renal Physiology (Williams and Watkins, Baltimore 1972).

McGregor, A.L. and Duplessis, D.J.: A Synposis of Surgical Anatomy, 10th Ed. (Wright, Bristol 1969).

Hutch, J.A.: Anatomy and Physiology of the Bladder, Trigone and Urethra (Butterworths, New York 1972).

Pott, P.: The Chirurgical Works of Percival Pott, Vol. 2 (Lowndes, London, 1779).

Wright, S.: Applied Physiology, 9th Ed. (Oxford, London 1952).

Chapter III

Diagnosis and Investigation of Genitourinary Disease

An adequate history and a thorough physical examination enables many urological diagnoses to be made. This is emphasised in the section on inguino-scrotal swellings.

Special investigations have greatly increased the accuracy of clinical diagnosis although their usefulness, risks and costs should always be considered. The continuing development of sophisticated special investigations has not replaced careful history taking and examination findings, nor the special doctor-patient relationship, which is essential and requires a combination of mature common sense, responsibility and scientific knowledge.

One special investigation, urodynamics, is discussed separately, in chapter IV.

The Patient History

Patients commonly present to urologists complaining of difficulty with micturition, pain, haematuria, a swelling or a urethral discharge. There is much to be gained by allowing the patient to describe his own problems before asking direct questions.

General Considerations

The age, marital status, previous medical and surgical problems, including venereal disease and any suspicion of tuberculosis, present and past drug therapy, cigarette smoking habits and alcohol intake, family history, fluid intake, past and present occupation, and present level of physical and mental activity are essential items of information. The link between cigarette smoking, analine dye contact and carcinoma of the bladder is now well established. In women the date of the last menstrual period must be known and indicated to the radiologist before any x-ray examinations are undertaken. Any past history of abnormal bleeding must be fully investigated before surgical procedures are carried out.

Haematuria

All patients who present with macroscopic haematuria, or with microscopic haematuria greater than 20,000 red blood cells per ml, require both radiological outlining and direct visualisation of all of the urinary system, irrespective of their age or other symptoms (see chapter VI).

Pain

Renal and Ureteric Pain: Renal and ureteric pain is usually due to obstruction (see chapters IX and XII) but may be due to infection or neoplasia. The pain may be acute or chronic. Acute renal and ureteric colic is discussed in chapter XII, page 210. Chronic renal pain produces a dull loin ache, usually with anterior radiation and aggravated by jolting movements.

Bladder Pain: Acute obstructive bladder pain indicates that both the bladder musculature and nerves are healthy and, provided that the obstruction can be corrected (see chapter X), will function well after surgical correction, while chronic pain, or no pain in the presence of a large distended bladder, usually indicates the reverse.

Chronic obstructive bladder pain is felt supra-pubically whilst bladder outlet inflammatory pain, due to infection, calculus or neoplasm, produces a constant desire to void. An intense supra-pubic and penile desire to void, with associated frequency of micturition and, often, terminal haematuria, is termed *strangury*.

Prostate Pain: Prostatic pain may be acute but is usually chronic and due to inflammation. It is felt in the perineum and occasionally in the rectum and related areas.

Urethral Pain: Urethral pain may be chronic but in females, is usually acute-on-chronic and caused by inflammation. Sterile or infected non-obstructive urethro-trigonitis (see p. 136) is the most commonly referred urological problem in our community. The pain may be accompanied by scalding or burning depending upon the degree of inflammation present.

Back Pain: Lower tract genitourinary neoplasms are common and metastases, particularly from carcinoma of the prostate, often spread to the vertebrae and present as back pain. Paraplegia may result from a failure to investigate such pain. Most patients presenting with back pain, as an isolated symptom, have back strain and not genitourinary pathology.

Inguino-scrotal Pain: Torsion of the testis, or its appendages, may result in scrotal and/or referred abdominal pain in males, usually under the age of 21 years, whilst inflammatory epididymo-orchitis commonly produces intra-scrotal pain in older adults. Testicular neoplasms (p. 184) are rare but commonly present with scrotal pain. Idiopathic scrotal oedema and the rare scrotal fat necrosis are other causes of scrotal pain in children (see below).

Inguinal pain may be due to an obstructed or strangulated inguinal femoral hernia or to inflammation of the related drainage lymph glands from a primary infected source.

Frequency/Nocturia

Frequency is a common presenting symptom and, if associated with lower genitourinary tract infection, sterile or neoplastic inflammation, occurs together with urgency, scalding, burning, or even strangury. Frequency as a solitary symptom is most commonly due to anxiety but may be due to local disease which reduces the bladder capacity such as neoplasia, tuberculosis, interstitial cystitis or irradiation, or to general diseases, such as congestive cardiac failure, diabetes or to malfunction of the pituitary and adrenal glands (p. 45).

With a fluid intake of 1,500ml per day most healthy younger adults void 4 to 6 times whilst awake, and rarely at night.

Urgency-frequency and Strangury

As indicated previously inflammatory lesions of the bladder and/or bladder outlet produce a hypersensitive and painful pattern of micturition.

Incontinence

Urinary incontinence (see also chapter XV) may result from:

a) *Bladder outlet, external sphincter and or posterior pubo-urethral ligament weakness caused by:*
Congenital abnormality
Childbirth trauma
Post-surgical trauma
Pelvic fracture trauma
Infection

and/or,

b) *Detrusor malfunction resulting from:*
Infection
Neoplasm
Neurological causes
Anxiety

or,

c) *Congenital or acquired anatomical abnormalities such as:*
Ectopic ureter
Vesico-vaginal fistula, etc.

Incontinence may present as one of the following 3 types.

Stress Incontinence: Increasing the intra-abdominal pressure in the presence of an inefficient bladder outlet or external sphincteric mechanism may result in incontinence of urine. The symptom is common in women, particularly after childbirth or other damage to the pelvic floor and bladder supports (p. 355).

Urgency Incontinence: Severe urgency-frequency of micturition may result in incontinence, in the presence of a normal bladder outlet and sphincteric mechanism, and is independent of any increase in the intra-abdominal pressure.

Overflow Incontinence: Chronic retention of urine, in the presence of a large, insensitive, distended bladder and a weak bladder outlet and sphincteric mechanism, may result in continual or intermittent incontinence due to mechanical overflow. This condition is often wrongly attributed to senility.

Post-micturition dribbling may be due to overflow incontinence but more commonly is not a result of organic disease but inability to empty the bulbous urethra at the end of micturition. It is effectively treated by backwards ➡ forwards finger-stripping of all the anterior urethra at the completion of micturition.

Dysuria

Difficult micturition is not always due to mechanical and/or infective causes (chaps. V, X). Hesitancy is the most important symptom in assessing bladder outlet obstruction (p. 248).

Enuresis	Children who are incontinent at night, but dry during the day, and who have no detectable genitourinary abnormalities are termed enuretic (see p. 318).
Inguino-scrotal Swellings	See below.
Urethral Discharge	See chapter XIX.
Haemospermia	As an isolated symptom this condition is not uncommon and often causes considerable concern. It results from the rupture of a seminal vesicle, prostatic or posterior urethral vein. Reassurance and temporary abstinence is all that is necessary for a spontaneous resolution.
Pneumaturia	A vesico-intestinal (usually colonic) fistula, or a recent cysto-urethroscopy, may result in the passage of air bubbles in the urine. Large fistulae may result in the passage of both air and faecal material.
Dyspepsia and Nausea	The related nerve supply of the kidney, retro-peritoneal tissue and upper gut may result in a pelvi-ureteric hydronephrosis or a retro-peritoneal tumour presenting with dyspepsia and/or nausea (p. 274).
General Symptoms of Uraemia	Patients with long standing chronic retention of urine may admit to little difficulty voiding, even though their bladder is grossly distended. They may present with weight loss, anaemia, hypertension, fluid retention and a uraemic breath (see chapter XVI).
Impotence and Ejaculation Problems	See chapter XX.
Chyluria	Obstruction of the renal lymphatics may result in the passage of white, lymph-laden urine (p. 284).

Physical Examination

A thorough physical examination implies in particular a general estimation of the patient's cardiovascular, respiratory and neurological state, together with a specific examination of the genitourinary system, and must include both a microscopic and chemical analysis of the urine and measurement of the blood pressure.

Specific genitourinary examination includes smelling the breath for the odour of uraemia and examining the tongue and eye-balls for evidence of dehydration. Abdominal, back, scrotal and perineal inspection, palpation, percussion and auscultation are conducted in a systematic manner. Inspection is often more revealing, particularly in children, than palpation. Auscultation over the aorta and renal arteries may reveal a bruit indicating renal artery stenosis, a renal arterio-venous fistula, or even a large renal artery aneurysm.

Kidney

Apart from the lower pole of the right kidney it is usually not possible to palpate normal kidneys unless they have doubled in size.

Enlarged kidneys often retain their shape, are ballotable, and move downwards on respiration, unless they are fixed to the surrounding tissues by severe inflammation or extensive neoplasia. Inflammation, obstruction, neoplasia or trauma may produce pain on palpation and reflex abdominal muscle guarding, with consequent palpation difficulty.

Ureter

A giant mega-ureter may be palpable but is usually mistaken for bowel.

Bladder and Bimanual Pelvic Examination

The adult bladder cannot be palpated unless it is distended. Bladder distension, as with all pelvic masses, cannot be 'got below' and, when the bladder is emptied, the mass disappears.

Acute bladder distension is easily visible and palpable but chronic bladder distension, although percussible, is often difficult to visualise and to palpate (p. 240).

A bimanual pelvic examination may indicate the presence of a pelvic tumour or a bladder calculus but, unless the patient is thin and very cooperative, such an examination usually requires a general relaxant anaesthetic and an empty bladder for accurate definition.

Prostate and Seminal Vesicles

This examination is peformed with the patient in the left or right lateral position with the hips and knees flexed and the buttocks on the edge of the bed. The prostate is easily palpable per rectum but the seminal vesicles are not unless they are chronically inflamed. The rectal mucosa should be carefully palpated for hardness or irregularity suggestive of a neoplasm.

Palpation of the prostate should determine:

  1) Character
     a) Rubbery — *Benign prostatomegaly*
     b) Firm — *Fibrous prostatitis*
     c) Hard — *Neoplasm. Prostatic calculi are hard but are usually moveable, multiple; and apparent on a straight pelvic x-ray*
     d) Firm/hard — *Possible fibrosis or tuberculosis*
     e) Soft — *Possible abscess or, extremely rarely, anaplastic neoplasm.*
  2) Size

Should the patient require a prostatectomy it is essential that an approximate estimate of the size of the gland be made (p. 240). Benign enlargements less than 60 grams in size, and all neoplastic enlargements, are best removed by endoscopic prostatectomy whilst greater benign enlargements are best removed by open prostatectomy. A distended bladder pushes the prostate inferiorly and may give a false impression of its size.

Inguino-scrotal Area

All inguino-scrotal examinations should be conducted with the patient standing and lying.

Systematic inspection, palpation, percussion, auscultation, transillumination and aspiration, if indicated, of swellings in this area are performed in order to answer the following diagnostic questions:

Can you get above the swelling?
If the answer is *No* or indefinite and the swelling is inguinal or inguino-scrotal then it may be:

a) *Indirect inguinal hernia* (p. 73). Such hernia protrude lateral to the inferior epigastric vessels and may enter the scrotum.

b) *Direct inguinal hernia* (p. 73). Such hernia protrude medial to the inferior epigastric vessels but rarely enter the scrotum.

c) *Pantaloon hernia.* Such hernia have combined indirect and direct protrusions. It is not always possible, particularly with large people and a large hernia, to distinguish clinically between the 3 types but, as they all require surgical correction, the precise diagnosis, and the appropriate surgical reconstruction of the abdominal wall, will be made at the time of operation.

d) *Femoral hernia* (p. 73). Such hernia protrude inferiorly to the inguinal ligament, through the saphenous opening and are usually covered with fat which, particularly in large females, may again make the clinical diagnosis difficult.

e) *Inguinal adenitis.* Inflamed lymph glands in this area are rarely difficult to diagnose although, in large people, a strangulated hernia must be excluded. Inguinal adenitis resolves after treatment of the primary focus of infection.

f) *Undescended testicle* (p. 349). An undescended testis may be visible and/or palpable and the scrotum on that side will be empty. The management is discussed in chapter XIV.

g) *Lipoma.* Lipoma often occur in this area and, if large, require excision.

h) *Saphena varix.* A large venous dilatation, at the junction of the femoral and long saphenous vein, is termed a saphena varix. When the patient coughs there is a palpable pulse and, on lying down, the dilatation disappears.

i) *Femoral artery aneurysm.* This condition is rare and the swelling is usually pulsatile and in the line of the femoral artery.

j) *Psoas abscess.* Although an extremely rare condition a tuberculous psoas abscess may present below the inguinal ligament.

If the answer to the question *Can you get above the swelling?* is *Yes* then the swelling is in the scrotum. Transillumination should indicate whether the swelling is solid or cystic and usually differentiates between a testicular and epididymal origin.

Is the scrotal swelling painful and of recent onset?
If the answer is *Yes* then the swelling may be:

a) *Testicular neoplasm* (p. 184). These are commonly painful and heavy but may be insensitive and small.

b) *Torsion of the testis* (p. 70, p. 350). This is really a torsion of the spermatic cord above the testis and epididymis. There is usually a recent severe onset of acute testicular or lower abdominal pain, nausea and/or vomiting, with a past history of similar but less severe episodes. Physical examination reveals a swollen, oedematous and red scrotal wall, within which the acutely painful testis inhibits palpation. Any male under the age of 21 years, presenting with such a history, requires an immediate open diagnostic, and possibly therapeutic, surgical exploration of the testis, manual reduction of the torsion and posterior scrotal wall fixation of both testes, if possible, or removal of the dead testis and fixation of the other side (Allan and Brown, 1966).

c) *Torsion of the testicular appendages.* The history and examination findings are similar to those found in torsion of the testis but are less severe and it is often possible to palpate the tender torted appendage accurately (figs. 81-82). Immediate diagnostic open surgical exploration of the testis is performed both in order to differentiate the condition from torsion of the spermatic cord and to enable excision of the torted appendage to be carried out. The condition is usually bilateral and therefore requires associated exploration of the second testis and prophylactic removal of any appendages.

d) *Acute epididymitis and orchitis* (p. 70).

e) *Idiopathic scrotal oedema or scrotal fat necrosis.* Young children may develop a minimally painful, oedematous, red scrotal wall and related skin, with normal intra-scrotal contents, of unknown aetiology. The condition resolves satisfactorily and can be observed without surgical exploration. Fat necrosis presents as a painful small mass in the scrotal wall, usually in fat boys who have recently bathed in cold water. It resolves with rest.

f) *Haematocele* (p. 312). The non-surgical or surgical traumatic history is usually diagnostic but if there is no history of trauma, or the haematocele is large, then the scrotum is surgically explored both to eliminate the possibility of a testicular neoplasm and achieve a more rapid convalescence.

Is the scrotal swelling non-painful? If the answer is *Yes* then the swelling may be:
a) *Testicular neoplasm.* These may be painless (p. 184).

b) *Hydrocele* (p. 28). An excessive amount of clear tunica vaginalis fluid produces a hydrocele. The most common, *idiopathic* hydrocele, often requires surgical excision in view of its size. An *inflammatory* hydrocele usually resolves with satisfactory treatment of the cause of the epididymo-orchitis. Unless the testis and epididymis can be accurately palpated then the surrounding hydrocele must be aspirated and the fluid examined microscopically for possible malignant cells (*neoplastic* hydrocele) or excised so that an adequate examination can be made. *Congenital* hydrocele is discussed on p. 28. A persistent processus vaginalis may result in a hydrocele collection of peritoneal fluid. Ligation of the connection is performed if it has not closed by the age of 2 years. An *encysted* hydrocele is excised if it is of sufficient size to cause discomfort. Congestive cardiac failure, renal failure, or the rare filarial lymphatic obstruction may produce *bilateral* hydroceles.

c) *Epididymal cysts.* Clear fluid cystic changes within the head of the epididymis are common in young men although the aetiology is unknown. Inspection, palpation and transillumination indicates that the testis is situated below the cysts which are transilluminable. Very large cysts are surgically excised but with small cysts only reassurance of the patient is required.

d) *Spermatocele.* An enlarged epididymal cyst containing opaque (spermatozoa) fluid is termed a spermatocele. The condition occurs in older men, is often bilateral, and only requires surgical excision if it becomes inconveniently large.

e) *Sperm granuloma and granulomatous orchitis.* Sperm extravasation may rarely produce a chronic inflammatory 'foreign body' granuloma, which is only diagnosed by open surgical exploration, indicated because of the possibility of a testicular neoplasm. Granulomatous orchitis is also a rare inflammatory condition of unknown aetiology and cannot be diagnosed clinically.

f) *Testicular gumma.* This extremely rare consequence of tertiary syphilis may present as a painless testicular lump and is usually only diagnosed when surgical exploration has been performed because of the possibility of a testicular neoplasm.

g) *Varicocele* (p. 72, 169, 375).

Penis and Urethra

Congenital abnormalities such as hypospadias or phimosis (p. 346) or acquired lesions such as Peyronie's disease (p. 66) may be detected whilst a urethral stricture, diverticulum or discharge may be palpated or seen.

Perineum

Swellings, nodules, ulcers or rashes should be diagnosed and treated if necessary, and the anal and peri-anal appearance and tone recorded. In children the area should be carefully examined for worms (p. 317).

Vagina, Cervix and Female Urethra

Adults: With the patient in the dorsal position inspection of the vulva will show any abnormalities such as inflammation, dystrophies, cysts, warts or neoplasms. Separation of the labia minora exposes the vaginal introitus and urethral meatus. The patient is requested to strain and cough and the extent of any cysto-urethrocele prolapse, or stress incontinence, demonstrated. Caruncles (p. 155) and urethral prolapses are common in the elderly.

Female stress incontinence of urine results from congenital and/or acquired bladder outlet muscle sphincteric inefficiency and/or congenital and/or acquired posterior pubo-urethral (p. 64) ligamentous deficiency or damage. Increased urethral mobility is usually found in patients with weak posterior pubo-urethral ligaments. Using a male olivary tipped urethral sound, careful multiple point bladder neck and proximal urethra upward support is applied whilst the patient increases her intra-abdominal pressure. The muscular or ligamentous areas responsible for the stress incontinence can then be identified. The history and these physical examination findings greatly influence the decision to operate and the choice of a particular operation (p. 358).

After the examination in the dorsal position the patient is then turned to the left lateral position and, with the aid of a Sim's speculum, the vagina and cervix are inspected. In particular, discharges from this area are noted:

1) A *slight, white, non-irritating* vaginal discharge usually indicates secretion from the glands of the cervix and requires no treatment.

2) A clear or *coloured irritating* discharge (p. 382) from the vagina or cervix may result from:
   a) *Candidiasis (monilia).* The main symptom is pruritus and signs vary from a minimal to an obvious 'cheesey' discharge, with the occasional presence of white plaques. If pruritus is present, without a discharge or white plaque formation, then a culture of this area commonly

reveals monilial infection. Recurrent infections are common in diabetics.

b) *Trichomoniasis.* A profuse frothy discharge, with red vaginal walls, is commonly found with trichomonal infections. Motile trichomonads are seen by mixing a drop of the discharge with normal saline and examining under a microscope.

c) *Haemophilus vaginalis.* The discharge is usually grey in colour and often malodorous. Microscopy of a drop of discharge mixed with saline shows vaginal squamous cells stippled with the bacteria.

d) *Senile vaginitis.* This is occasionally associated with a varying degree of purulent discharge.

e) *Herpes genitalis.* The vesicles and/or shallow ulcers may result in a thin clear discharge but often only red inflamed areas are seen.

Any urethral discharge merits the exclusion of gonorrhoea and other venereal diseases by examination of swabs taken from the urethra and the endo-cervix (chapter XIX). Inspection of the cervix may reveal child-birth lacerations, acute infections with a purulent discharge, or chronic cervicitis, with a red 'erosion' and a thick muco-purulent discharge. Nabothian follicles, polyps, or a neoplasm may be present. Taking a smear for cervical cytology is a routine part of any gynaecological examination.

The patient now resumes the dorsal position and a bimanual examination is performed. This indicates the size, regularity, consistency and mobility of the uterus, and may also reveal other pelvic masses, such as an ovarian cyst, or inflammatory tenderness.

Gynaecological examinations, in particular, should be carried out in the presence of a third party, such as a nurse, both for added assistance and medico-legal reasons.

Children: Vaginal examinations, particularly in the presence of vulvovaginitis, are difficult in children and may require a general anaesthetic.

Urine Examination

Human urine is an excellent medium for bacterial growth (Asscher et al., 1966). The laboratory-detected presence of bacteriuria indicates that either the patient has a urinary tract infection or that the urine specimen has been contaminated upon leaving the bladder. Such contamination is common in view of:

a) The organisms which normally live in the external urinary meatus and related areas
b) The difficulties of obtaining mid-stream specimens of urine in children and women
c) The delays which sometimes occur between collecting the specimen and examining it in the laboratory.

Kass (1956) used the term 'significant bacteriuria' to distinguish between true urinary tract infection and contamination. Significant bacteriuria implies the presence of more than 100,000 organisms per ml of urine. This is discussed further in chapter V.

Collection of Urine Specimens

The collection of specimens in young children and neonates is difficult and requires specialised, experienced nursing staff. This has led to the maxim, 'Send the child to the laboratory not the urine specimen' (see chapter XIV tables I and II).

Bladder catheterisation, under strictly aseptic conditions, provides an uncontaminated bladder urine specimen but, even with cooperative adult women, also requires experienced staff. Bladder catheterisation is traumatic and difficult in young children.

Suprapubic bladder aspiration is a safe (Pryles et al., 1959) and efficient procedure for obtaining uncontaminated specimens of urine and is particularly suitable for children, cases presenting diagnostic difficulty, or where post-gynaecological or obstetric vulval and vaginal contamination exists.

Visual Examination of the Urine Specimen

In order to prevent the multiplication of contaminated organisms the urine should be microscopically examined and cultured immediately after voiding (p. 317). If this is not possible then the urine should be stored at 4°C until such an examination can be made.

A macroscopically cloudy specimen may indicate infection or phosphatic material which, unlike infection, dissolves on acidification. Infected urine usually smells of ammonia. Methylene blue may colour the urine green whilst beetroot and rhubarb may produce a pink urine. Red blood cells (see chapter VI) and haemoglobin will change the urine to a red colour and phenazopyridine produces a yellow-orange colour. Acute porphyrinuria is rare but may be suspected when the patient's urine becomes deep red on standing for several minutes. Melanin, bile pigments, phenol and methyldopa will often produce a brown or black urine.

Urinary Dip-strip Testing

Metabolites: The specific gravity of the urine sample is determined and, using chemical dip strips, an indication as to whether the urine contains blood, protein, sugar and ketones is obtained, together with an estimation of the pH. There is a relatively high uric acid content in urine in our community and thus the urine is usually acidic.

Organisms: 'Dipslide' and 'strip' diagnostic methods of chemically identifying urinary tract infection are cheap and can be used in the patient's home and subsequently brought to the laboratory. The tests are of value in certain situations but do not replace the professional accuracy of fresh microscopically examined specimens.

Microscopy

The urine may be examined with or without centrifuging but far more information is obtained from a centrifuged specimen (fig. 84). Approximately 10ml of urine is centrifuged in a conical tube at 1,500 revolutions per minute for 5 minutes. The urine is decanted from the tube until approximately 0.5ml of concentrated sediment remains. One drop of this sediment is transferred to a clean microscope slide and covered with a cover slip before being microscopically examined, under reduced illumination, using low and then high power. It is usually not necessary to stain the centrifuged specimen as the urinary constituents mentioned below can be easily seen in a fresh centrifuged specimen. A Sternheimer-Malbin stain does display the centrifuged contents more vividly and, because of its alcohol content, enables preservation of the specimen should this be necessary. A Gram stain enables an accurate distinction to be made between Gram-negative and

84 Microscopy findings in urine sediment.

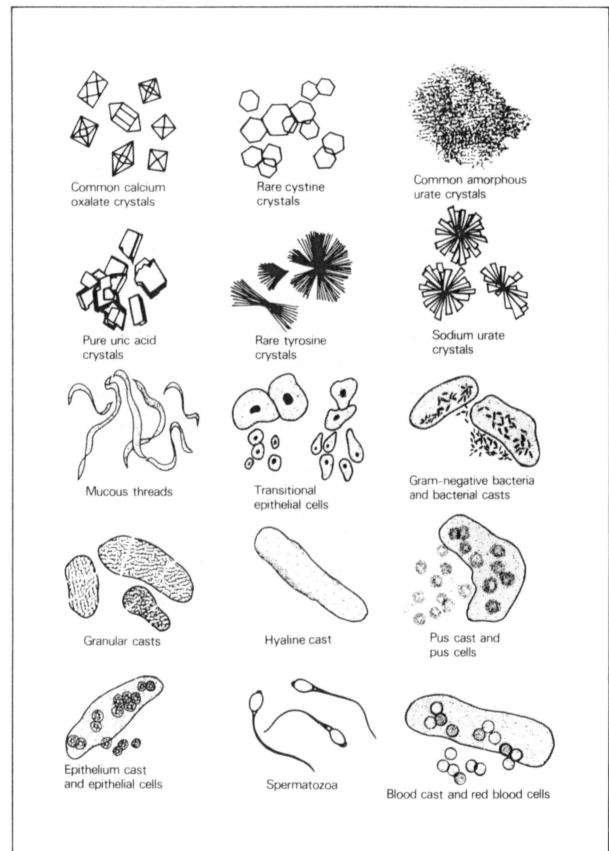

Common calcium
oxalate crystals

Rare cystine
crystals

Common amorphous
urate crystals

Pure uric acid
crystals

Rare tyrosine
crystals

Sodium urate
crystals

Mucous threads

Transitional
epithelial cells

Gram-negative bacteria
and bacterial casts

Granular casts

Hyaline cast

Pus cast and
pus cells

Epithelium cast
and epithelial cells

Spermatozoa

Blood cast and red blood cells

Gram-positive organisms but is rarely necessary as almost all rod-shaped organisms detected in an unstained specimen are Gram-negative and all cocci Gram-positive.

Organisms: Gram-negative infections are very common and are discussed in detail in chapter V.

Should tuberculosis (p. 148) be suspected then the centrifuged specimen is treated with acid fuchsine, heated, washed with alcohol and acid and then counterstained with malachite green. This is the Ziehl-Neelsen stain, which identifies acid-fast organisms, but does not specifically identify *Mycobacterium tuberculosis*. A positive Ziehl-Neelsen identification requires a subsequent laboratory culture and/or a guinea pig inoculation test before genitourinary tuberculosis can be confirmed.

Trichomonal or monilial infections may occasionally be detected and, extremely rarely outside tropical countries, the ova of Schistosomia may be found in travellers who have visited endemic bilharziasis areas.

Cells: Red blood and pus cells may occasionally be seen in urine but they fragment rapidly and this emphasises the need for specimens to be fresh or refrigerated. *The presence of 1 or 2 red or pus cells per HPF is abnormal and necessitates quantitative urine counts.* A recurrent red blood cell quantitative count greater than 20,000 per ml requires further investigations (p. 162) but with lesser, asymptomatic counts they are not justified (Syme, 1979).

Normal centrifuged urine contains less than 2,000 leucocytes per ml. Higher counts may be suggestive of vaginal or preputial contamination or of tuberculosis, as yet unidentified infection, or glomerulonephritis, and also require further investigation (McGuckin et al., 1978).

Staining of the centrifuged deposit by the Papanicolaou technique may reveal neoplastic genitourinary mucosal cells. The identification of these cells requires some expertise and is used to follow patients with previously diagnosed and treated transitional cell carcinomas of the urothelium (Weller and Greene, 1966).

Crystals: Urinary crystals have distinct shapes (fig. 84).

Casts: Urinary casts (p. 85) are fragile and best detected in uncentrifuged urine. They may be:

   a) Granular — *desquamated tubular or pus cells*
   b) Hyaline — *excessive protein loss*
   c) Haematin — *red blood cell loss.*

Table I. Radiation doses resulting from investigative techniques. (Average human background radiation 100 millirads per year)

Investigation	Radiation dose (millirads)
Intravenous pyelogram	720
Computerised tomography (kidney)	4,000
Renal angiography	2,000
Renal scan	200

**Special
Investigations**

Special investigations are never performed 'routinely' — this is wasteful of intellect, time and money — but are selectively performed, dependent upon the clinical findings and suspicions.

There is now general agreement (Morgan, 1979) that all levels of radiation are potentially dangerous to humans. This fact must be kept in mind when advising patients to undergo sophisticated radiological investigation. The average human background radiation dose is of the order of 100 millirad per year and the additional radiation dose associated with the various procedures discussed in this section is shown in table I. Renal ultrasound investigations do not involve radiation and as far as is known have no side effects.

Serum Analysis

The serum concentration of various substances indicates both the quality of renal function and, occasionally, the presence of various diseases. Normal serum levels relevant to genitourinary disease, and the likely implications of abnormal levels, are shown in table II.

Urine Analysis

The urinary excretion rate of various substances may also indicate both the quality of renal function and the presence of diseases such as hyperparathyroidism, hyperuricaemia, congenital oxaluria, cystinuria, Cushing's disease, Conn's syndrome or phaeochromocytoma (p. 374).

Table II. Normal values, and implications of abnormal values, of serum constituents relevant to genitourinary disease

Serum constituent	Likely implication	
normal level	raised level	lowered level
Urea Adults 2-8.5mmol/L Infants 1.3-4.2mmol/L	Renal failure, dehydration	
Creatinine 0.04-0.12mmol/L	Renal failure, dehydration	Fluid retention
Potassium 3.5-5mmol/L	Renal failure, adrenal hyperplasia or neoplasm	Some large bowel neoplasms and vomiting
Sodium 134-146mmol/L	Renal failure, Cushing's syndrome or Conn's syndrome	Addison's disease
Chloride 98-110mmol/L	Renal failure	Vomiting
CO₂ content 22-32mmol/L	Renal failure	Vomiting
Total proteins 60-80g/L	Dehydration	Overhydration, malnutrition
Calcium (avoid blood stasis) 2.1-2.6mmol/L	Hyperparathyroidism	Hypoparathyroidism
Phosphate 0.7-1.3mmol/L	Excessive intake	Hyperparathyroidism
Testosterone (plasma) Males 10-42mmol/L Females 1-3mmol/L		Occasionally infertility and impotence
Urate 0.15-0.44mmol/L	Hyperuricaemia	
Acid phosphatase (prostatic) Less than 0.8 U/L (37°C)	Prostatic carcinoma	
Acid phosphatase (total) Less than 12U/L	Prostatic carcinoma	
Alkaline phosphatase Less than 110U/L		
Prolactin Males 6-20ng/ml Females 12-25ng/ml	Occasionally impotence (p. 391)	
Renal renin (depends on sodium intake, posture and other drug therapy) Recumbent 1.4-5.5mmol/L/3 hours Ambulant 3.5-12mmol/L/3 hours	Renal hypertension	
α-Fetoprotein (AFP) (an expensive test) < 40ng/ml	Carcinoma of testis and other malignancies (liver)	
Human chorionic gonadotrophin (see table III)		
Follicle stimulating hormone Males: 0.5-4.1mU/ml	Testicular teratoma, sometimes	Hypopituitary disorders (p. 376)
Females: follicular 0.5-6mU/ml luteal 0.5-4mU/ml mid-cycle 4-15mU/ml post-menopausal > 10mU/ml		
Luteinising hormone Males: 1-5mU/ml	Testicular teratoma, sometimes	Hypopituitary disorders (p. 376)
Cyclical, females: 0.5-5mU/ml		

Glomerular Filtration Rate

The detection of oxalates and cystine is expensive and certainly not justified routinely (see chapter IX). Urate and phosphate excretion levels are particularly related to diet and this must be controlled before these levels are estimated. The constituents and values for normal urine, which does *not* contain protein, glucose or ketones, are listed in table III.

Inulin clearance is the most accurate method of measuring the glomerular filtration rate but, because it is less time consuming, creatinine clearance values are used. This test is explained in detail on page 44.

Renal Tubular Function

See also chapter II.

Tubular Concentration Efficiency: The ability to concentrate urine in response to water deprivation is an excellent test of renal tubular function. This is measured by the subcutaneous injection of 5 units of vasopressin tannate (an oily suspension which must be warmed and mixed before injecting) and measuring the fasting patient's urinary specific gravity over the next 12 hours.

Table III. Normal urinary values

Constituent	Normal value	Notes
Urea	200-600mmol/day	
Creatinine	10-25mmol/day	
Creatinine clearance	80-120mls/min (0.68-1.33mls/sec/m²)	
Potassium	45-80mmol/L	Urinary sodium and potassium levels are of value in managing acute renal failure and differentiating between prerenal and renal failure (chap. XVI)
Sodium	75-200mmol/L	
Calcium	0.2-7mmol/day on a random diet	
Phosphate	27-39mmol/L	
Urate	1.6-6.6mmol/day	
Oxalate	< 0.35mmol/L	
Cystine	< 0.63mmol/day	
Vanillyl-mandelic acid (VMA)	40mmol/day	(See p. 374)
Androsterone Males Females	7-13μmol/day 4-9μmol/day	(See chapters XVIII, XX)
17-Hydroxy-cortico-steroids	< 330mmol/day measured as free cortisol	(See Cushing's disease, chapter XVII)
Aldosterone	10-40mmol/day (4-15μg/day) on 100mmol of sodium/day	(See Conn's syndrome, chapter XVII)
Human chorionic gonadotrophin (HCG)	< 300 IU/24 hours	

The concentrated urinary specific gravity in patients with normal renal tubular function may rise to a level of 1.030 or higher but tubular failure results in a fixed urinary specific gravity of about 1.010, which represents the specific gravity of the glomeruli filtrate.

Tubular Acidification Efficiency: The ability of the renal tubules to handle an acid load is essential for the preservation of the normal body acid-base balance. Gelatin capsules of ammonium chloride (0.1g per kg body weight) are taken with 1 litre of water over a 1 hour period, using the previous day's urinary excretion pH levels as a control. Normal renal tubules should respond to this acid load by secreting urine with a pH less than 5.5 over the next 6 hours.

Intravenous Pyelogram

An intravenous pyelogram is an essential investigation in all patients presenting with either haematuria or clinical renal colic. Intravenous iodine should never be administered to any patient who has experienced a previous allergic reaction. Because of the 1 in 100,000 risk of the contrast medium causing a major anaphylactic shock, resuscitation equipment should always be available and an initial small intravenous test dose should be given and the result assessed before injecting the remaining 40 to 60ml.

The contrast medium is filtered through the glomeruli and concentrated in the tubules before passing into the calyces, pelvis, ureters and bladder. This enables both the function and the anatomy of the system to be assessed. A greater concentration of the dye is achieved by dehydrating the patient, using contrast medium which contains 3 atoms of iodine in each molecule, and by applying abdominal compression during the investigation in order partly to obstruct the system. There is little to be gained from attempting intravenous pyelography examination in the presence of gross renal failure as the kidneys are unable to concentrate the dye.

An intravenous pyelogram has 3 stages:

1. A full length *straight abdominal and pelvic x-ray* is taken in order to detect the presence of urinary calculi (radio-opaque in 94% of cases in our community), skeletal abnormalities, and soft tissue outlines such as renal or bladder shadows (fig. 85).

2. The *injection* stage produces 2 phases:

The Nephrogram: As the contrast medium fills the glomeruli and tubules opacification of the renal parenchyma occurs at a rate dependent upon the renal blood supply, glomerular function and the capacity of the tubules to reabsorb water. If the kidney is not obstructed the medium rapidly fills the collecting system and enters the bladder. Should the kidney be obstructed then the medium may remain proximal to the level of the obstruction for hours or days. The radiologist will vary the dose of injected contrast medium and the timing of his x-rays, depending upon these various changes. For greater detail the focal length of the x-rays may be altered, using a section of the kidney which is sharply in focus compared with its surroundings. Such x-rays are termed *tomograms* (fig. 86).

85 A straight abdominal and pelvic x-ray. Numerous calcifications are present which may represent calculi, phleboliths or mesenteric lymph glands. The bladder and psoas muscle soft tissue outlines are seen but the film is not focused sufficiently to assess the renal outlines. The skeletal structures seen are normal.

86 Nephrogram. Normal nephrograms, taken 30 seconds after intravenous injection of the medium, which has opacified the nephron system but has not yet entered the calyceal-pelvi-ureteric collecting system.

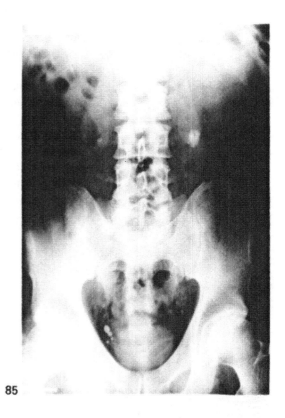

85

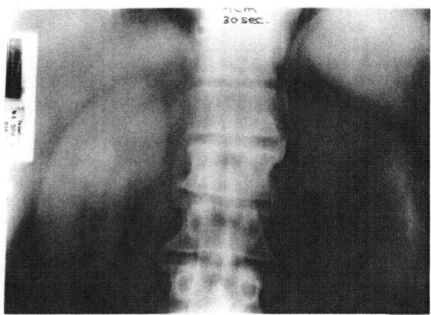

86

The Calyceal-pelvi-ureterogram: As the contrast medium leaves the renal parenchyma it enters the collecting system and both the anatomical outlining of this system and the efficiency of delivery to the bladder is estimated and abnormalities noted (fig. 87). Continual peristalsis of the ureter often means that its whole length is not displayed in a single x-ray. In a normal, although slightly dehydrated system, provided the patient is mobile, the upper urinary tract should be anatomically normal and free of dye within 1.5 hours. There should be no intra-luminal filling defects.

3) The third stage of the intravenous pyelogram is that of *residual urine estimation* (fig. 88).

An intravenous pyelogram is an excellent method of diagnosing upper urinary tract mechanical and functional abnormalities but, because usually only 40ml of contrast medium is ejected — being less than a tenth of the adult bladder capacity — the resultant cystogram is not usually of sufficient quality to enable intra-vesical pathology to be interpreted accurately, apart from large tumours or calculi, which present as constant filling defects. During this partial cystogram phase an attempt is made to interpret the degree of residual bladder urine which may be present but, unless the residue is gross, this may be inaccurate, as many people have difficulty voiding in the unfamiliar surroundings of a busy x-ray department.

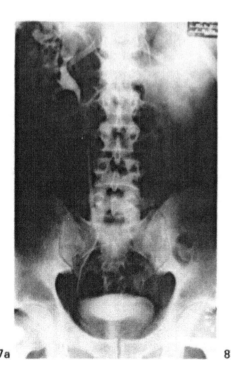 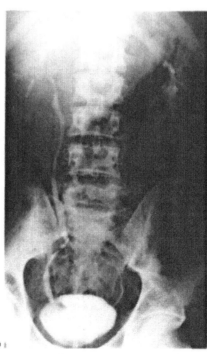 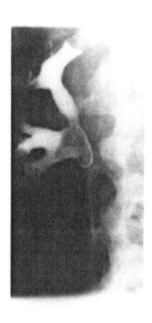

87a   87b   87c

Calyceal-pelvi-ureterograms

87a A normal calyceal-pelvi-ureterogram on the right side but a grossly obstructed nephrogram on the left side.

87b A moth-eaten right calyceal-pelvic system together with an early vesico-ureteric stricture: highly suggestive of tuberculosis.

87c Non-opaque calyceal and pelvic filling defects due to neoplasms or uric acid calculi.

88 Intravenous pyelogram. Post-micturition intravenous pyelogram indicating a moderate residual bladder urine, a heavily trabeculated bladder wall and a large pulsion diverticulum.

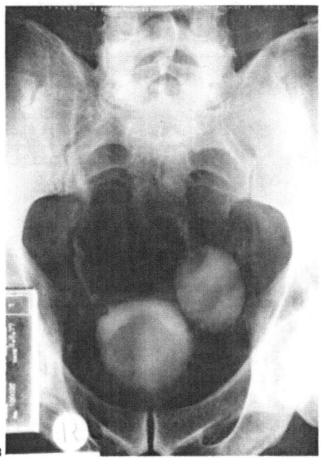

Other Investigations for Renal Function, Space Occupying Lesions and Filling Defects

Several special investigations developed during the past 20 years have greatly assisted the accurate diagnosis of renal space occupying lesions and constant filling defects (fig. 89).

Ultrasound, Renal Cyst Aspiration and Cystogram: Ultrasound utilises soundwaves of a high frequency (2 million cycles per second) produced and received by a transducer, which interprets the echoes of the soundwaves as they pass through tissue interfaces of differing density. The echoes are converted into electricity and displayed on an oscilloscope screen; this oscilloscope screen tracing can be made permanent by using a Polaroid camera, which produces a negative (black dots) and a positive (white dots) image. Ultrasound diagnosis is particularly useful in deciding whether a mass lesion in the kidney is cystic or solid. Should the lesion be entirely echo-free then a simple benign renal cyst (p. 32) or a dilated, non-functioning half of a bifid system (figs. 6 and 7) are the most likely diagnoses, although an extremely small proportion of apparently benign renal cystic lesions are malignant with either a carcinomatous nodule on the wall of the cyst, a cystic adenocarcinoma, or a very necrotic haemorrhagic centre of a carcinoma appearing as an echo-free mass (Ambrose et al., 1977). Because of this slight risk all moderate to large renal cysts should be completely aspirated under local anaesthetic, the fluid sent for cytological examination, and a cystogram performed through the aspirating needle (figs. 90-91).

Renal ultrasound examinations are carried out with the patient in the prone or supine (particularly for the right kidney, where the liver is translucent and there is no bowel gas) position and transverse and longitudinal views taken. If the lesion is found to be solid it is almost certainly a neoplasm or, on extremely rare occasions, a renal carbuncle (p. 132), hamartoma or other

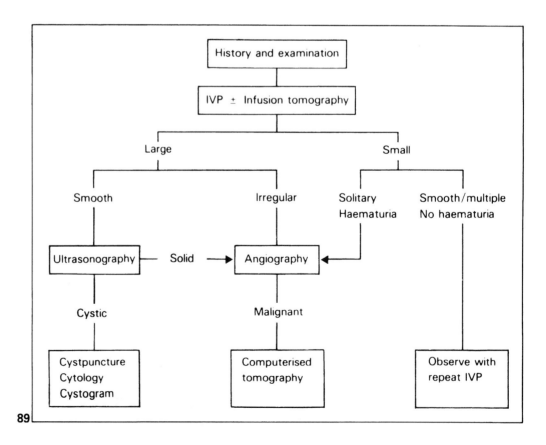

Renal space occupying lesions

89 An investigation plan.

90a An intravenous pyelogram reveals a large asymptomatic left renal space occupying lesion in a 50-year-old man presenting with mild dysuria.

90b A longitudinal ultra-sound examination confirms the smooth lesion to be a benign cyst. No treatment was advised.

91a An intravenous pyelogram reveals numerous space occupying renal lesions, with a particularly large, smooth right-sided lesion.

91b A transverse ultrasound examination shows all the space occupying lesions are benign cysts, the large right cyst was aspirated and cytology and the cystogram confirmed its benign character.

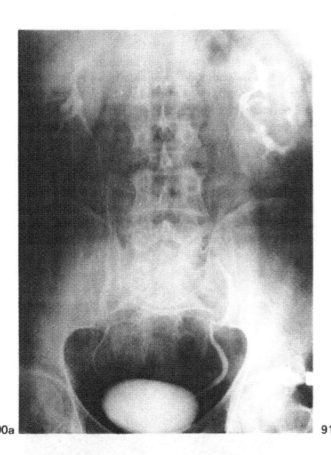

90a

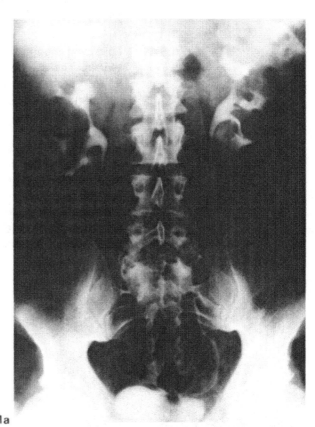

91a

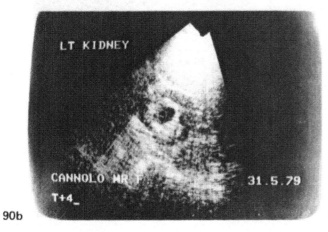

90b

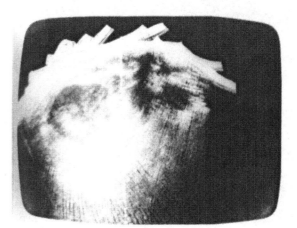

91b

benign tumour. The rare *angiomyolipoma* can usually be diagnosed with great accuracy (Baron et al., 1977) because of its characteristic lipoma element echoes and its angiographic pattern (p. 170). Should a solid renal mass, or a relatively small single cystic lesion be found, then renal angiography is performed, both in order to assist the diagnosis and to indicate the pattern of the major blood vessels, which assists technically any subsequent surgical procedure.

Renal Angiography: The introduction of contrast medium directly into the renal artery, through a percutaneous puncture of the femoral artery, and the subsequent outlining of the renal vascular system and parenchyma provides an excellent means of identifying renal vascular abnormalities such as stenosis, aneurysm (beware of a constant smooth filling defect in the superior aspects of the renal pelvis) or arteriovenous malformations, as well as differentiating between a neoplasm and a benign cyst or tumour (figs. 92-94).

Following injection of the contrast medium x-rays are taken at 1 second intervals. The arterial phase of the examination delineates the renal artery whilst the nephrogram phase, which normally begins within 5 seconds of injection, may identify renal parenchymal abnormalities. The calyceal-pelvi-ureterogram phase may indicate mechanical and/or functional obstruction to the system.

Angiography for renal neoplasm usually reveals many bizarre, poorly muscularised primitive vessels; these pool medium within their thin walls and fail to contract to intravenously administered adrenaline, in contrast to the vessels surrounding a benign renal cyst which, although stretched, have an otherwise normal appearance and contract vigorously to intravenously administered adrenaline.

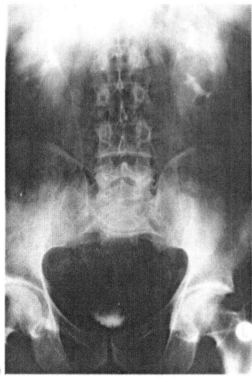

92a

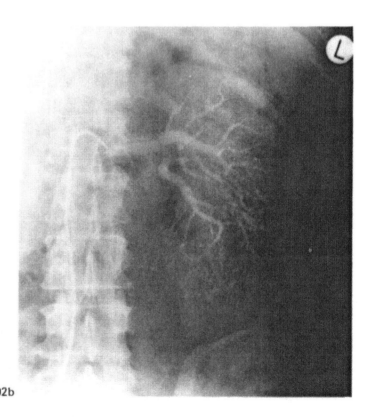

92b

Renal angiography

92a A 58-year old man presented with painless haematuria. An intravenous pyelogram reveals an irregular space occupying lesion within the lower half of the left kidney.

92b A left selective renal angiogram confirms the clinical diagnosis of renal adenocarcinoma. Note the bizarre, poorly muscularised, primitive neoplastic vessels, which fail to contract following intravenously injected adrenaline.

93a A smooth asymptomatic left renal space occupying lesion detected in an intravenous pyelogram in a patient with severe hypertension.

93b The left selective renal angiogram revealed that the space occupying lesion was a moderately large benign left renal cyst. No treatment was advised.

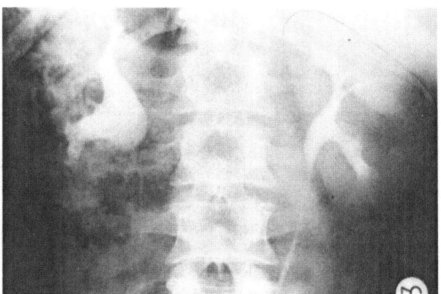

93a

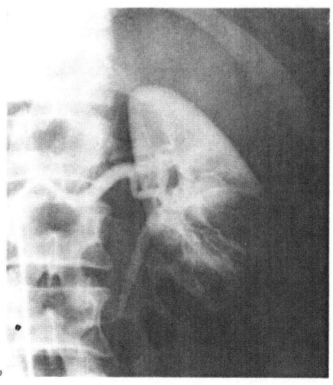

93b

Rarely, renal neoplasms, such as an *oncocytoma* (p. 169), may exhibit a stretched but relatively normal angiographic appearance (Wright and Walker, 1975). A renal *carbuncle* is a very rare lesion usually with a characteristic angiographic appearance showing inflamed renal vessels pushed aside by the abscess which, together with its clinical presentation and course, usually enables diagnostic distinction from a neoplasm.

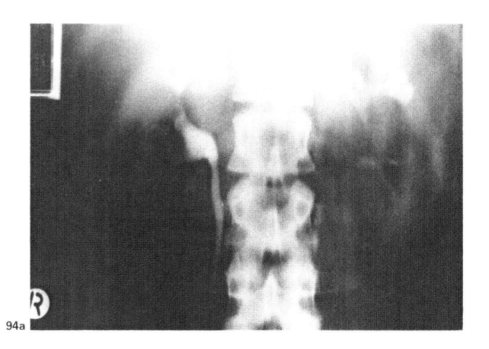

94a

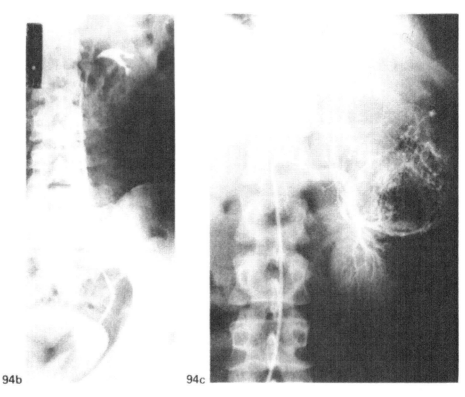

94b   94c

Renal angiography and computerised tomography

94a A 34-year-old woman presented with clot retention of urine. An intravenous pyelogram revealed an irregular space occupying renal lesion. Panendoscopy revealed no lower genitourinary tract abnormality other than the blood clot. Bleeding was observed to be coming from the left ureteric orifice.

94b A left retrograde pyelo-ureterogram revealed a normal left ureter but did not fill all the pelvi-calyceal system.

94c Left renal selective angiogram revealed an adenocarcinoma which was treated by radical nephrectomy.

94d Computerised tomography study clearly revealed the large solid neoplasm and assisted preoperative staging by displaying the absence of involved para-aortic lymph nodes.

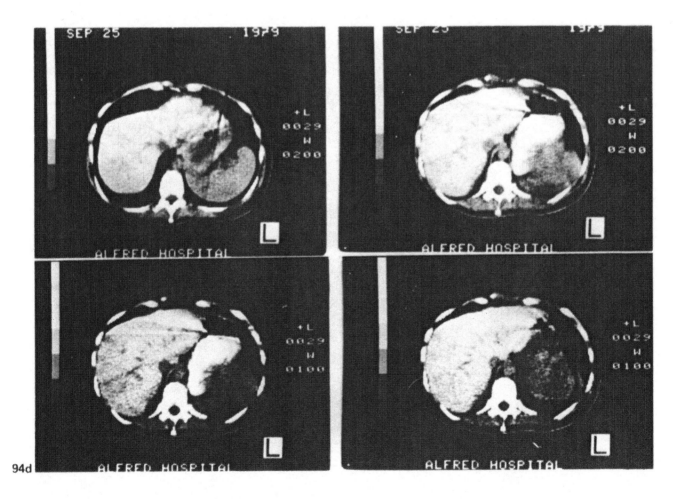

94d

Venogram: Outlining of the minor and major venous drainage of the kidney may illustrate benign or neoplastic obstruction and this aids both the diagnosis and management of such conditions (fig. 95-96).

Catheterisation of the femoral vein and subsequent entry into the right renal or left suprarenal vein, using image intensifier screening, enables *venous renin levels* to be determined in suspected cases of renal hypertension or Conn's syndrome (p. 46, 372).

Computerised Tomography: Computerised tomography is of considerable diagnostic significance in selected patients and was regarded as such a significant advance that the 1979 Nobel Prize for Medicine was awarded to its co-inventors, Dr Godfrey Hounsfield and Dr Allan Cormack.

Renal venography

95 A normal venogram in a 38-year-old man with a testicular teratoma. Note the associated intravenous pyelogram and lymphangiogram.

96 An abnormal venogram due to a right renal adenocarcinoma thrombous invasion.

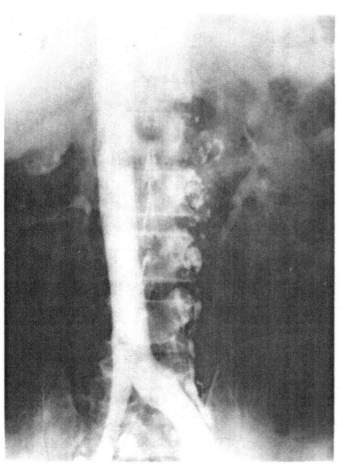

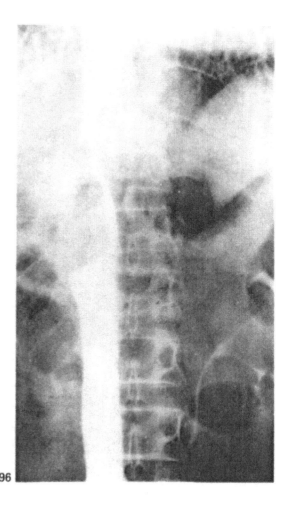

95   96

Ultrasound differentiates solid from cystic structures but computerised tomography demonstrates and differentiates such radiographic tissue densities in a far more precise manner (fig. 97-99) and provides the most accurate means of diagnosing unusual renal tumours, such as lipoma, liposarcoma and hamartoma (chapter VII). The multiple tomographic sections, usually about 13mm thick, demonstrate coronal sectional anatomy. The ultrasound examination costs less than a quarter of a computerised tomography study and, as the ultrasound examination is more than adequate for distinguishing between most cystic and solid lesions, it is used initially, tomography being retained for the more difficult diagnosis. As computerised tomography does not provide sufficient information concerning the vascular pattern of a tumour it has not replaced angiography, nor does it replace the cytological information derived from cyst puncture.

Computerised tomography is also of value in detecting the presence of both local neoplastic extension and metastatic lymph gland involvement in genitourinary neoplasia and is now an essential preoperative investigation in all such patients (figs. 94d, 98b, 99).

Renal cyst confirmed by ultrasound and computerised tomography
97a A 70-year-old man presented with a large left renal mass.

97b An intravenous pyelogram suggested that it was a renal cyst (see over).

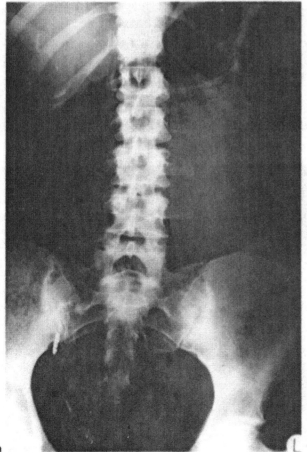

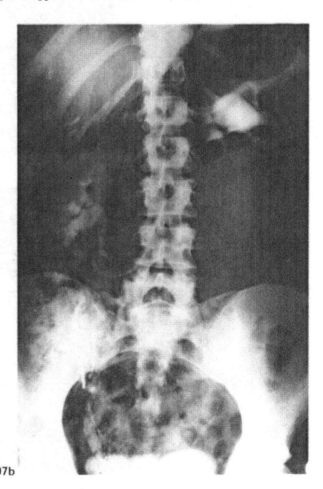

97a   L 97b

Renal cyst confirmed by ultrasound and computerised tomography (continued)
97c This was confirmed by longitudinal ultrasound.

97d Further confirmation by computerised tomography studies, where the cyst is displayed as a grey shadow. Note the smaller cyst in the right kidney. The large cyst was aspirated and the resultant cystogram confirmed its benign character.

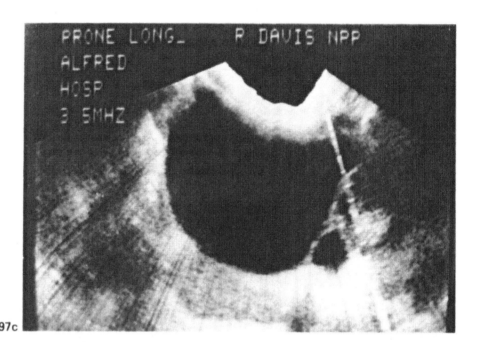

97c

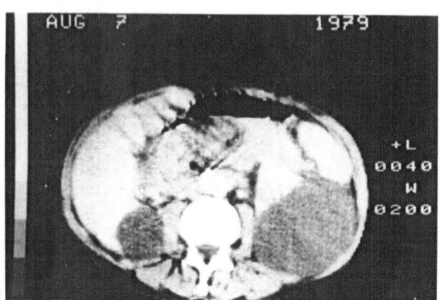

97d

Renal tumour confirmed by computerised tomography

98a An intravenous pyelogram of a 51-year-old man who presented with painless haematuria. The pyelogram revealed a large irregular space occupying lesion within the left kidney.

98b Computerised tomography confirmed the diagnosis of renal adenocarcinoma and also disclosed large metastatic para-aortic lymph node involvement. A difficult radical left nephrectomy was performed.

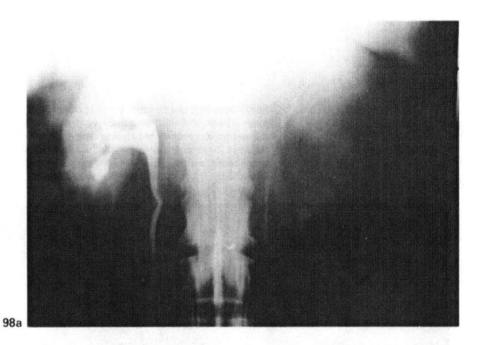

98a

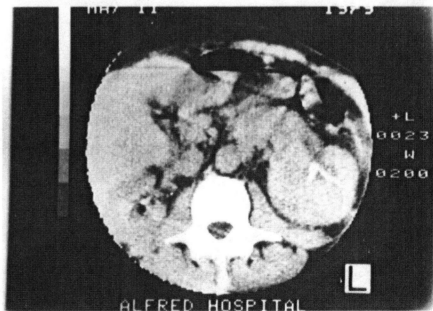

98b

Radio-isotope Studies: Radio-isotope studies are of particular value in patients who are allergic to iodine.

The Renogram: Renal function can be measured safely and non-invasively (Koff et al., 1979) by the intravenous injection of radioactive compounds, such as technetium, and using a gamma camera and computerised recording to graph the number of counts from the kidney per unit of time. A normal renogram has 3 phases (fig. 100):

Vascular: This measures the blood flow to the kidney.

Secretory: This phase measures the glomerular filtration and tubular excretion of the hippuran and corresponds to the nephrogram injection phase of an intravenous pyelogram.

Renal tumour confirmed by computerised tomography (continued)
99 A 50-year-old man presented with painless haematuria. An intravenous pyelogram showed no abnormality but an assessment panendoscopy revealed the presence of a clinical stage II, grade II-III posterior bladder wall neoplasm. Computerised tomography of the pelvis confirmed the presence of the neoplasm but did not reveal any involved metastatic lymph nodes. Note the different transverse levels.

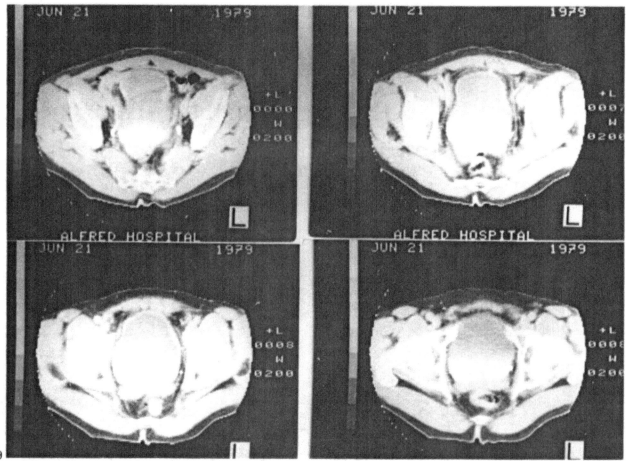

Excretion: In this the efficiency of the calyceal-pelvi-ureteric collecting system is measured.

Renograms are of particular value in detecting and following the progress of patients with either upper urinary tract obstruction or trauma. Portable machines enable the investigation to be performed at the bedside in a quick and safe manner.

Renal scanning: The distinction between anatomically solid and cystic renal space occupying lesions can also be made by intravenously injecting gamma radio-active chlormerodrin [197]Hg and detecting the uniformity or otherwise of the renal gamma ray emissions by external scintillation counting

100 The 3 phases of a renogram. Showing both normal and obstructed renal patterns.

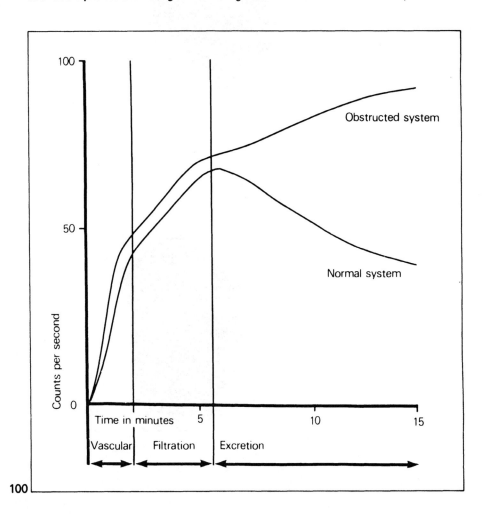

and subsequent photographic reproduction (figs. 101, 102). Schlegel et al. (1979) have described an accurate and rapid method of estimating renal plasma flow, and filtration fraction and rate, using radio-labelled hippuran and iron ascorbate.

Renal scanning does not give the accuracy of anatomical diagnosis achieved by intravenous pyelography-tomography, ultrasound, angiography or computerised axial tomography but is of considerable value in detecting bone and other tissue malignant metastases and in diagnosing intravenous pyelogram-nonfunctioning kidneys (Lome et al., 1979).

Renal scanning
101 A normal system.

102 A large benign right renal cyst.

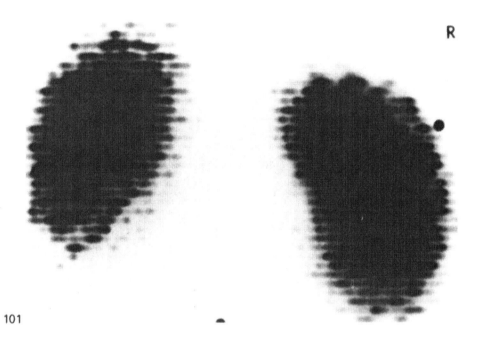

R

101

L   R

102

Perirenal Air Insufflation: This investigation is performed when an adrenal tumour is suspected. Air or oxygen is introduced into the space between the rectum and sacrum by a needle guided by a finger in the rectum. X-rays are taken every 10 minutes with the patient erect. The air provides a dark contrast medium outlining both the adrenal glands and the kidneys on each side (fig. 103). Insufflation should not proceed unless, by aspiration, it is shown that the needle is not sited in a pelvic vessel (Ransom et al., 1956). Non-invasive, more accurate, computerised tomography has replaced perirenal air insufflation in most centres.

Percutaneous Antegrade Pyelography: Percutaneous antegrade pyelography (fig. 104) is performed by passing a 20 gauge spinal needle through the skin, under local anaesthesia, into the renal pelvis and then outlining the pelvi-calyceal-ureteric system with contrast medium (Casey and Goodwin, 1955).

The procedure is of great value in demonstrating a level of obstruction when this cannot be shown by intravenous pyelography or retrograde pyelo-ureterogram (see fig. 126b) but it is essential that either preliminary straight abdominal x-rays, limited intravenous pyelograms, radio-isotope studies, ultrasound or computerised tomography have demonstrated both the precise site of the renal pelvis and the fact that it is distended. Prior to injection of any contrast medium urine should be aspirated.

103 Peri-renal air insufflation. The clinical impression of a large left adrenal phaeochromocytoma is confirmed.

104 Antegrade pyelography. A 50-year-old woman underwent a right hemi-colectomy operation. Three weeks later she presented with persistent aching right loin pain. A grossly obstructed poorly functioning right kidney was diagnosed by intravenous pyelography and the site of obstruction confirmed by antegrade pyelography. Note the needle entering the pelvis.

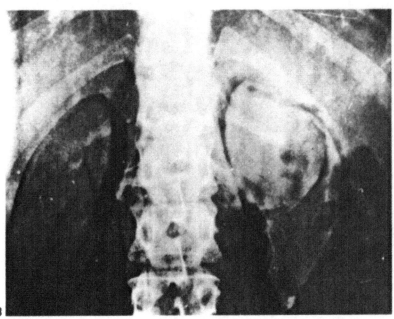

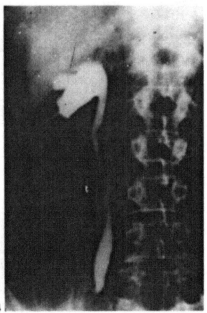

103

104

Percutaneous nephrostomy (p. 204) is now commonly used to relieve acute or chronic upper urinary tract obstruction of urine, dilate uretero-ileal strictures (p. 119), dissolve certain selected renal calculi (p. 226) and even remove some impacted calculi (Smith et al., 1979).

Whitaker's Test: Several chapters in this book emphasise that a dilated system does not necessarily imply an obstructed system. Whitaker's test is based on the fact that an obstructed system requires an increased proximal pressure to maintain the normal flow rate. The test is used in an endeavour to differentiate between dilatation and obstruction and is described on p. 121.

Figure 105a-f shows the result of several of the investigations described in this section performed in a 42-year-old man who presented with painless haematuria; they highlight some of the problems encountered in arriving at an accurate diagnosis in some cases of renal space occupying lesions.

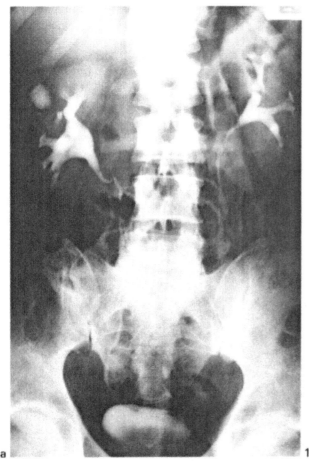

105a

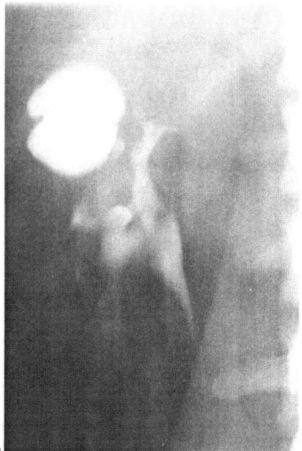

105b

Diagnostic difficulties
105a A 42-year-old man presented with painless haematuria. An intravenous pyelogram revealed a space occupying lesion of the right kidney.

105b An infusion tomogram magnified the outline of the lesion.

105c An ultrasound study suggested the lesion was cystic (see over).

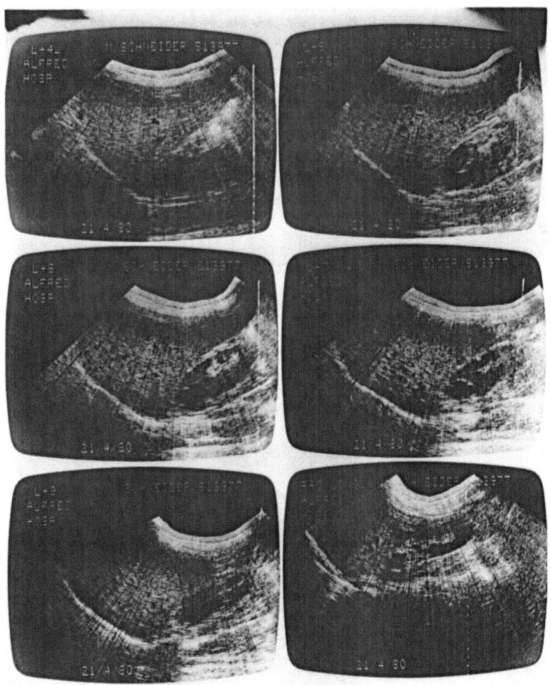

105c

*Lower System
Investigations*

Cysto-urethroscopy: *Cystoscopy* is the term used to describe optical instrument visualisation of the bladder wall and outlet by utilising telescopes with a visual field varying between 30° and 120°. Genitourinary assessment of this area includes such visualisation, together with an associated urethroscopy, utilising a visual field between 0 and 30° inspection of the genitalia and a bimanual examination of the pelvis.

Cysto-urethroscopy is best performed under general anaesthesia although local anaesthesia is used when it is estimated that therapeutic or extensive diagnostic manipulations will not be necessary or there are general medical reasons inhibiting general anaesthesia.

Many patients undergoing cysto-urethroscopy require a preliminary intravenous pyelogram examination to exclude probable or silent upper tract pathology and to thereby indicate whether or not retrograde pyelo-ureterograms and/or upper urine collection specimen studies are necessary at the time of the procedure.

Upper urine collection specimens can be obtained from either system and microscopically and chemically examined. This procedure is used to localise urinary tract infections and may be of value in differentiating between a

Diagnostic difficulties (continued)
105d A right selective renal angiogram showed a non-neoplastic vessel pattern.

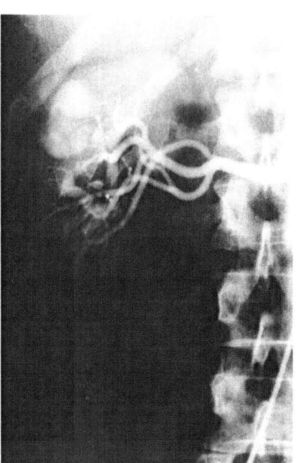

105d

non-opaque filling defect in the renal pelvis or ureter by microscopic examination of the specimen for malignant cells or uric acid crystals.

The associated use of an image screening intensifier enables an appreciation of the calyceal-pelvi-ureteric conducting efficiency and often helps to identify obstruction as well as assisting in differentiating between a non-opaque calculus and a neoplasm.

Diagnostic difficulties (contined)
105e,f Computerised tomography again suggested a benign cystic lesion. As the studies had not completely excluded a malignancy and he had presented with haematuria, the patient was cysto-urethroscoped. Two small papillomas were found on the trigone. Subsequent cyst puncture of the renal large calyceal diverticulum revealed no abnormal cells.

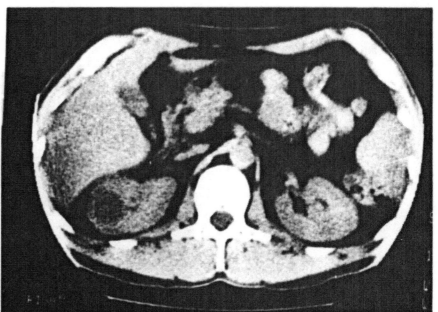

105e

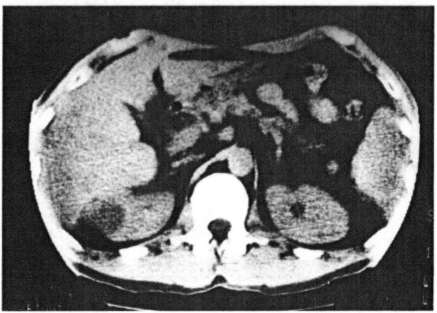

105f

The development of modern concentrated contrast media and techniques such as hyperconcentration and high dose infusion pyelography have resulted in far fewer indications for *retrograde pyelo-ureterograms.*

Modern cystoscopes are now made of either stainless steel alloy with an insulated tip or a metal inner tube with an outer non-conducting smooth teflon coating (fig. 106). The original Nitze (1889) glass lens system has been replaced with a series of solid glass rods, which greatly increase the optical resolution and contrast by utilising both the considerable modern

106 Cystoresectoscopes. A modern cystoresectoscope set, with a light source in the background connected to a working resectoscope with its adjacent introducing sheath and obturator. A paediatric resectoscope is shown in the foreground.

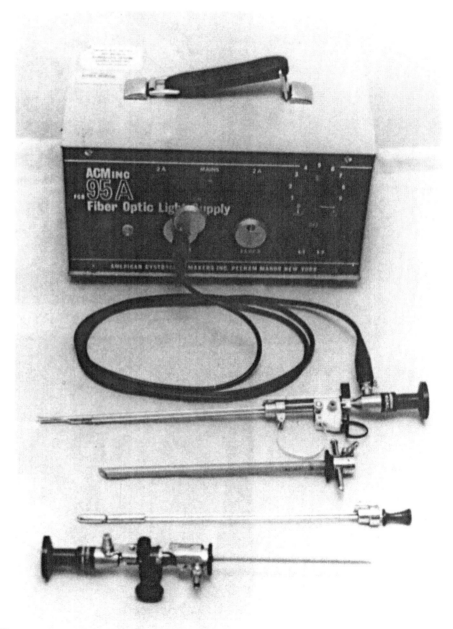

engineering advances involved in grinding and coating such rods and by reducing the air space between the glass. These improvements provided a wider viewing angle with a lens system which occupies less space and therefore enables reduction in the absolute diameter of the instrument. The modern light source consists of similar glass fibres which pass inside the telescope and conduct light from an externally generated power source. This provides brilliant illumination, sufficient even to enable photography or television transmission to be carried out. The variety and quality of equipment now enables such procedures to be performed on newly born children, although this may require an external bulbous urethrotomy for newly born males.

Indications for Cysto-urethroscopy

a) *Haematuria:* All patients who experience macroscopic haematuria or asymptomatic recurrent microscopic haematuria greater than 20,000 red blood cells per ml require radiological outlining of the upper system and cysto-urethroscopic visualisation of the lower system, irrespective of their age, in order to detect and treat possible life-threatening pathology such as carcinoma. (See chapter VI.)

b) *Urinary tract infection:* cysto-urethroscopy enables:

   i) an attempted accurate diagnosis of the cause and/or localisation of the site of infection
   ii) a distinction to be made between those situations which are actually or potentially capable of causing permanent renal and/or other tissue damage and those which are not
   iii) occasional simultaneous surgical correction or palliation of the cause. (See chapter V.)

c) *Lower urinary tract obstruction of urine:* The diagnosis and usually the treatment of lower urinary tract obstruction of urine requires cysto-urethroscopy (chapter X).

d) *Bladder calculi:* Bladder calculi are not always radio-opaque (chapter IX) and cystoscopy may establish the diagnosis. An endoscopic lithotrite may be used to crush such calculi and to irrigate the fragments from the bladder.

e) *Ureteric calculi:* These may be endoscopically extracted if they are below 0.5cm in size, impacted in the lower third of the ureter and causing persistent or recurrent pain. (See chapter IX.)

f) *Upper urinary tract obstruction of urine:* Retrograde pyelo-ureterograms may identify the site and the pathology of the obstruction. A Braasch bulb catheter (fig. 107) is inserted into the ureteric orifice and subsequent injection of contrast medium outlines the upper system.

g) *Removal of foreign bodies* (see p. 155).

h) *Infertility:* Catheterisation of the ejaculatory ducts and subsequent study of vaso-seminal vesiculograms may assist in the diagnosis and treatment of infertility (p. 378).

Complications of Cysto-urethroscopy: All surgical procedures have complications; the incidence of serious complications during and following diagnostic cysto-urethroscopy is extremely low but increases when extensive cutting procedures are performed.

Urinary tract infection, bacteraemia/septicaemia, intravascular haemolysis and blood loss are the major early complications whilst urethral stricture is the major long term complication (p. 252).

Cystogram: Complete distension of the bladder with contrast medium inserted through a small urethral catheter gives a more accurate outlining of the bladder mucosa than intravenous pyelography and may reveal diverticula or constant filling defects (fig. 108-109), such as a neoplasm or non-opaque calculi, but rarely provides as much information as a telescopic examination.

Voiding cystograms are of greater value in detecting the presence of vesico-ureteric reflux (p. 136), posterior urethral valves (p. 22, p. 338) or in assessing female stress incontinence (p. 356). In infants the bladder is emptied by supra-pubic compression with the operator wearing a lead-lined glove.

107 A Braasch bulb retrograde ureteric catheter. Note the arrow-shaped tip, which retains the catheter in the distal ureter during the injection studies.

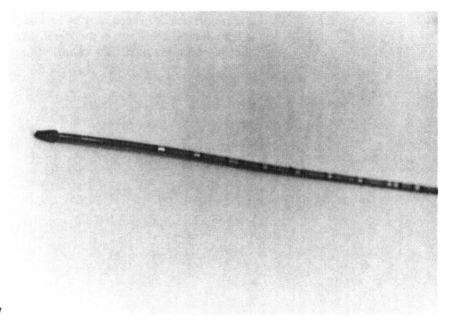

Cystograms

108 A constant left-sided filling defect consistent with a bladder neoplasm.

109a A 28-year-old woman who presented with recurrent urinary tract infections was found to have a solitary dilated left system.

109b A micturating cysto-urethrogram revealed grade III vesico-ureteric reflux, which was corrected by anti-reflux surgery.

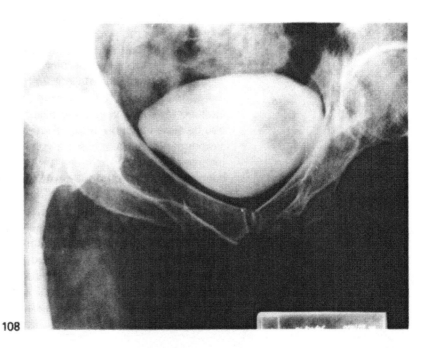

108

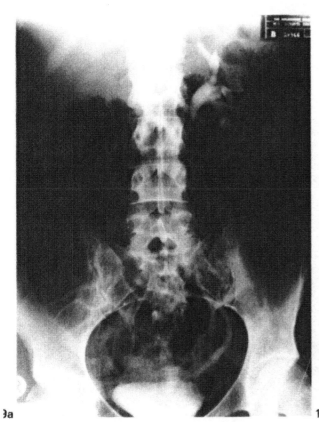

9a

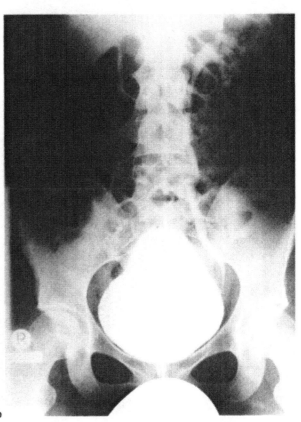

109b

Cine-cysto-urethrography: This provides a film of bladder filling and emptying and is occasionally of value in assessing functional bladder outlet obstruction.

Urethrogram: Visualisation of the urethra can be achieved by the introduction of 25ml of a radio-opaque viscous medium 'Umbradil' (Astra) via a nozzle inserted into the external urinary meatus. Urethral strictures, ruptures, diverticula, neoplasms or fistulae may be detected (figs. 110-111).

Urethral Discharge: See chapter XIX.

Lymphangiography: Lymphangiography is used in an endeavour to detect neoplastic lymph gland metastases or benign obstruction. Evans blue dye is injected intradermally into the first web space of each foot. Within an hour the subcutaneous lymphatics of both lower limbs are usually sufficiently outlined to enable surgical exposure, cannulation and subsequent introduction by slow injection pump of contrast medium. As the medium enters the lymph glands metastases may be identified as filling defects (fig. 112). The technique is time consuming and often difficult to interpret and has largely been replaced by computerised tomography.

Perineal Prostatic Needle Biopsy: In order to confirm the clinical suspicion of a prostatic carcinoma a needle biopsy may be necessary (p. 182). A spinal or general anaesthetic is administered and a Vim-Silverman (Franklin modification) needle passed through the perineal body, directed by a finger in the rectum, until the hard prostatic area is reached and a core tissue extraction made for microscopical examination. Haemorrhage and penetration of the rectum or bladder are very rare complications of this procedure.

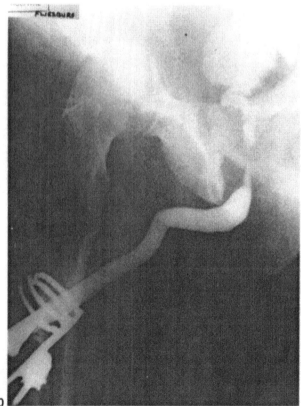

110

Urethrograms

110 A normal urethrogram. Note the extended penis and the thick dye, containing 1% neomycin, entering the bladder.

111 In this 38-year-old man the dye cannot pass into the posterior urethra because of a gross stricture of unknown but presumed traumatic origin.

112 A lymphangiogram. In a man of 55 with a known right-sided infiltrating bladder neoplasm, a large metastatic pelvic lymph node is disclosed.

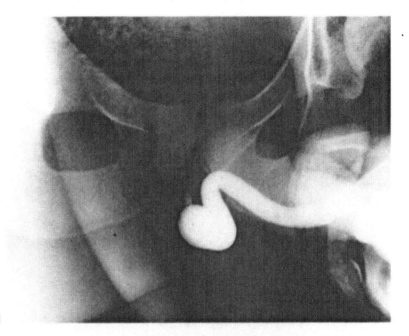

111

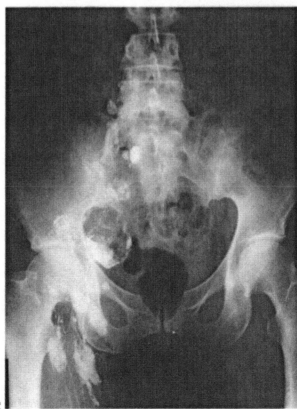

112

**General
Investigations**

Patients with urological problems are often in the older age group at their initial consultation and usually require an electrocardiograph tracing and an assessment of their pulmonary function, together with a full blood examination . A chest x-ray is an essential investigation in all patients undergoing a general anaesthetic for major surgery and a necessary annual investigation in all patients over the age of 45 years, particularly tobacco smokers. A chest x-ray may disclose primary or secondary heart or lung disease, including neoplastic metastases (fig. 113). Peri-renal neoplastic infiltration or inflammation may result in elevation and/or fixation of the diaphragm.

Other specialised investigations such as tuberculosis culture and guinea pig inoculation, bleeding and coagulation times, platelet counts, malarial blood smears and a renal biopsy may be necessary, dependent upon the particular clinical situation.

113 Annual chest x-ray. Asymptomatic 'cannon-ball' metastases from an asymptomatic renal adenocarcinoma, in a 50-year-old man.

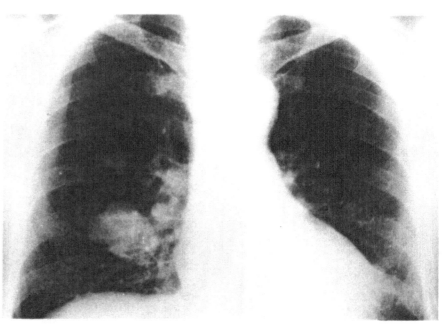

113

References

Ambrose, S.S.; Lewis, E.L.; O'Brien, D.P.; Walton, K.N. and Ross, J.R.: Unsuspected renal tumours associated with renal cysts. Journal of Urology 117: 704 (1977).

Allan, W.R. and Brown, R.B.: Torsion of the testis: A review of 58 cases. British Medical Journal 1: 1396 (1966).

Asscher, A.W.; Sussman, N.; Waters, W.E.; Davis, R.H. and Chick, S.: Urine as a medium for bacterial growth. Lancet 2: 1037 (1966).

Barnett, E. and Morley, P.: Diagnostic ultrasound in renal disease. British Medical Bulletin 28: 196 (1972).

Baron, M.; Lester, E. and Brendler, H.: Preoperative diagnosis of renal angiomyolipoma. Journal of Urology 117: 701 (1977).

Casey, W.C. and Goodwin, W.E.: Percutaneous antegrade pyelography and hydronephrosis. Journal of Urology 74: 164 (1955).

Davies, P.; Woods, K.A.; Evans, C.M.; Gray, W.M. and Kulatilake, A.E.: The value of provocative and acute urography in patients with intermittent loin pain. British Journal of Urology 50: 227 (1978).

Harrison, L.H. and Boyce, W.H.: Image intensification fluoroscopy. Transactions of the American Association of Genitourinary Surgeons 56: 55 (1975).

Kass, E.H.: Asymptomatic infection of the urinary tract. Transactions of the Association of American Physicians 69: 56 (1956).

Koff, S.A.; Thrall, J.H. and Keyes, J.W. Jnr: Diuretic radionuclide urography: A non-invasive method for evaluating nephroureteral dilatation. Journal of Urology 122: 451 (1979).

Lome, L.G.; Pinsk, S. and Levy, L.: Dynamic renal scan in the non-visualising kidney. Journal of Urology 121: 148 (1979).

McGuckin, M.; Cohen, L. and MacGregor, R.R.: Significances of pyuria in the urinary sediment. Journal of Urology 120: 452 (1978).

Morgan, K.Z.: How dangerous is low-level radiation? New Scientist 82: 18 (1979).

Pryles, C.V.; Atkin, M.D.; Morse, T.S. and Welch, K.J.: Comparative bacteriologic study of urine obtained from children by percutaneous suprapubic aspiration of the bladder and by catheter. Paediatrics 24: 983 (1959).

Ransom, C.L.; Landes, R.R. and McLelland, A.: Air embolism following retroperitoneal pneumatography. A nationwide survey. Journal of Urology 76: 664 (1956).

Schlegel, J.U.; Halikiopoulos, H.L. and Prima, R.: Determination of filtration fraction using the gamma scintillation camera. Journal of Urology 122: 447 (1979).

Sklaroff, D.M. and Berkn Kravitz, C.: The renal scintigram in urological work up. Journal of the American Medical Association 178: 418 (1961).

Smith, A.D.; Lange, P.H. and Fraley, E.E.: Applications of percutaneous nephrostomy. New challenges and opportunities in endo-urology. Journal of Urology 121: 382 (1979).

Syme, R.R.A.: The significance of asymptomatic microscopic haematuria. British Journal of Urology 51: 425 (1979).

Wright, F.W. and Walker, M.M.: The radiological diagnosis of avascular renal tumours. British Journal of Urology 47: 253 (1975).

Further Reading

Emmett, J.L. and Witten, D.M.: Clinical Urography: An atlas and textbook of roentgenologic diagnosis (Saunders, Philadelphia 1971).

Gow, J.G. and Hopkins, H.H.: Handbook of Urological Endoscopy (Churchill Livingstone, London 1978).

Murphy, L.J.T.: The History of Urology (Charles C.Thomas, Springfield 1972).

Nitze, M.: Lehrbuch der Kystoskopie (Bergman, Wiesbaden, 1889).

Stanley, R.J.; Sagel, S.S. and Fiar, W.R.: Computerised tomography of the genito-urinary tract. Journal of Urology 119: 780 (1978).

Weller, J.M. and Greene, J.A. Jnr: Examination of the Urine (Appleton-Century-Crofts, New York 1966).

Chapter IV

Urodynamics

Urodynamics is the study of the flow of urine from the renal papilla to outside the body. It can be divided into the study of the upper urinary tract, the renal calyces, pelvis and ureter, and the study of the bladder and its outflow mechanism.

Upper Urinary Tract Urodynamics

The history of the investigation of the dynamics of the upper urinary tract falls into two distinct eras. First, there was a period of intensive experimental investigation. The pioneers in this field were Kiil (1957), Struthers (1969) and Boyarsky (1972). There was then a lull while some of this basic physiological information was fed into clinical practice by such workers as Ross and his colleagues (1972) and Backlund and Reuterskiold (1969). The second era was heralded by the appreciation that not all dilated upper tracts were obstructed and that a careful look at the dynamics might help to distinguish the obstructed from the unobstructed system. Early studies were performed at the time of operation in such conditions as hydronephrosis (Johnston, 1969) and mega-ureter (Backlund and Reuterskiold, 1969). What was then needed was a preoperative diagnostic study that could decide if indeed an operation was necessary.

It was in the late 1960's that it became clear that the renal pelvis could be punctured safely and, following this, antegrade pyelography (p. 107) became popular as both a therapeutic and diagnostic technique. The method also provided ready access to the kidney for urodynamic studies. This was an important advance because it then became possible to make an accurate diagnosis as to the site and degree of obstruction (Whitaker, 1973).

Purpose of Dynamic Studies

Measurement of Activity: Dynamics can be useful in two respects. First, a simple method of measuring pressure via a thin tube can tell whether there is any spontaneous activity in the upper urinary tract by measuring changes in the pressure. This can be useful when planning an operation on a wide system: for instance, after a period of severe obstruction it is helpful to know that the system has regained tone before undertaking reconstructive surgery. The introduction of contrast medium via the same fine tube and examination with fluoroscopy will give information as to whether these spontaneous contractions are producing any useful ureteric motility with propulsion of a bolus.

Also, measurements of pressure, together with electromyography and histology, have shown that there are *pacemaker cells* in the pelvicalyceal system that initiate the spread of electrical and muscular activity.

Detection of Obstruction: Secondly, dynamic studies can provide the all important answer to the question of whether or not the upper tract is obstructed, and the use of dynamics in this respect is discussed more fully below.

Dynamic Diagnosis of Upper Urinary Tract Obstruction

Before making the diagnosis of an obstruction we must be clear as to what we mean by the term obstruction as applied to the ureter and renal pelvis. In simple terms it means an impediment to flow, but when analysed in dynamic terms obstruction is best defined as a situation where there is an abnormally high pressure within the system to transmit the usual flow through it. There will, of course, be times when the kidney is no longer capable of producing a high pressure and the result will then be a lower flow than usual. It is clear then that both pressure and flow must be estimated if the degree of obstruction is to be critically evaluated.

Alternative Investigations: Dynamic studies have proved necessary because, in difficult cases of obstruction, almost all other forms of investigation including radiology and isotope studies fail to give the necessary information concerning the two parameters of pressure and flow. A urogram, a retrograde ureterogram and a probe renogram all have these limitations, although individually they may provide information about morphology, motility and function.

Recently, more sophisticated types of isotopic study have been introduced in which the differential transit times have been compared between the renal parenchyma and collecting system (Whitfield et al., 1978). Such studies have the great advantage that they are less invasive than dynamic studies, but they need to undergo further evaluation before it can be shown that they can replace a dynamic assessment.

Technique: In 1969 Johnston showed that the renal pelvis could be perfused, at the time of operation, to simulate a rapid diuresis and that the pressure measured through a separate tube could give useful information on whether or not an obstruction was present. Similar studies were performed by Backlund and Reuterskiold (1969) in both animals and children. The pressure/flow perfusion studies that are now used as a diagnostic technique in many centres (Whitaker's test, p. 108) are based on this same principle, but have 2 distinct advantages (Whitaker, 1979). First, only one cannula is necessary for both the perfusion and the pressure measurement and, secondly, the cannula can be introduced into the renal pelvis percutaneously so that the presence or absence of obstruction can be confirmed before deciding whether or not an operation is necessary.

A thin cannula, mounted on a needle, is introduced into the renal pelvis, or a dilated calyx, by direct percutaneous puncture (fig. 114). This is most simply performed under x-ray control after the administration of an intravenous injection of contrast medium. In small children a general anaesthetic is preferable, but in older children and adults local anaesthetic is sufficient.

The cannula is then attached to a perfusion pump that will deliver at a rate of both 10 and 5ml per minute. Through a side arm the pressure is measured via a transducer and recorded on a simple one channel recorder. It is essential also to measure the bladder pressure via a urethral catheter and this can be recorded via the same transducer, intermittently, on the same recording. The upper tract is then perfused initially at 10ml per minute, with either contrast medium or saline, and the pressure within the renal pelvis is continuously recorded. After the study is complete the renal pelvis is aspirated, the cannula removed, and the patient returned to bed for 24 hours.

Interpretation: It now seems clear that a normal urinary tract can tolerate 10ml per minute with no greater pressure drop between the renal pelvis and bladder than 12 to 15cm of water. If the pressure rises above this level, but then equilibrates at between 15 and 30cm of water, a moderate degree of obstruction is present. If the pressure is higher than this, or tends to continuously rise and not reach an equilibrium, a severe obstruction is present.

Complications: The complications from this type of study are few and not serious. A minor degree of extravasation is not unusual and may produce a little discomfort. We have not encountered severe haemorrhage, but a little haematuria for a few hours is not unusual.

114 The Whitaker test. A diagrammatic illustration.

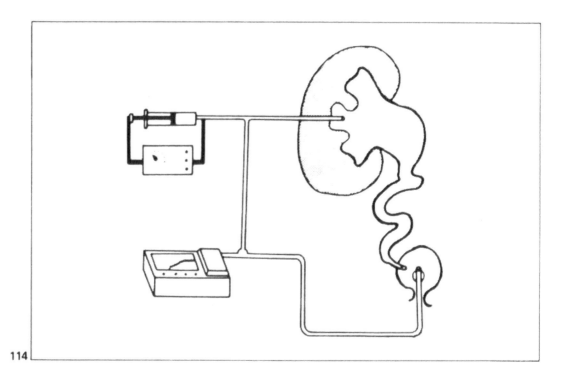

114

Indications for and Accuracy of Test: The only situation in which this study fails to indicate obstruction is in intermittent hydronephrosis (2 cases in nearly 200 studies in the writer's series). If the pelvi-ureteric junction is not obstructed at the time of the study then clearly the intra-renal pressure will be within normal limits. In these cases the only satisfactory diagnostic method is a urography during an attack of pain.

A knowledge of the bladder pressure is essential to distinguish between upper tract dilatation due to uretero-vesical junction obstruction and to bladder outlfow obstruction.

This method of investigation is reliable and, at times, indispensable when other methods of investigation have failed to elucidate the problem in difficult cases of equivocal obstruction with dilatation but no vesico-ureteric reflux.

Lower Urinary Tract Urodynamics

Lower urinary tract urodynamics are concerned with the flow of urine into and out of the bladder and urethra.

The ancients thought the bladder was an inert sac and the urine was expelled by abdominal pressure and it was not until the pioneer work of Mosso and Pellocani in 1882 that the contractile power of the bladder wall was demonstrated. Over the next 75 years intermittent reports of bladder dynamics appeared but it was not until modern electronics had developed to a stage which allowed measurement of bladder pressure, with little interference with the normal mechanism of micturition, that the possibility of applying these research procedures to clinical problems in urology was considered.

In the late 1950's von Garrelts of Stockholm (von Garrelts, 1956, 1957) introduced a method of measuring bladder pressure and urine flow which formed the basis of all subsequent investigations. He also demonstrated the application of these techniques to the clinical problems of prostatic disease and urethral stricture. Since then there has been a gradual but steadily increasing interest in urodynamics both from a research and clinical aspect.

Clinical urodynamics is concerned with the measurement of the physiological changes in the bladder and urethra during filling and voiding. Certain measurements are fundamental and each is discussed below.

Bladder Pressure

The pressure in the bladder has 2 components, the intrinsic pressure produced by the bladder wall and external or abdominal pressure. Bladder pressure is the most fundamental measurement in lower tract urodynamics and can be measured by a variety of different techniques.

a) *Use of an indwelling urethral catheter.* The commonest and generally the most satisfactory method, this obviously produces some obstruction to the lumen of the urethra during micturition but this effect is small and the safety and convenience of the method amply compensate for this disadvantage.

b) *Suprapubic puncture* to record bladder pressure has the advantage that the urethral mechanism is left unaffected but it is used chiefly in children.

c) Entirely *intravesical measuring devices* have been described but are complicated and have not found general favour.

Usually water-filled catheters are used with an external transducer but tiny transducers mounted on the tip of the catheter have been devised and proved reliable.

The Cystometrogram

This is the oldest standard procedure in urodynamics and cystometry has been in clinical use for over 50 years. Fluid or gas is instilled into the bladder and the pressure developed during filling is measured.

Technique: The apparatus employed ranges from a simple T-tube manometer to complicated electronic recording devices. The rate at which the bladder is filled seems to be unimportant, within fairly wide limits, but in-flow rates of 25 to 50ml/minute are commonly used. The pressure is recorded and related to the volume of fluid in the bladder.

Interpretation: The cystometrogram may in fact measure 2 different properties of the bladder: first, the physical characteristics of the bladder wall, and secondly, the physiological reaction of the detrusor muscle and its neurological connections. The normal cystometrogram consists of a very flat pressure curve with little rise in bladder pressure until capacity is almost reached. Abnormal rises in the pressure curve may indicate an abnormality called *instability of the bladder muscle.* In severe cases this may be induced by filling the bladder slowly and is often associated with incontinence, or leakage of urine, but in milder cases the instability may only be demonstrated by getting the patient to cough or strain or by tilting the patient from the horizontal to the upright position. Usually no cause can be found for this abnormality but it may be associated with upper motor neurone lesions such as occur in multiple sclerosis or spinal injuries (p. 266).

Reliability: The cystometrogram is a reasonably consistent measure of bladder capacity and detrusor response to filling but may be *modified* by a number of factors, such as the temperature of the filling fluid, the psychological state of the patient, the number of times it is repeated and the presence of complications such as bladder stone or infection.

Micturition Studies

Recording of pressure and flow events during micturition can reveal much useful information of clinical relevance. However, it must be realised that all methods of measuring bladder pressure during micturition involve some interference with the normal micturition mechanisms and must always be interpreted with caution.

Urinary Flow Rate

The rate of flow of urine is the most easily recorded of all micturition events and a variety of different types of instrument of very varying complexity have been devised to record this measurement. Electronic derivatives can be employed to yield instantaneous flow rates and are particularly useful in patients who have an interrupted flow (fig. 115).

Von Garrelts (1956, 1957) described the various types of flow in normal as well as pathological conditions of the urinary tract. However, there is a wide variation in individual cases so a single flow rate may have little clinical significance. Flow rates for bladder volumes under 150ml in the adult are unreliable (fig. 116). However, in general terms, flow rates over 15ml/second in the male exclude obstruction whereas those under 10ml/second are often associated with obstruction. In the female, flow rates tend to be rather higher than in the male.

Urinary flow rates
115 Plot of volume against time.

116 Normal and abnormal patterns.

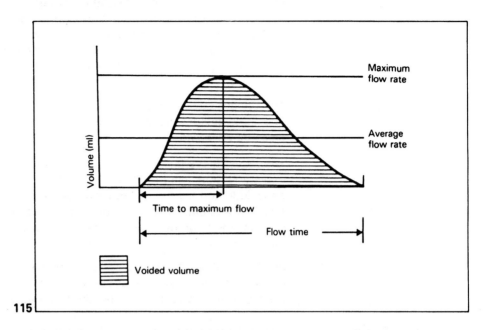

115

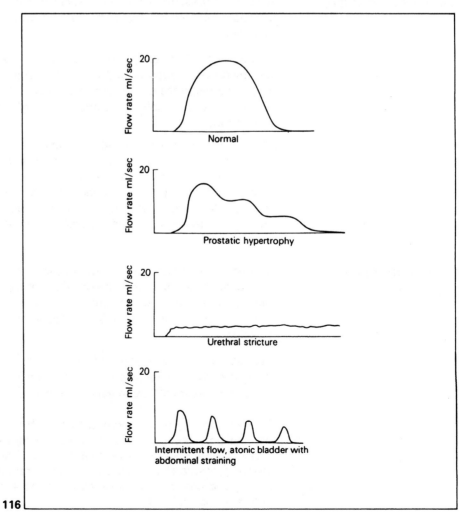

116

The chief advantage of urinary flow rate measurement is that it is simple and reproducible and does not involve any instrumentation of the urinary tract. By performing sequential flow rates the effects of such procedures as prostatectomy or urethral dilatation for stricture may be assessed (p. 244, 254). Flow rates may be used to determine the timing of urethral dilatation in stricture cases and the author has devised a simple uro-flowmeter consisting of a plastic funnel in the barrel of the syringe which will accurately record a single flow rate and help to determine when urethral dilatation is necessary.

The Urinary Stream

The urinary stream has been studied by cinematography, spectroscopy, direct and indirect pressure measurements and, since time immemorial, by personal observation.

The study of the urinary stream in the female is difficult but in the male is easier and represents the force left in the urine after urethral resistance has been deducted from the bladder pressure. Unfortunately, the most important factor altering the characteristics of the urinary stream is the external meatus, for a narrow meatus may give an excellent projection despite a poor flow rate.

External meatal stenosis presents few diagnostic problems in the male although it is not always realised that the effective diameter of the external meatus in the adult male is only 3mm or equivalent to 11 French gauge.

Micturition Pressure

This is the pressure within the bladder during voiding and can be measured by suprapubic or more commonly by a transurethral pressure catheter in the bladder.

In urethral obstruction there is commonly a rise in the bladder pressure during micturition accompanied by a fall in the urinary flow rate. This represents the response of the detrusor muscle to urethral obstruction and is frequently accompanied by trabeculation of the bladder wall visualised by cystoscopy.

In conditions where the muscle of the bladder wall fails the pressure curve during micturition may be flat or nonexistent. Under these circumstances micturition may be initiated by increases in the intra-abdominal pressure produced by voluntary abdominal muscle. Such micturition by straining is usually intermittent for it is difficult for voluntary straining to produce a sustained stream. Thus it is important to measure intra-abdominal as well as intra-vesical pressure.

Intra-abdominal Pressure

This pressure, which acts on the bladder itself and on the proximal urethra, is a variable factor in micturition. Normal micturition is possible and frequently occurs without any change in the intra-abdominal pressure. However, changes in the intra-abdominal pressure may profoundly alter bladder function.

True abdominal pressure is difficult to measure and, usually, rectal pressure measured by a water filled rectal balloon is taken to represent intra-abdominal pressure although some authors have used intra-gastric balloons.

True *detrusor pressure* represents total bladder pressure minus intra-abdominal pressure and is now reasonably easily measured using bladder and rectal catheters and electronic subtraction. However, this refinement is not vital as pressure changes produced by abdominal muscles are usually short lasting and can be differentiated from the slow rise and fall produced by detrusor contractions.

Urethral Pressure Profile

Originally described in 1969 by Brown and Wickham, this measurement has been extensively studied without any very firm conclusions having emerged (fig. 117).

A fine urethral catheter with side holes located a little distance from the tip is perfused with fluid at a slow rate (2ml/min) and withdrawn along the length of the urethra as the pressure in the catheter is measured. At points of urethral narrowing, such as the sphincter or a urethral stricture, the pressure measured will rise. The magnitude of the rise at sphincter level can be enhanced by a voluntary squeezing of the pelvic muscle. The urethral pressure profile has been shown to produce consistent results that can be modified by drug treatment. In the female a low profile is often associated with a low urethral resistance and incontinence. In the male the pressure profile can be used to demonstrate anterior urethral strictures but these are better demonstrated by a urethrogram. It is, however, of considerable help in neurological disorders affecting the bladder and sphincter region where it can be used to demonstrate the effect of drug or nerve blockades.

Electromyography

These rather complicated techniques can be applied to the sphincter region or the detrusor muscle. They remain a research technique but are of value in assessing some of the problems of neurological disorders of the bladder and urethral function.

117 Urethral pressure profile.

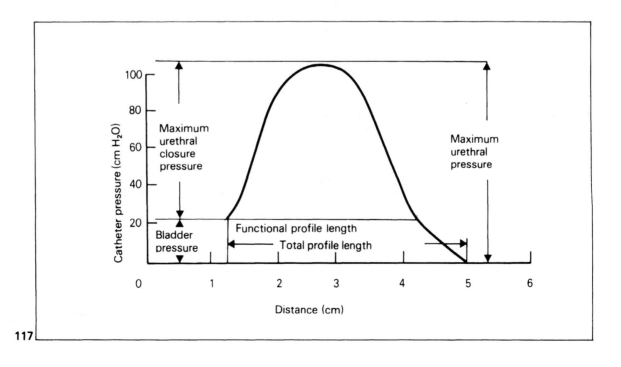

117

Indications for Urodynamic Studies

Studies of lower urinary tract dynamics have increased our knowledge of disorders of micturition a great deal over recent years and have provided endless occupational therapy for academic urologists. In some instances they have contributed to the diagnosis and treatment of urological disorders, often in a negative way by demonstration of the absence of urethral obstruction. This may be a positive benefit to the patient who may well be saved unnecessary surgical procedures.

The apparatus is expensive and the procedures are time consuming. They are also very limited in value unless the clinician concerned takes an active interest in the performance and interpretation of the studies. It seems probable that for the moment such studies should be performed only in urological units with an active interest but the lessons learnt may often be applied to urological practice elsewhere.

The indications for urodynamic studies will vary depending on local circumstances and the particular research interests of the unit. Their value is now well proven in demonstrating the presence or absence of urethral obstruction and the study and treatment of bladder instability.

References

Backlund, L. and Reuterskiold, A.G.: The abnormal ureter in children. 1. Perfusion studies on the wide non-refluxing ureter. Scandinavian Journal of Urology and Nephrology 3: 219 (1969).

Bosky, S. and Labay, P.: Ureteral Dynamics (Williams and Wilkins, Baltimore 1972).

Brown, M. and Wickham, J.E.A.: The urethral pressure profile. British Journal of Urology 41: 211 (1969).

Johnston, J.H.: The pathogenesis of hydronephrosis in children. British Journal of Urology 41: 724 (1969).

Kiil, F.: The Function of the Ureter and Renal Pelvis (University Press, Oslo 1957).

Mosso, A. and Pellacani, P.: Surles fonctions de la vessie. Archives of Italian Biology 97: 127, 291, 323 (1882).

Ross, J.A.; Edmond, P. and Kirkland, I.S.: Behaviour of the Human Ureter in Health and Disease (Churchill Livingstone, Edinburgh 1972).

Struthers, N.W.: The role of manometry in the investigation of pelvi-ureteral function. British Journal of Urology 41: 129 (1969).

von Garrelts, B.: Analysis of micturition. Acta Chirurgica Scandinavica 112: 326 (1956).

von Garrelts, B.: Intravesical pressure and urinary flow in normal subjects. Acta Chirurgica Scandinavica 114: 49 (1957).

Whitaker, R.H.: Methods of assessing obstruction in dilated ureters. British Journal of Urology 45: 15 (1973).

Whitaker, R.H.: The Whitaker test. Urologic Clinics of North America 6: 529-539 (1979).

Whitfield, H.N.; Britton, K.E.; Hendry, W.F.; Nimmon, C.C. and Wickham, J.E.A.: The distinction between obstructive uropathy and nephropathy by radioisotope transit times. British Journal of Urology 50: 433 (1978).

Further Reading

Backman, K-A.: Micturition in normal women. Acta Chirurgica Scandinavica 130: 357 (1965); 132: 413 (1966); 132: 403 (1966).

Gierup, J. Micturition studies in infants and children. Scandanavian Journal of Urology and Nephrology Suppl. 5 (1970).

Hjalmas, K.: Micturition in infants and children with normal lower urinary tract. Scandinavian Journal of Urology and Nephrology Suppl. 37 (1976).

Smith, J.C.: Urethral resistance to micturition. British Journal of Urology 4: 125 (1968).

Chapter V

Infection and Dysuria

Urinary tract infections are common and result from a variety of causes but many patients, particularly children, present with symptoms and signs of infection although subsequent investigation reveals a sterile urine. The cause of the infection, or the symptoms and signs of infection, must be determined if treatment is to be successful.

This chapter deals first with genitourinary infection other than that caused by tuberculosis, then with tubercular infection, and finally with infective and non-infective dysuria. Venereal causes of urethritis are discussed in detail in chapter XIX and epididymal and testicular inflammations and infections are discussed in chapters II (p. 70) and III (p. 80).

Genitourinary Tract Infections

Urinary tract infections are very common with a high incidence in women, presumably because of their shorter urethra and its relationship to sexual intercourse and both vaginal inflammation and contamination.

General Aspects

Urinary tract infection occurs in all age groups but there are 3 peak periods of presentation:

1) During the first 6 years of life, because of the anatomy and hygiene of young girls (p. 316) and the presence of male and female congenital abnormalities (chapter I).
2) At the time of sexual activity and childbirth
3) After the age of 55 years in males, as a result of mechanical and/or functional urinary tract obstruction (chaps X and XI).

Urinary tract infections can result in permanent renal (chapter XVI) and other genitourinary tissue damage and this is particularly evident in the presence of renal obstruction or vesicoureteric reflux. In view of this potential all children who experience one episode of infection and all adults with recurrent infection should be thoroughly investigated in order that the cause can be diagnosed and, if possible, corrected.

Diagnostic Methods

The early diagnosis and correction of potentially serious causes of urinary tract infection provides one of the major challenges of modern preventive medicine.

History and Physical Examination: All patients with symptoms and signs suggestive of a urinary tract infection require a full history taking and thorough general examination.

Symptoms and signs: The symptoms and signs of urinary tract infection result from inflammation of the affected area or areas. Renal inflammation may cause loin pain and tenderness to palpation whilst bladder, prostatic and urethral inflammation are characterised by suprapubic pain, perineal pain, micturition and/or post-micturition painful dysuria and/or haematuria.

In children general signs dominate the clinical presentation whilst in adults local symptoms and signs are more common.

Loin pain as an isolated symptom/sign: The majority of patients presenting with loin pain as a solitary symptom have back strain and not urinary tract infection.

Dysuria as an isolated symptom: Although many patients presenting with dysuria, with or without haematuria, are subsequently found to have a urinary tract infection, some have a sterile urine (p. 154) or a venereal urethritis.

Urine Examination: All patients presenting with symptoms and signs suggestive of a urinary tract infection should undergo a microscopic, chemical and, if necessary, culture examination of the urine in order to determine whether or not infection is present. The laboratory detected presence of bacteriuria indicates that either the patient has a urinary tract infection or that the urine specimen has been contaminated after leaving the bladder. Such contamination is common in view of:

1) The organisms which normally live in the external urinary meatus and related areas
2) The difficulties of obtaining mid-stream specimens of urine in children and women
3) The delays which sometimes occur between collecting the specimen and examining it in the laboratory.

Kass (1956) used the term 'significant bacteriuria' to distinguish between true urinary tract infection and contamination. Significant bacteriuria implies the presence of more than 100.000 organisms per ml of urine. This count could only occur under conditions of gross contamination. Most urinary tract infections are due to a single bacterial strain.

The presence of less than 100,000 organisms per ml of urine does not mean that the urine is uninfected. Chronic renal infection, patients receiving chemotherapy at the time of culture, and conditions of extreme diuresis, may all produce an 'insignificant bacteriuria'.

A full account of the techniques of urine collection and examination will be found on p. 84, and 316.

Asymptomatic Bacteriuria: There is considerable evidence (Kunin and Paquin, 1965) that asymptomatic bacteriuria in young school girls can indicate the presence of gross genitourinary abnormalities. These workers found that:
1) Vescio-ureteric reflux was present in 23% of such young girls
2) The intravenous pyelogram was abnormal in 22%.

Kass (1960) stressed that 20% of pregnant women with asymptomatic bacteriuria developed acute pyelonephritis during pregnancy but that this could be prevented by treating the asymptomatic bacteriuria when it was originally diagnosed.

Norden and Kass (1968) stressed the importance of asymptomatic pregnancy bacteriuria which has an incidence of up to 10% (Polk, 1959). Kincaid-Smith and Bullen (1975) investigated such patients after delivery and found that the intravenous pyelogram was abnormal in 51% and that there was a significant renal size difference in 45%.

Screening tests for asymptomatic bacteriuria: Wide scale screening tests for asymptomatic bacteriuria are expensive and in the light of present knowledge can only be justified in the 2 high-risk groups mentioned above.

Further Investigations: The diagnosis of urinary tract infections depends not only upon the clinical and urine examination findings but also upon the radiological and endoscopic findings (see below).

Bacteriology

More Common Organisms: The organisms most commonly responsible for urinary tract infections are *Escherichiae coli,* Klebsiella, *Proteus mirabilis, Streptococcus faecalis,* Micrococci and *Pseudomonas aeruginosa. Esch. coli,* Klebsiella and *Strep. faecalis* infections are common in those cases without detectable upper or lower genitourinary tract abnormalities whilst Proteus and Pseudomonas infections are usually found in patients following hospitalisation, in those who have had repeated antibiotic therapy or in those with a present or past history of a large renal calculus. *Staphylococcus aureus* may cause urinary tract infections, particularly in ill, hospitalised patients and is also responsible for the rare renal carbuncle (see below). *Staphylococcus albus* is another uncommon cause of urinary tract infection in debilitated patients.

Fungal infections are uncommon but occur in diabetics, patients in poor general health or in those receiving immunosuppressive, cytotoxic or toxic bone marrow drugs.

Less Common Infections: In addition to tuberculosis other rare *granulomatous* infections include, *malakoplakia,* an extremely rare coliform infection which results in the formation of multiple honeycombed granulomatous renal abscesses forming within and outside the kidney. The condition is thought to result from a particularly virulent *E. coli* infection and a nephrectomy is usually required. Malakoplakia can also occur in the bladder, testis and epididymis (Melicow, 1957).

Schistosomiasis and *brucellosis* infections are extremely rare in developed countries but, very rarely, renal *hydatid* disease occurs (fig. 118). The disease is usually diagnosed by a positive intradermal Casoni skin test but a negative result does not exclude the infection. A nephrectomy is usually necessary.

Urinary pH and Other Considerations: Most organisms that invade the urinary tract survive better in an alkaline than an acid urine. Most of the successful chemotherapeutic drugs act more effectively in an acid medium. Many Gram-negative bacteria produce *bacteriocins* which inhibit the growth of other different species.

Most Gram-negative organisms produce *endotoxins* which, if released into the circulatory system in moderate amounts, will produce severe shock. This situation can occur spontaneously but more commonly follows operative or postoperative trauma, where very large numbers of bacteria may suddenly enter the circulation.

Methods of Invasion: *Ascent through the urethra:* This theory is supported by the dominance of gut organisms. causing urinary tract infection and by their known colonisation of the vagina and external urinary meatal area (Cox, 1966; Marsh et al., 1972). Their subsequent introduction into the bladder could occur under circumstances such as sexual intercourse, urological instrumentation, and even by spontaneous movement (Mayo and Hinman, 1973). Such ascent would be favoured by primary inflammatory pathology in this area such as the 'urethral syndrome' (see below). Stamey has shown that bladder bacterial invasion can often be predicted by the initial appearance of such organisms within the vagina before they are even located within the bladder (Stamey et al., 1971).

Vesico-ureteric reflux: This represents the most commonly known form of preventable permanent renal damage within the community (p. 135, 334).

Haematogenous infection: Organisms may enter the kidney through the circulation but they rarely establish a colony unless the kidney is abnormal and/or the patient is generally unwell or a severe diabetic.

Overwhelming local renal tissue necrosis may result in the formation of a *renal carbuncle* (Craven et al., 1974). This rare condition usually presents as an initial septicaemia with local renal pain and tenderness and a high fever. The responsible organism is usually *Staph. aureus,* but is rarely found in the urine as the lesion does not usually communicate with the drainage system. The clinical diagnosis is confirmed by a characteristic renal angiogram (p. 98) and the carbuncle usually responds well to high dose chemotherapy, although it may be necessary to surgically drain the collection or to perform a nephrectomy.

Infection by direct extension: This can occur from locally related infective sources, or possibly from the gut via the lymphatics, although there is no evidence to support this theory.

Results in Untreated Urinary Tract Infection

Such infections may resolve, scar or suppurate (renal carbuncle, prostatic abscess) and/or aid the formation of urinary calculi. Renal scarring may produce effects ranging from a small scar in the renal cortex (with or without widening of the related calyx, dependent upon both the site of the fibrosis and whether or not associated papillary necrosis has occurred) to severe generalised fibrosis resulting in a contracted, poorly functioning kidney (see chapters XVI, XVII). Bladder tissue sloughing and destruction may result in future calculus formation by providing the primary nucleus. Urethral infections may produce a stricture (p. 252).

Proteus (urea splitting) renal infections, by raising the urinary pH (p. 210), may encourage the formation of phosphatic calculi, as may other Gram-negative organisms.

Particular organisms may produce a possible antigen-antibody local tissue response which, in the kidney, may result in the formation of a thick, non-opaque, mucous material termed a *matrix calculus*. This matrix can also act as a nidus for stone formation and may calcify rapidly if the infection is not treated efficiently (p. 210).

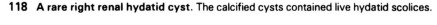

118 A rare right renal hydatid cyst. The calcified cysts contained live hydatid scolices.

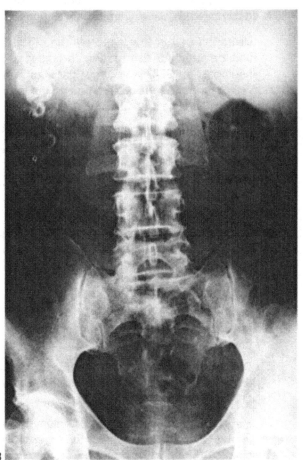

118

Investigations

All children and young adults with one proven episode of urinary tract infection and all patients with recurrent infection or recurrent symptoms require further investigation in order to:

1) Attempt to localise and diagnose the cause of the infection (Fairley et al., 1967)
2) Determine those infections actually or potentially capable of causing permanent renal and/or other tissue damage
3) Instigate simultaneous therapy (occasionally).

As indicated above, many patients who present with symptoms and signs of possible urinary tract infection, but in whom urinary examinations have failed to reveal any evidence of infection, may also require further investigations. All children and all pregnant women with asymptomatic bacteriuria also require further investigation as previously indicated.

Chapter III should be consulted for details of the essential investigations listed below.

Static and Voiding Cysto-urethrograms: Vesico-ureteric reflux is common in children and for this reason a voiding cysto-urethrogram often reveals this potentially serious abnormality. As renal fibrosis may take many years to develop gross reflux may be present without the intravenous pyelogram indicating upper tract abnormality. A voiding cysto-urethrogram should always be performed as the first diagnostic investigation in children and young adults (fig. 119).

Intravenous Pyelogram: Anatomical and functional abnormalities of the kidney may be revealed (fig. 120). Ureteric and bladder abnormalities may be diagnosed or suspected, although the small amount of dye intravenously injected usually limits the diagnostic accuracy of the cystogram.

Dilatation of the lower ureters (fig. 119a) upper and lower pole pulsation and/or infective destruction, or the presence of a pelvi-ureteric hydro-nephrosis (p. 274) in younger patients, may also suggest the presence of vesico-ureteric reflux; dilatation of the lower ureters, in older patients suggests mechanical or functional obstruction (fig. 121).

Cysto-urethroscopy: This provides an accurate diagnostic assessment of the lower genitourinary system and occasionally enables a simultaneous correction of abnormalities. Localisation of the source of infection is often possible (Stamey et al., 1965; Fairley et al., 1967) and pyelo-ureterograms may detail upper tract pathology.

Selective Renal Angiography: This may be necessary when space occupying lesions of the kidney are present or when poor renal function provides an inadequate anatomical and/or physiological intravenous pyelogram or retrograde pyelo-ureterogram details.

Haemagglutination Test: A high *E. coli* O serotype titre (> 1:640) may indicate renal infection whilst a low titre (< 1:320) may indicate lower tract infection. These findings are of some value in managing patients with chronic infective pyelonephritis.

Cystometrogram and Urine Flow Studies: These may be of value in diagnosing a neurogenic bladder presenting with urinary tract infection (see chapters IV and XI.)

Renal Biopsy: This may be of value in differentiating between chronic infective pyelonephritis and other chronic destructive renal diseases (see chap. XVI) and in selecting appropriate therapy for these patients.

Vesico-ureteric reflux as a cause of urinary infection

119a A 28-year-old man presented with a urinary tract infection. An intravenous pyelogram revealed a solitary left system with a dilated lower ureter.

119b A voiding cystogram reveals grade I vesico-ureteric reflux. Surgical correction was not advised.

120 A 30-year-old woman presented with a urinary tract infection. The voiding cystogram was normal but the left system, in particular, is highly suggestive of previous vesico-ureteric reflux. Note the marked blunting of the upper and lower calyces.

121 A 62-year-old man presented with severe dysuria without haematuria. The intravenous pyelogram revealed dilated, tortuous, terminally uplifted ureters, suggesting that a known benign prostatomegaly was responsible, but panendoscopy revealed numerous bladder neoplasms.

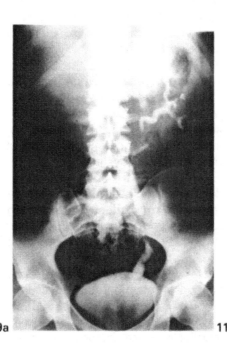

119a

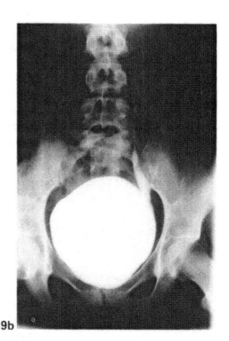

119b

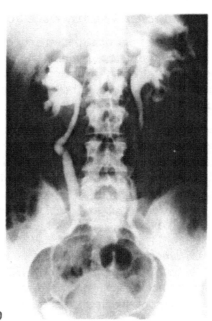

120

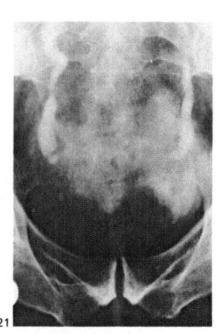

121

Diagnostic Results

The investigation of subjects with symptoms and signs of urinary infection, with or without evidence of infection on urine microscopy or culture, reveals two groups of patients, those with infection and those in whom no infecting organism is detected.

Infected Group: *Acute urethro-trigonitis (female) or posterior urethritis/prostatitis (male) and acute pyelonephritis:* In view of their similar development it is not surprising that both sexes suffer inflammatory episodes in these areas. The shorter female urethra and resultant external proximity accounts for the higher female prevalence.

The onset of sexual activity (honeymoon cystitis), childbirth or first use of the contraceptive pill often initiates acute infective dysuric episodes. However, this precipitating history is often lacking and the precise means by which organisms enter the posterior urethra and bladder is unknown. Venereal urethritis is discussed in chapter XIX. Acute pyelonephritis, in the absence of vesico-ureteric reflux, other types of obstruction, or primary renal disease, is uncommon.

Chronic urethro-trigonitis (female) or chronic prostatitis (male): Chronic urethro-trigonitis and chronic prostatitis result from repeated episodes of infective and non-infective inflammation in the proximal urethra and embryologically related bladder trigone. Rarely chronic prostatitis may be tuberculous. Acute-on-chronic episodes of infection are responsible for subsequent attacks of dysuria.

In females there is no sharp dividing line between those patients suffering from acute-on-chronic infective urethro-trigonitis and those suffering from the 'urethral syndrome', whilst in males, particularly diabetics, chronic non-infective prostatic inflammation is not uncommon (see below).

Vesico-ureteric reflux: Severe vesico-ureteric reflux destroys renal tissue by a combination of infection, back pressure and, in some instances, by exacerbating latent pelvi-ureteric obstruction (p. 274). It is the most commonly known preventable cause of permanent renal damage in the community and its accurate diagnosis and treatment are essential

Chronic renal infection: This may result from:

1) Upper urinary tract obstruction and/or other renal abnormalities such as calculus formation, scarring and/or papillary necrosis
2) Chronic or atrophic pyelonephritis in which no apparent primary defect in the system, other than the presence of the infection, is found.

It is now known that many patients who in previous years were diagnosed as having developed 'idiopathic' chronic pyelonephritis sustained their renal destruction because of vesico-ureteric reflux (Hodson, 1959). Some of the histological architecture of chronic pyelonephritis may represent an autoimmune response to intermittent bacterial infection. Chronic pyelonephritis may also result from diabetes, analgesic abuse (Dawborn et al., 1966) or from sickle cell disease.

Xanthogranulomatous pyelonephritis: This is a rare renal tissue response to chronic infection (Hatch and Cockett, 1964). The kidney assumes a hard yellow appearance which, microscopically, consists of chronic fibrous tissue and numerous macrophages containing large quantities of fat. The pathogenesis is unknown and the condition may be confused with a renal neoplasm although the angiogram of the latter is usually diagnostic (see chapter III; p. 96).

Cystitis: A severe cystitis may involve the trigone but cystitis and urethro-trigonitis are best considered as separate clinical conditions.

Infected cystitis may result from lower genitourinary tract mechanical or neurogenic obstructive causes such as prostatomegaly, neurogenic bladder or a urethral stricture. Less common causes include bladder neoplasm, foreign bodies, calculi, tuberculosis, diabetes, debilitating diseases, vesico-intestinal and vesico-vaginal fistulae and rarely, bilharziasis (El-Badawi, 1966), leukoplakia (O'Flynn and Mullaney, 1967), and malakoplakia (Melicow, 1957) which are all discussed further under Dysuria. Sterile, or secondarily infected chemical cystitis, may result from bubble baths (Roberts, 1967) or excessive vigorous applications of antiseptic vaginal preparations. Drugs such as cyclophosphamide (Anderson et al., 1967) can also cause a severe, vascular, secondarily infected cystitis.

Phosphatic encrusted cystitis (Letcher and Matheson, 1935) results from a pseudomonas or proteus infection, which produces an alkaline urine due to the splitting of urea (see chapter IX). Endoscopic resection of the plaques, chemotherapy, and acidification of the urine may resolve the condition.

Cystitis emphysematosa results from a Gram-negative infection, which ferments glucose, to produce gas which is found within the lumen of the bladder or within its wall. This produces a cobble-stone radiological or cystoscopy appearance. The condition is not uncommon in elderly patients and/or severe diabetics and usually requires no treatment other than correction of the infection.

Abacterial cystitis: In 1940, Moore first described a rare, acute, non-infective cystitis in young, ill, non-febrile, patients whose intravenous pyelogram showed features similar to genitourinary tuberculosis (see below) but where no infective agent was found. The urine microscopy revealed numerous pus and red cells but no organisms. The condition responds well to tetracycline therapy (Doyle et al., 1977) but its aetiology is still unknown. Abacterial cystitis should not be diagnosed unless repeated attempts to detect tuberculosis and/or other organisms have failed.

Non-infected Group: *Paediatric sham syndrome:* This term was originally used by Stephens et al. (1966), to describe those non-infected children who present with frequency and urgency, wetting and, often, behavioural problems. The children are usually tense and nervous and only rarely are local tissue abnormalities found (p. 320).

Paediatric vulvovaginitis: This is the most common gynaecological problem in children and may result from the short perineum, nearby anus, thin labia and absence of pubic hair, the lack of oestrogen which results in a neutral pH, and a thin vaginal mucosa. Poor toilet hygiene, foreign body insertion, pinworm or monilia infestation or previously unsuspected diabetes mellitus are other causes.

The child presents with a combination of vaginal and vulval itching, discomfort and dysuria. Local examination is often difficult and is best achieved by sitting the child, with outstretched legs, on the mother's lap.

Parting the labia usually enables a clinical diagnosis of primary vulvitis with secondary vaginitis or *vice versa* to be made. A rectal examination is difficult to achieve but improves the view of the vagina and may detect a foreign body. Vaginal secretions are gently aspirated with a sterile medicine dropper and microscopically examined for possible monilial infestation. Transparent perianal tape swabs are examined on several occasions for the presence of pinworm. If no causative agent is found the condition is diagnosed as nonspecific vulvovaginitis.

Urethral syndrome: The urethral syndrome is very common and is characterised by intermittent or, less commonly, persistent frequency dysuria in the presence of a sterile urine (see below). Pyuria and microscopic haematuria may be present together with a chronic urethro-trigonitis in the female or a posterior urethritis/prostatitis in the male.

The aetiology is unknown but is related to local anatomy, tissue irritation during and after sexual intercourse, vaginitis, allergic tissue responses and personality problems.

Although the paediatric sham syndrome, nonspecific paediatric vulvovaginitis and the urethral syndrome are non-infective conditions the breakdown of natural host defensive mechanisms in this area may result in a secondary infection.

Other causes: Uninfected cystitis may result from neoplasm, interstitial cystitis (Hunner, 1914; Badenoch, 1971), cyclophosphamide or irradiation therapy (p. 312).

Treatment of the Infected Group

As stated, it is essential that an accurate diagnosis of the cause of the infection and/or the symptoms and signs be made prior to instigating treatment. This diagnosis can be made on clinical grounds but usually requires radiological and endoscopic investigation.

It is difficult to assess the results of various drug treatments of 'urinary tract infection' in many published papers as often there is no indication given as to the precise cause of the infection.

Treatment depends upon:

1) The cause
2) Whether cure or palliation is indicated
3) The efficiency of the defensive host factors.

Drug and Other Therapy for Acute Infections: It is not necessary to await the results of a urine culture and sensitivity examination before starting symptomatic females with *acute urethro-trigonitis* or males with *acute urethritis/prostatitis* on appropriate therapy, although this does provide more satisfactory short and long term treatment by ensuring that the most advantageous drug is used; however it is *mandatory* that urine specimens be forwarded to the laboratory before such treatment is started.

The choice of drug depends upon sensitivity patterns, the past and present clinical situation, recent experience, side effects and cost.

Synergistic (*in vivo*) sulphamethoxazole and trimethoprim (*co-trimoxazole*) disrupt bacterial folate metabolism and are commonly used (2 tablets twice daily for 5 days) to treat acute urethro-trigonitis and/or posterior urethritis/prostatitis despite the relatively high incidence of hypersensitivity, nausea, vomiting and haematological abnormalities, including the very rare Stevens-Johnson syndrome. *Ampicillin* (500mg 6-hourly for 3 days) also provides effective therapy within this group but skin rashes, hypersensitivity and diarrhoea are common. *Amoxycillin* (250mg 8-hourly for 3 days) is as effective as ampicillin with fewer side effects.

Nitrofurantoin (50mg 8-hourly for 7 days) is also highly effective within our community but hypersensitivity and nausea are common whilst pulmonary oedema and peripheral neuritis are rare complications. (Macrocrystalline nitrofurantoin causes fewer complications than the crystalline form).

Nalidixic acid (500mg 8-hourly for 10 days) is similarly, but rather less, effective. Cephalosporins (*cephalexin* 250mg 6-hourly for 6 days) inhibit bacterial cell-wall synthesis and are bactericidally effective, particularly against Coliform, Proteus and Klebsiella organisms but may also cause hypersensitivity reactions and diarrhoea.

Single dose antibacterial treatment is effective and cheap (Bailey, 1979) and has the added advantages that the patient is known to have taken the drug, there are fewer side effects and less emergence of resistant organisms than with multiple dose regimens. Amoxycillin, 3g for adults (100mg/kg for children); co-trimoxazole 2.88g for adults (0.72-1.44g for children) and kanamycin, 500mg intramuscularly for adults, have all been shown to be at least as effective as longer term therapy and are therefore ideally suited for domiciliary practice.

Immediate *parenteral* treatment is indicated in the seriously systemically ill patient. Ampicillin, 2g intravenously and gentamicin 1.5mg/kg intravenously are given simultaneously, with subsequent therapy being determined by the clinical situation, precise drug sensitivity patterns and the development of possible side effects. Other aminoglycoside drugs, such as tobramycin and sisomicin may be used but all have some degree of nephrotoxicity and ototoxicity and require daily serum level measurements during their use. The combination of renal failure and urinary tract infection increases the incidence of such side effects while producing inadequate urinary concentrations. Nitrofurantoin is absolutely contraindicated under these circumstances as it is poorly excreted and soon produces a neurotoxic effect. Similarly, tetracyclines are contraindicated as they increase the azotaemic process and satisfactory urine concentrations are never achieved with nalidixic acid.

Drug treatment should be associated with a daily *fluid intake* of at least 4 litres as this results in frequent bladder emptying.

Urinary alkalinisation is of value in relieving symptoms but it may occasionally aid bacterial growth and also inhibit the efficacy of drugs such as mandelamine. Urinary alkalinisation on its own has no place in the treatment of urinary tract infection but it assists the action of co-trimoxazole and the aminoglycosides.

Severe acute prostatitis may produce retention of urine and require temporary bladder catheterisation, in addition to appropriate chemotherapeutic treatment and, rarely, surgical drainage of a prostatic abscess.

Follow-up: Repeat urine microscopy and culture examination is performed 7 days after cessation of the drug therapy and repeated if symptoms recur.

Chronic Female Urethro-trigonitis

If urinary tract infection is detected then it is treated as previously indicated. Some patients benefit from long term courses of chemotherapy even though infection is not always detected.

The incidence of future episodes of acute-on-chronic urethro-trigonitis can often be reduced by maintaining a daily fluid intake of 4 litres, liberally applying 0.5% cetrimide cream to the peri-urethral area prior to sexual intercourse and the immediate premenstrual period and by post-coital micturition and 48-hour nitrofurantoin therapy. Associated vaginal infections and inflammations (chapter XIX) must be adequately treated.

Recurrent infections, in the presence of an otherwise normal urinary system and failing to respond to the above measures, often benefit, after bacteriological proof of cure of the presenting infection has been obtained, from a 6 to 12 months course of nitrofurantoin 50mg, co-trimoxazole half a tablet, nalidixic acid 500mg or methenamine mandelate 2g — taken as a single nightly dose. Methenamine mandelate may cause nausea and gastric discomfort in susceptible patients. Long term nitrofurantoin and nalidixic acid therapy have been shown to induce the development of resistant bacteria by the transfer of R factor and long term co-trimoxazole may also produce this effect (O'Grady et al., 1973). Cycloserine, 250mg twice daily for 10 days, also inhibits bacterial cell-wall synthesis but, in view of its occasionally serious complications of nervous system disturbance, liver damage and dermatitis, it should only be used in selected patients when other drugs have failed and the organism has been shown to be sensitive to the drug.

Division of the anterior bridge of the hymen on either side of the external urethral meatus may assist post-coital initiated infections (Blackledge, 1979), as may correction of gynaecological abnormalities such as prolapse and cervicitis. Specific endoscopic surgery including urethral and bladder neck dilatation, trigonal diathermy, resection or diathermy of bladder neck inflammatory polyps, bladder distension, 'Elase'[1] and neomycin mucosal irrigation, or correction of local abnormalities such as a urethral caruncle or prolapsed urethral mucosa may also provide benefit as may the stabilisation of detrusor instability (Pengelly et al., 1978). Fungal infections of the bladder often respond to neomycin mucosal irrigation but may require additional amphotericin therapy as well as correction of any local or general abnormality such as diabetes.

Chronic Prostatitis

Granato et al. (1973), have shown that co-trimoxazole gives satisfactory therapeutic prostate gland tissue levels but the author's results using this drug have been disappointing. Long term nitrofurantoin therapy, posterior urethral and bladder neck dilatation, posterior urethral irrigation with 'Elase'[1] and neomycin solution and, occasionally, prostatic massage (see p. 159) are also of value in selected patients.

Vesico-ureteric Reflux

A congenitally short sub-mucosal ureter is responsible for 90% of cases of reflux the remainder being due to acquired lower genitourinary tract obstructive or inflammatory conditions. Acquired causes of reflux need correction of the primary cause which usually results in cessation of the reflux.

1 'Elase' (Parke Davis)

Congenital vesico-ureteric reflux requires immediate surgical correction or continued observation dependent upon:

1) Rate of recurrent infections
2) Total renal function and scarring
3) Severity of the reflux
4) Severity of the endoscopic findings
5) Age
6) Sex
7) The likely adequacy of follow-up supervision.

Provided that careful clinical, radiological and endoscopic criteria are used for patient selection the results of anti-reflux surgery are excellent, with elimination of the reflux and intravenous pyelogram improvement occurring in 90% of children. (p. 334).

Chronic Renal Infection

If possible the cause of the infection and/or obstruction must be corrected (e.g. surgical removal of a staghorn calculus or a nephro-ureterectomy for a grossly diseased tuberculous kidney).

Chronic or atrophic pyelonephritis, of unknown aetiology, requires treatment of any infection detected, though this is rare. Severe unilateral chronic atrophic pyelonephritis, in the presence of a normal contralateral system, may justify nephrectomy, particularly if renovascular hypertension is detected (see chapter XVII), whilst severe bilateral chronic or atrophic pyelonephritis calls for renal failure management, which may necessitate renal homotransplantation (see chapter XVI).

Specific Cystitis

Surgical and/or medical treatment is determined by the particular aetiological cause (see also Dysuria).

Treatment of the Non-infected Group

Paediatric Sham Syndrome. *Psychotherapy:* Many of these children have behavioural problems and often they, and their parents, require psychotherapeutic advice.

Drug treatment: Hyoscine methobromide, 2.5mg twice daily or imipramine, 25 to 50mg at night, are occasionally of value.

Other measures: Frequent voiding and high fluid intake inhibit the colonisation of the bladder and urethra by infective organisms and prevent possible secondary infection occurring.

Paediatric Vulvovaginitis. *Perineal hygiene:* Severe nonspecific vulvovaginitis requires alternate 4-hourly 15 minute non-soap saline baths and wet compresses. The vulva should be gently patted dry and the area exposed, air dried and cooled for the next hour. If underclothing is used then it should be regularly changed and consist of moisture absorbing cotton material. In addition a wide air circulating dress or skirt should be worn.

After resolution of the severe inflammation hygienic aids such as instruction in the adoption of a 'forwards-to-backwards' toilet technique, rather than the reverse, wash-away showers, rather than baths, and the use of cotton rather than fluffy underpants together with barrier cream application to the area after showering and a high fluid intake, which encourages regular frequent voiding, all assist in preventing recurrent inflammation.

Foreign body in the vagina: The detection or suspicion of such an object, which is commonly found to be toilet paper, necessitates a full vaginal examination under general anaesthetic in order to remove all of the material and to detect any serious associated lesion such as a neoplasm.

Pinworm infestation: Piperazine syrup, given as a daily dose of 65mg/kg for 7 days, is not only effective against pinworm but also against roundworm. Other children in the family should also be treated. In addition the child should be instructed not to scratch the area and to carefully wash both hands and nails after using the toilet and again before eating food. Bedclothes should be regularly cleaned and aired and the child should wear cotton panties to bed.

Other causes of paediatric vulvovaginitis: Streptococcal vaginitis occasionally results from an upper ear, throat or respiratory infection whilst gonorrhoeal vaginitis is rare (p. 382).

Trauma, neoplasms, syphilis, trichomoniasis, prolapsed urethra or allergic tissue responses are other, uncommon, causes of paediatric vulvovaginitis. See also chapter XIV.

Urethral Syndrome: Many patients with the urethral syndrome are tense and nervous and require mature counselling and, occasionally, relaxant drug therapy. They often have a dry, easily inflamed vaginal mucosa, which benefits from regular liberal lubrication, particularly prior to sexual intercourse and the menstrual period. Advice against excessive douching or strong antiseptic baths should be given.

By definition infection is not present in the urethral syndrome but secondary infection does occur in view of the primary inflammatory tissue changes and, if detected, is treated as indicated above.

Other anti-inflammatory therapy includes those urethral, bladder, vaginal and perineal measures discussed under the treatment of chronic urethro-trigonitis. As indicated, there is often no sharp dividing line between chronic urethro-trigonitis and the urethral syndrome. (See also Dysuria section.)

Dysuria from Other Non-infected Causes of Urethritis and Cystitis: Treatment of these conditions is discussed later in this chapter.

Catheter, Operative and Postoperative Infection

There are many reasons for bladder catheter drainage (see chapter X) and aseptic insertion techniques, with a carefully cleaned, continually closed drainage system are mandatory.

Urological operations must often be carried out in the presence of infection and the operation itself may introduce infection. The immediate and major infective risk to the patient results from bacteraemia and this is prophylactically controlled by the 1-hour preoperative intravenous administration of appropriate broad spectrum chemotherapy (p. 249). The urinary tract infection resulting from or exacerbated by such procedures may require additional supportive chemotherapy but such infections often resolve spontaneously if successful surgery has been achieved.

Defensive Host Factors

Hydrodynamics: If the bacterial multiplication rate in urine falls below their rate of destruction by death and 'washout' then the bacteria will diminish in numbers (O'Grady and Cattell, 1966). Upper tract perfusion is usually more regular than lower tract perfusion although this varies considerably. Wolin (1971) found that 1% of young women claimed to void only once in 24 hours. Local areas of obstruction may interfere with flow rates whilst incompetent vesico-ureteric junctions will also inhibit a uni-directional perfusion flow. Animal experiments and theoretical calculations (O'Grady et al., 1968; Shand et al., 1970) have shown that a high flow rate considerably reduces the number of bacteria in the system if:

a) Reproduction rate is low
b) Bladder emptying occurs frequently and regularly (Cox and Hinman, 1961)
c) The residual bladder volume is normal (not greater tham 1ml).

The clinical implications of these findings are that all patients with urinary tract infection should:

a) Drink as much bland fluid as is possible
b) Ensure frequent and regular bladder emptying.

Urine Composition: Normal urine is an excellent culture medium but there is evidence that:

a) A *high protein intake* produces an acid urine and buffers animals against experimentally induced pyelonephritis (North and Miller, 1966).
b) The normal *urinary pH* varies between 4.5 and 8. *E. coli* organisms are inhibited by growth below pH 5.5. At this low pH organic acids such as hippuric and mandelic can penetrate cell membranes and become bacteriostatic; advantage is taken of this knowledge in the use of mandelamine therapy.

Healthy Tissue Factors: Healthy genitourinary tissue resists the invasion of pathogenic bacteria by destroying organisms with a *factor* produced from the urothelium (Norden et al., 1968).

Excessive immunoglobulins (secretor IgA) may be produced by the bladder mucosa (Kaufman et al., 1970) and together with IgE (Burdon, 1973) would also assist in the destruction of invading organisms.

Stamey et al. (1968) have shown that the normal male *prostatic fluid* exhibits antibacterial properties.

Long Term Follow-up Treatment

Follow-up treatment is essential for patients with established permanent renal damage or those with the potential for developing such pathology. Long term follow-up is also of considerable assistance to those with 'nuisance value' local bladder outlet and/or urethral infective or non-infective symptoms as it enables more efficient continuity of treatment.

Genitourinary Tuberculosis

Genitourinary tuberculosis accounts for a major part of extrapulmonary tuberculosis; both the urinary tract and genital organs can be affected by the disease or either the urinary tract or genital organs alone. Tuberculosis of the genitourinary tract has not decreased in incidence, as have other forms of tuberculosis, and this trend is expected to continue.

Genitourinary tuberculosis is a great imitator and the early lesion is easily missed; it is essential to investigate any patient with unexplained genitourinary symptoms and signs for the disease. Modern chemotherapy is successful in treating most early cases provided that it is taken for 2 years, but there are definite indications for surgical intervention, particularly in advanced cases.

Incidence

Although the incidence of pulmonary tuberculosis (Campbell, 1974) in affluent countries has decreased this is not so in poorer countries where the disease, in its many forms, still causes much morbidity. Genitourinary tuberculosis is now the most frequent form of extra-pulmonary tuberculosis and this may be due to the fact that this particular form of the disease usually manifests itself about 10 years after a pulmonary tuberculosis infection; it may also partly reflect the incidence of resistant acid-fast bacilli to the standard triple therapy fromerly used.

Pathology

Genitourinary tuberculosis must be considered to be a local manifestation of a generalised tuberculous infection; the primary focus is usually in the lungs but occasionally in infected bronchial or mesenteric lymph nodes.

Tuberculosis of the Kidney: During the active phase of the disease blood-borne dissemination of the tubercle bacilli occurs and showers of organisms are seeded into the tiny capillary glomerular tufts of both kidneys where the formation of microscopic tubercles will occur if the organisms survive. Most of these cortical lesions resolve (Medlar et al., 1949) but some expand and are sloughed into the collecting system of the nephrons producing tuberculous bacilluria and pyuria. In some patients tuberculous bacilli and debris become trapped in the narrow loops of Henle and eventually form caseous tubercles in the medulla. These tubercles increase in size, coalesce, liquefy and may erode into the papilla from where ulceration into the calyx occurs, producing the typical ulcerocavenous type of tuberculous lesion. Once the infection progresses to this degree the tissues never heal spontaneously and the process may progress rapidly causing extensive destruction of the kidney (figs. 122, 123).

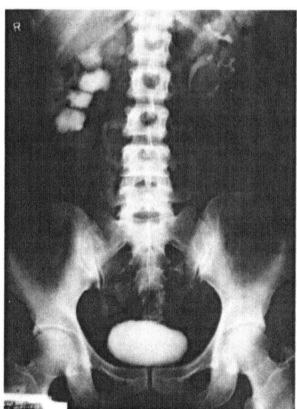

122a

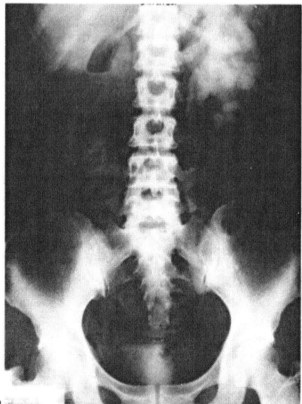

122b

Renal tuberculosis

122a Serial intravenous pyelograms showing rapid progression of bilateral tuberculosis which was not diagnosed when the patient had a right upper ureterolithotomy operation.

122b Tuberculosis was diagnosed 2 years later and chemotherapy begun.

122c The right kidney is shown to be functioning again but both kidneys have lost considerable cortex

123 Caseous renal tuberculosis.

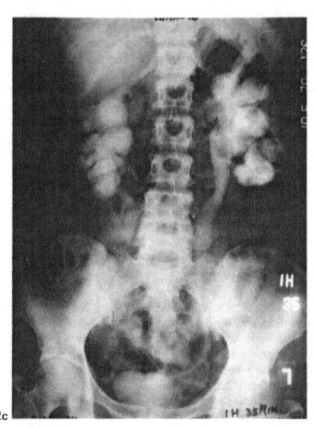

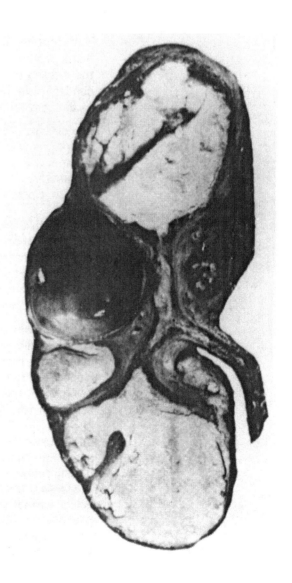

122c   123

Tuberculosis of the ureter is secondary to disease progression in the kidney. Tubercles are formed as a result of implantation of tuberculous bacilli in the wall of the ureter, or as a downward sub-mucosal extension of the tuberculous infection from the renal pelvis. Depending upon the extent and degree of involvement, ulceration of the ureteric mucosa, irregular ureteric wall thickening and/or ureteric fibrosis may occur. Strictures occur most commonly at the lower end of the ureter, occasionally in the middle and/or at the pelvi-ureteric junction. When the tuberculosis process is established the ureteric wall becomes thick and rigid (fig. 124).

Tuberculosis of the Bladder: Involvement of bladder is secondary to renal tuberculosis; spread to the bladder occurs both by ureteric descent implantation of tubercle bacilli and by direct extension from an infected ureter. The disease process starts around a ureteric orifice and, as the disease spreads, a patchy cystitis occurs throughout the bladder. Tubercles are rare in the bladder. With increasing inflammation and fibrosis the ureteric orifice dilates, assuming a 'golf hole' appearance, and the bladder contour becomes distorted. In the later stages the bladder may become severely contracted with a capacity of less than 50ml and vesico-ureteric reflux occurs through the now incompetent golf hole orifices into dilated tuberculous ureters. At this stage the disease process has become irreversible by chemotherapy and corrective surgery is necessary to preserve renal function (fig. 124).

Tuberculosis of the Prostate: Genital tuberculosis occurs in at least two-thirds of male patients with renal tuberculosis. Most authorities agree that the disease process starts in the prostatic ducts which have become secondarily infected from bacilli in the urine. From the prostate spread occurs to the seminal vesicles and epididymis.

The disease process in the prostate may be silent and chronic, causing no symptoms and resulting in a resolved fibrosis and nodularity; however, in patients with poor resistance and infected with virulent organisms, a rapidly progressive course may result in abscess formation, caseation and perineal sinuses. Spread rapidly occurs to the seminal vesicles and epididymis.

One has to think of the possibility of tuberculosis of the prostate if the rectal examination reveals hard-firm prostatic nodules with irregular surfaces or a very soft area with fluctuation. A urethrogram may reveal para-urethral sacs or diverticulae; the prostatic secretion should be examined for acid-fast bacilli and a histological diagnosis, with a needle biopsy, may be necessary to exclude malignancy.

Tuberculosis of the Epididymis: Even though the incidence of tuberculous epididymitis has been reported to be rare it is advisable to check carefully as many cases are misdiagnosed or not even considered. Tuberculous epididymitis is most frequent in the 30 to 40-year-old age group, being most unusual before 20 years. Almost all genital tuberculosis presents clinically as a tuberculous epididymitis.

Tuberculous involvement of the epididymis usually occurs by retrograde extension along the vas deferens. The first changes in the epididymis are usually found in the tail; the early lesions are usually small, rounded, cold abscesses, but occasionally the entire epididymis is replaced by tuberculous caseation and associated necrosis may occur. In about 30% of patients the inflammation spreads to the testis and sometimes to the tunica vaginalis. Fistula formation occurred in most patients before the advent of chemotherapy.

Tuberculosis of the Urethra: This is rare and usually presents as single or multiple strictures (see below).

Diagnosis

Symptoms and Signs: The sex and age incidence of genitourinary tuberculosis is similar to pulmonary tuberculosis. Males are affected more than females in a ratio of 2:1 and most of the patients are in the 20 to 40 year age group. A past history of pulmonary tuberculosis in any patients with unexplained genitourinary symptoms and signs should make one consider the possibility of tuberculosis.

Symptoms are mostly nonspecific and the typical general symptoms of tuberculosis such as malaise, loss of weight, fever and night sweating are common. Asymptomatic pyuria may be the only finding. Loin pain occurs in about 20% of cases. Haematuria is seen in only 10% of patients.

Frequency of micturition, both by day and night, with only slight dysuria (see section 3) which has not responded to previous antibiotic or anti-inflammatory treatment, is a common symptom, as are suprapubic pain and urgency. Many women have been diagnosed and treated for the 'urethral syndrome' and men for 'chronic prostatitis' for many years before the diagnosis of tuberculosis was eventually made. A small percentage of patients present with urolithiasis and/or renal failure.

Tuberculosis of the ureter
124a A delayed intravenous pyelogram showing an obstructed right kidney due to a tuberculous stricture of the mid-ureter; the left kidney is non-functioning.

124b The cystogram shows a small contracted bladder and gross reflux into a thick rigid ureter.

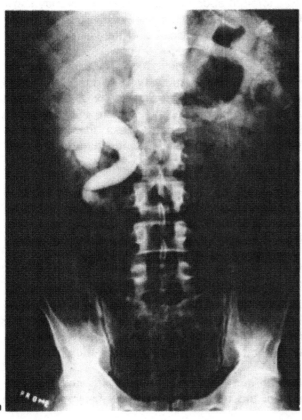

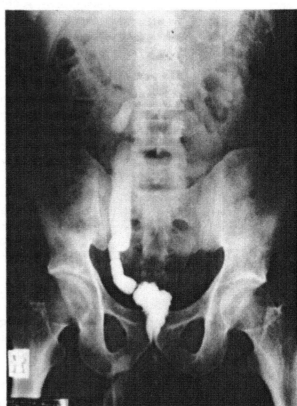

124a   124b

Haemospermia and a decrease in the ejaculatory fluid are uncommon presenting symptoms. Swelling, thickening and/or tenderness of the epididymis and thickening of the vas deferens may also be found. Scrotal sinuses are now rare. Induration and nodularity or a soft area with fluctuation in the prostate gland, and a hardening palpability of the seminal vesicles, also suggest a tuberculous involvement (p. 79).

Investigations. *Mantoux skin test:* A positive test is suggestive, but a negative reaction does not exclude tuberculosis.

Urine examination: An acid urine containing numerous white blood cells, a few red blood cells and no growth or organisms on repeated culture is a characteristic finding in tuberculosis and is an indication for further investigation.

Fresh early morning specimens of urine should be sent for smear, culture sensitivity tests and guinea pig or hamster inoculation. At least 6 such specimens should be tested as it has been shown that in only 50% of patients who excrete mycobacteria is the culture positive after the first 3 specimens have been tested.

Occasionally the urine culture may be repeatedly negative and treatment has to be started based on the clinical symptoms and signs, the results of tissue biopsy and/or the important x-ray findings.

Blood tests: A full blood examination, erythrocyte sedimentation rate, renal and liver function studies are essential preliminary investigations. Liver function studies are particularly necessary before beginning antituberculous drug therapy.

Radiography: A chest and a straight abdominal and pelvic x-ray may show a pulmonary lesion and/or tuberculous calcification in the lung or kidney and in abdominal lymph nodes, seminal vesicles and the vas deferens.

An *intravenous pyelogram* is an essential investigation. The early tubercular lesions show a loss of minor calyceal cupping with an irregular eroded appearance; progression of the disease is indicated by a moth-eaten appearance leading to a distortion of the calyceal system with cavitation and parenchymal caseation (fig. 124). In late cases the intravenous pyelogram may show hydro-uretero-nephrosis, ureteric strictures and even a functionless kidney.

Retrograde pyelo-ureterograms are not now commonly required, because of the sophistication of intravenous pyelography (p. 90). In some situations however, particularly where the kidneys are poorly functioning, retograde pyelo-ureterograms, using a Braasch bulb catheter and radiological screening, may be necessary to delineate the underlying pathology.

Antegrade pyelography is occasionally used in those cases where nephrostomy diversion (see chapter VIII) has been performed and is particularly useful in visualising the degree and level of ureteric obstruction especially when combined with screening (fig. 126b). *Cysto-urethrograms* outline the bladder size and indicate the presence of vesico-ureteric reflux (fig. 124b).

Cysto-urethroscopy: Classical text-book appearances are not frequent. When present they consist of tubercles and tuberculous ulceration, which appears as multiple, small, yellow-grey nodules with hyperaemic peripheral zones, initially situated around a ureteric orifice; later a patchy cystitis with areas of normal bladder wall between the areas of cystitis occurs. The more usual appearance is ureteric orifice hyperaemia and associated bullous oedema and later a generalised, patchy cystitis. With increasing ureteral involvement shortening of the sub-mucosal ureter occurs, causing retraction of the orifice and often vesico-ureteric reflux.

Management

With the advent of modern antituberculous drugs the chances of cure have increased and the incidence of surgical intervention has decreased (Cooper and Robinson, 1972).

The disease is infectious and should be reported and preventive action taken to avoid community spread. Although the patients do not have to be isolated they should have separate toilet facilities.

During the initial stages of treatment patients are hospitalised for rest and ease of investigation but, with the excellent early anti-infectious results using modern chemotherapy, most patients can now be treated as ambulant outpatients.

Medical Therapy: Chronic diseases require chronic treatment. Genitourinary tuberculosis requires long term chemotherapy.

Triple drug regimens are used in various combinations; most authorities now prefer the modern combination of isoniazid, rifampicin and ethambutol, in preference to the old regimen of streptomycin, para-amino salicylic acid (PAS) and isoniazid. This modern initial triple drug treatment is used to avoid development of resistant strains of acid-fast bacilli. Regular sensitivity tests will show whether to continue the same drug combination or to change to alternative drugs. The dosage depends on body weight:

    Isoniazid: 5 to 8mg/kg/day
    Rifampicin: 8 to 10mg/kg/day
    Ethambutol: 25mg/kg/day.

It is extremely important to obtain a sufficiently high concentration of drugs in the tissues. This initial dose is used for at least 90 days and, rarely, up to 6 months. A maintenance dose is given for a period of 2 years after the last positive histological examination or culture; for maintenance, a rifampicin-ethambutol or rifampicin-isoniazid or ethambutol-isoniazid combination may be used. The dosage of ethambutol should be reduced to 20mg/kg/day to avoid eye complications but a dose level below this is ineffective. Other drugs used include,

    Streptomycin: 15mg/kg/day
    PAS: 200mg/kg/day
    Cycloserine: 15mg/kg/day
    Pyrazinamide: 35mg/kg/day

The above dosages are for those patients with normal renal and liver function.

If the former standard regimen of streptomycin 1g intra-muscularly daily, isoniazid 300mg daily and PAS 12 to 15g daily is used, this triple therapy should be given daily for 3 to 6 months, followed by PAS and isoniazid daily for 2 years.

Side effects: All antituberculous drugs have side effects. Before starting treatment a full blood examination, liver and renal function tests and examination of the ear, nose, throat and eyes are essential; care should be exercised in prescribing these drugs in cases of renal failure and liver dysfunction.

Isoniazid can cause allergic hepatitis and other side effects on the central and peripheral nervous system.

Rifampicin may destroy blood and liver cells and may cause fetal abnormalities. *Ethambutol* may cause damage to the optic nerve and cases of blindness have been reported. Regular eye examination during therapy is essential. *Streptomycin* is ototoxic and nephrotoxic; *PAS* and *pyrazinamides* are toxic to the liver.

Results: The results of treatment depend upon 3 factors:

    a) The presenting state of the disease
    b) The response to the combined therapy
    c) A regular intake of the drugs by the patient and full cooperation concerning regular follow-up attendances and other medical advice.

If these factors are favourable the results will be excellent and only rarely will patients show a positive urine culture after 90 days of triple drug therapy. However, it is important to remember that even though the urine culture may be negative mycobacteria may still be excreted in the urine, so that frequent and long term checks of the urine are necessary. In males the conversion may be delayed because of the poor perfusion of the drugs within the prostate and epididymis.

During the early stages of treatment regular intravenous pyelograms are essential in order to evaluate the urinary tract progressively. Treatment will not prevent stricture formation throughout the system and may encourage it (fig. 125). This is particularly important in the small lumen ureter where rapid scarring may occur, occasionally without symptoms or signs, sufficient to destroy the kidney.

Steroids: The use of steroids in the management of genitourinary tuberculosis in an endeavour to lessen the incidence of fibrosis is controversial. Oral prednisolone may be of some benefit.

Surgery: There are definite indications for surgical intervention in the treatment of genitourinary tuberculosis. The timing of the surgery is important and its role must be considered in the conjunction with the general status of the patient, the stage of chemotherapy and the degree of renal function.

Drug treatment-induced tuberculous stricture

125a An intravenous pyelogram of early right renal tuberculosis. Note the minimal low right vesico-ureteric stricture.

125b Six weeks after beginning antituberculous drug therapy the vesico-ureteric stricture has rapidly progressed. Regular intravenous pyelogram monitoring of such patients is essential in order to prevent possible silent auto-nephrectomy. (Courtesy of Mr R.B. Brown).

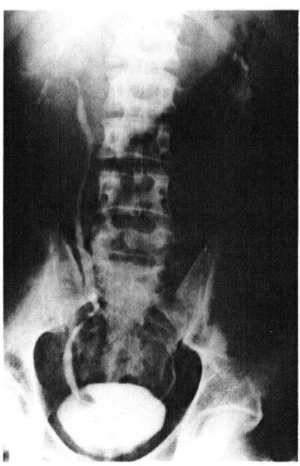

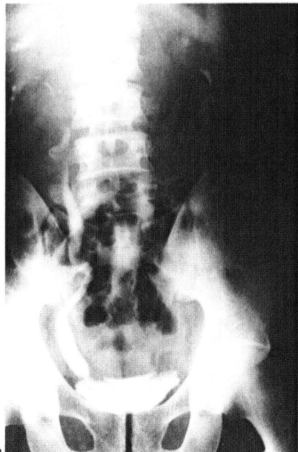

125a   125b

The incidence of surgical intervention is now less than 15% including extirpative and reconstructive surgery. The principle of surgical treatment is to preserve as much renal and bladder function as is possible (fig. 126).

Extirpative surgery includes total or partial nephrectomy (Hanley, 1970), epididymectomy and cavernotomy to remove diseased and functionless tissue. These forms of surgery should only be considered after at least 3 months of triple drug therapy.

Reconstructive surgery may be necessary for the management of urethral and ureteral strictures and bladder contractures (Gow, 1976). If possible surgery should be performed only after at least 2 years of drug treatment. As indicated previously this is not always possible as an acute obstruction requires immediate relief.

Most ureteral strictures involve the distal ureter and are best treated by reimplantation into the bladder, although this procedure may be very difficult in patients who have thick rigid ureters and small contracted bladders. In such cases it may only be possible to do a direct mucosa to mucosa anastomosis instead of using an anti-reflux tunnel technique (p. 52).

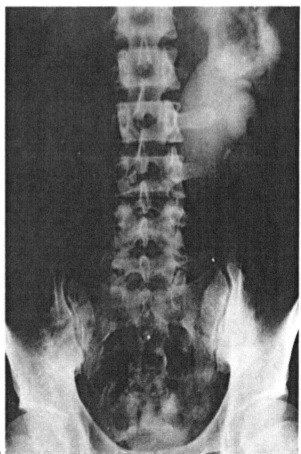

126a

Surgery in genitourinary tuberculosis

126a A 28-year-old man presented with renal failure. A high dose intravenous pyelogram showed a non-functioning right kidney and grossly hydronephrotic left kidney.

126b An emergency left-sided nephrostomy was performed and the antegrade ureterogram displayed a gross stricture at the distal end of the left ureter. The urine grew acid-fast bacilli.

126c A micturating cysto-urethrogram revealed a small contracted bladder.

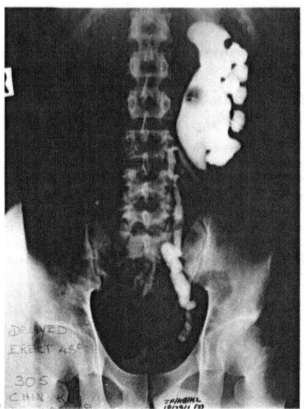

126b

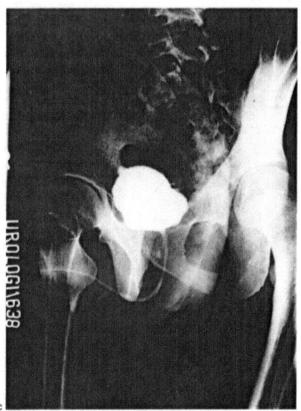

126c

Strictures involving the pelvi-ureteric junction may require a pyeloplasty operation, whilst those involving the middle third of the ureter may require excision, with a resultant re-anastomosis of the relatively healthy ureter or using an intubated Davis (1951) ureterotomy operation.

Severely contracted bladders may benefit from various enlargement operations using patches of ileum, colon or caecum (Shirley and Mirelman, 1978). Grossly contracted bladders may require urinary diversion using cutaneous ureterostomy, ileal conduit, uretero-sigmoidostomy or rectal bladder procedures (see chapter VIII).

Prognosis

Since the advent of earlier diagnosis and modern triple drug therapy, infection persisting after the 2-year period of chemotherapy has been completed is rare and most patients are able to be fully rehabilitated.
Patients presenting with advanced disease and secondary complications require a combination of surgery and antituberculosis treatment and do not have as good a prognosis as the group presenting earlier.

Dysuria

Dysuria is the most common disease affecting the genitourinary system. The common causes include urinary tract infection, the urethral syndrome, lower urinary tract retention of urine and prostatism, venereal and non-venereal urethritis, urethral caruncle, urethral stricture, bladder and urethral calculi and bladder neoplasms. Lower tract causes are discussed here but it is important to remember that upper tract pathology may be silent and present with dysuria (p. 210).

Common Causes of Dysuria

Infected Urethro-trigonitis and Prostatitis: The most common causes of dysuria are acute and chronic infected urethro-trigonitis, especially in adult females. Infection due to bacteria is diagnosed by microscopy and culture of the urine and treated as indicated earlier.

The Urethral Syndrome: This common form of dysuria is discussed on p. 138.

Lower Urinary Tract Retention of Urine and Prostatism: These causes of dysuria are discussed in chapter X.

Urethritis: Gonococcal and nonspecific-urethritis have become more common in the last decade with the availability of the contraceptive pill, altered community standards, increased international travel and increased homosexuality (see chapter XIX).

Urethritis can result from trauma (see chapter XIII) or allergy, particularly to rubber materials such as a contraceptive sheath or a rubber indwelling catheter. For this reason silastic catheters are always used for long term urinary drainage.

Uncommon causes of urethritis include trichomonas, moniliasis, herpes simplex and other adeno-virus infections, local abnormalities such as urethral carcinoma, chemical urethritis and various diets, such as those containing a high oxalate or nitrate level and ingested chemicals, such as cantharides and turpentine. An initially sterile urethritis may develop a secondary infection. Urethritis is often associated with prostatic, epidiymal and/or bladder infection.

Bladder Neoplasms: Sterile or infected inflammation of the neoplastic tissues, particularly at the bladder outlet, may result in a mild or a very severe dysuria with strangury. This presentation is more common than generally appreciated (see fig. 121 and chapter VII).

Bladder and Low Ureteric Calculi: As discussed in chapter IX, a sterile dysuria due to inflammation of the bladder mucosa and/or the vesico-ureteric junction may result from the presence of bladder calculi or a low ureteric calculus.

Urethral Caruncle: This usually red, sessile, vascular, benign tumour occurs at the external urinary meatus of women over the age of 50 years and can cause severe dysuria. Diathermy excision usually cures the condition.

Prolapsed Urethral Mucosa: This may need to be excised if it is large or the cause of dysuric symptoms.

Procidenturia: This may also produce severe dysuria. Reduction of the prolapse followed by a repair operation usually relieves the urinary symptom.

Balanitis: When associated with phimosis balanitis can produce dysuria or even retention of urine (p. 232) and is cured by a circumcision (p. 348).

Less Common Causes of Dysuria

Faecal Impaction: This can produce dysuria and often contributes to retention of urine in an elderly patient. Disimpaction of the faeces may relieve the retention.

Foreign Bodies: Dysuria may result from the passage, often denied, of one of a seemingly endless variety of foreign bodies. Open or endoscopic surgical removal (p. 114) usually under a general anaesthetic, is often necessary.

Case History
A 19-year-old oarsman was training when he sat down forcibly on the boat's seat and thereafter suffered acute retention of urine. He did not seek medical advice but procured a plastic drinking straw from the local milk bar and passed this via his urethra into the bladder, thereby relieving his retention. Unfortunately, the straw disappeared inside the external meatus and, although this allowed him to void, he experienced considerable dysuria. Eventually, 2 months later, he could not empty

his bladder and was unsuccessful in relieving himself by endeavouring to pass a second plastic straw along the urethra. A straight abdominal x-ray at this time (fig. 127a) shows 2 large stones in the bladder and the plastic straws. A urethrogram (fig. 127b) shows the filling defects within the urethra due to the straws as well as the bladder calculi. There is free reflux up the right ureter, presumably due to the chronic infection which the foreign body has produced. The patient required a supra-pubic cystostomy for removal of the stones and the straws.

Tuberculosis. The incidence of tuberculosis has increased over the last few years in many countries because of immigration from areas where it is endemic. Severe symptoms of dysuria. and even strangury, can occur when tuberculosis affects the bladder. Treatment with anti-tuberculous drugs and surgery is most effective (p. 149).

Interstitial Cystitis: This condition is most commonly seen in women from the fifth decade onwards and the aetiology is unknown (Hunner, 1914). Often there is a history of gynaecological or pelvic surgery. The dysuria can be extremely debilitating.

Inspection of the bladder often shows the mucosa ulcerated in a patchy manner; the lesions, which are called Hunner's ulcers, bleed easily on distension of the bladder.

Treatment depends mainly on progressive dilatations of the bladder at regular intervals. Rarely severe chronic interstitial cystitis produces such a small capacity bladder that enlargement, utilising a small or large bowel cystoplasty operation, may be necessary (Shirley and Mirelman, 1978).

The Unstable or Irritable Bladder: Women are more commonly affected by this uncommon condition which can be diagnosed only by urodynamic studies. Patients experience dysuria due to abnormal contractions of the bladder detrusor, which leaves them with a feeling of unsatisfied micturition interpreted as a failure to empty the bladder, although this is not so.

Irradiation Cystitis: This is not common but is difficult to treat although careful fulguration of the inflamed bleeding areas or intra-vesical formalin instillation (Brown, 1969) may help (p. 312).

Vesico-intestinal and Vesico-vaginal Fistulae: These fistulae may result from neoplasia, deep x-ray therapy, obstructed labour or surgery. An infective dysuria may result. Treatment is directed at the cause (p. 310, 312).

Dysuria caused by foreign body
127a Plastic straw-induced bladder calculi in a patient presenting with dysuria.

127b A urethrogram shows the calculi as bladder filling defects and also demonstrates gross inflammatory right-sided vesico-ureteric reflux.

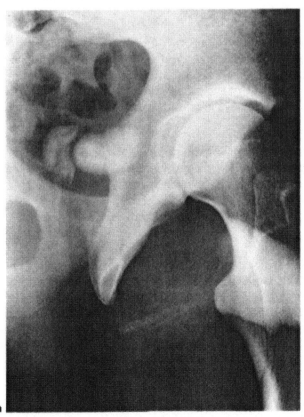
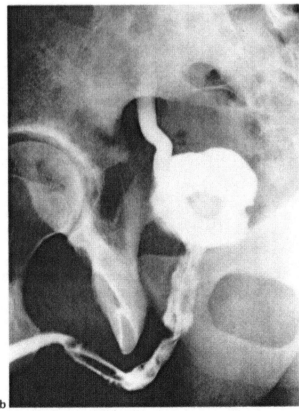

127a   127b

Rare Causes of
Dysuria

Drugs and Chemicals: Cyclophosphamide-induced cystitis can cause severe haemorrhagic dysuria. Bubble baths and exessive vigorous vaginal hygiene measures may result in a sterile or secondarily infected cysto-urethritis.

Ureterocele: If the ureterocele is large it may cause dysuria. The treatment is discussed in chapter XIV.

Leukoplakia: An increased thickness of the bladder wall mucosa, with squamous metaplasia, is a rare complication of chronic infection. Macroscopically the lesion is blue-grey and shaggy in appearance. The condition is pre-malignant and every attempt should be made to control the infection and to closely follow the progress of the lesion.

Schistosomiasis: In 1852 Bilharz discovered the worm *Schistosoma haematobium.* Bilharziasis (schistosomiasis) is the disease caused by this or one of the other, later-discovered, worms, *S. japonicum* or *S. mansoni.* In Egypt 40% of the population are still infected with these worms but the condition is relatively rare outside Africa, South America and parts of Asia.

The worms produce eggs which, on contact with water, liberate free-swimming miracidia which enter and live in the liver of the one of the variety of fresh-water snails able to act as intermediate hosts. The miracidia produce numerous 1mm cysts which contain many premature worms (*cercariae*), which penetrate human skin easily, enter the portal and pelvic venous systems via the lymphatics, and develop into mature worms which disseminate throughout the human body and excite chronic inflammatory reactions at their site of lodgement. A variety of chronic, pre-malignant inflammatory and granulomatous lesions results from this reaction and the cycle is perpetuated when the voided eggs attain their fresh-water snail intermediate host.

The only satisfactory solution to the problem of bilharzia would be the development of a specific vaccine. At present stibophen is the drug of choice (a total of 100ml is given on alternate days in 5ml doses). Antimony and potassium tartrate is also effective when given intravenously (a total dose of 1.6g is given on alternate days in gradually increasing doses up to a unit dose of 90mg).

Bilharzial infection may result in tubercles, nodules or papillomas of the bladder and cause intense dysuria. The diagnosis depends upon finding the ova in the urine (p. 86) or in the tissue following biopsy.

Abacterial, Phosphatic and Emphysematous Cystitis: These have been discussed on page 137.

Malakoplakia: See page 137. Dysuria may, very rarely, result from the presence of macroscopically sharply demarcated grey bladder sub-mucosal lymphocyte and malakoplakia cell granulomas. There is usually a history of urinary tract infection. Treatment consists of control of the infection and excision of the granulomas. Microscopic examination of the removed tissue reveals the characteristic intracellular calcified areas known as Michaelis-Guttman bodies.

Dysuria Associated with other Symptoms of Genitourinary Tract Disease

Haematuria, urethral bleeding and *urethral discharge* may all occur in association with dysuria. A feeling of *pressure,* resulting from the existence of a prolapse or a pelvic tumour, and *pneumaturia,* suggestive of a vesico-intestinal fistula, may also present with an associated dysuria.

Investigation of the Causes of Dysuria

Immediate History: Sex and age, and the length and severity of symptoms may all give clues to the cause of dysuria. It is common in a young female for recurrent urethro-trigonitis to cause painful dysuria, whereas persistent dysuria, without much pain, in an older man, is more likely to be due to prostatic obstruction. Prostatic obstruction due to carcinoma of the prostate tends to be associated with a shorter history of dysuria than does benign prostatic disease.

Past and Family History: A family or past history of tuberculosis calls for a careful search for acid-fast organisms in the urine. If a patient has lived in areas where bilharzia is present a search for this organism may also be indicated.

Previous surgical or self-instrumentation of the urinary tract may suggest the possibility of a urethral stricture or a retained foreign body.

Physical Examination: See chapter III page 78.

Urine Examination: See chapter III page 83.

Prostatic and Urethral Fluid Examination: Prostatic fluid, collected after a prostatic massage, is examined microscopically and then cultured for bacterial pathogens and other uncommon organisms such as Monilia, Trichomonas and Chlamydia. The *technique* of prostatic massage is important if an adequate specimen is to be obtained. The patient, in the left lateral position with both knees bent up towards the chin, holds a Petrie dish in such a way that any fluid presenting at the external meatus will drip into the dish. The examining finger is then inserted into the patient's rectum and each lateral lobe of the prostate is massaged in turn from the upper end of the prostate down towards the apex and medially. The finger is then passed firmly down the midline milking the collection along the urethra. If no fluid has been expressed by this method then the patient is turned on his back and the urethra is milked from the perineum to the external meatus.

Intravenous Pyelography: See chapter III page 90.

Cystourethroscopy: As indicated on page 110 a right-angled telescope enables the urologist to see almost all of the bladder mucosa whilst the fore-oblique telescope visualises the remainder of the bladder, including the bladder outlet and the whole length of the urethra.

Cysto-urethrograms: See chapter III page 114.

Barium Enema: This is a necessary investigation if a vesico-colic fistula is suspected. Dye passes more readily from the bowel to the bladder rather than the reverse.

Urodynamic Investigations: Cystometrograms, intra-vesicular pressure measurements, flow studies and urethral pressure profiles may be necessary in order to prove or exclude the presence of a neurogenic bladder. The investigations are discussed in chapter IV.

Ultrasound: Dysuria rarely results from an extrinsic pelvic tumour but ultrasound (p. 94) may be helpful in confirming this clinical impression and in differentiating between a solid and a cystic lesion.

Computerised Tomography: This expensive investigation (chapter III; p. 100) may assist in detecting and staging pelvic neoplasms by indicating their extension into local tissues and related lymph glands.

Summary

The cause of dysuria must be identified and a decision made as to whether palliative treatment should be given or curative treatment attempted.

References

Anderson, E.E.; Cobb, O.E. and Glenn, J.F.: Cyclophosphamide haemorrhagic cystitis. Journal of Urology 97: 857 (1967).

Badenoch, A.W.: Chronic interstitial cystitis. British Journal of Urology 43: 718 (1971).

Bailey, H.: Cyctitis emphysematosa. American Journal of Roentgenology 86: 850 (1961).

Bailey, R.R.: Single dose antibacterial treatment for uncomplicated urinary tract infections. Drugs 17: 219 (1979).

Blackledge, D.: A simple operation for postcoital urethrotrigonitis in women. Australia and New Zealand Journal of Obstetrics and Gynaecology 19: 123 (1979).

Brown, R.B.: A method of management of inoperable carcinoma of the bladder. Medical Journal of Australia 1: 23 (1969).

Burdon, S.W.: Immunoglobulins in the urinary tract; in Brumfitt and Asscher (Eds) Urinary Tract Infection, p.148 (Oxford, London 1973).

Campbell, I.A.: British thoracic and tuberculosis association review. Tubercle 4: 48 (1974).

Cooper, H.G. and Robinson, E.G.: Treatment of genitourinary tuberculosis: report after 24 years. Journal of Urology 108: 136 (1972).

Cox, C.E.: The urethra and its relationship to urinary tract infection: the flora of the normal female urethra. Southern Medical Journal 59: 621 (1966).

Cox, C.E. and Hinman, F. Jr.: Experiments with induced bacteriuria, vesical emptying and bacterial growth in the mechanism of bladder defence to infection. Journal of Urology 86: 739 (1961).

Davis, D.M.: Intubated ureterotomy. Journal of Urology 66: 71 (1951).

Dawborn, J.K.; Fairley, K.F.; Kincaid-Smith, P. and King, W.E.: The association of peptic ulceration, chronic renal disease and analgesic abuse. Quarterly Journal of Medicine 59: 69 (1966).

Doyle, P.T. Abercrombie, G.F.; Jenkins, J.D.; Svarkt, C.J. and Vinnicombe, J.: Abacterial cystitis. British Journal of Urology 49: 647 (1977).

El-Badawi, A.A.: Bilharzial polypi of the urinary bladder. British Journal of Urology 44: 561 (1966).

Fairley, K.F.; Bond, A.G.; Brown, R.B. and Habersberger, B.: Simple test to determine the site of urinary tract infections. Lancet 2: 7513 (1967).

Gow, J.G.: Genitourinary tuberculosis; in Blandy (Ed) Urology, p.226 (Blackwell, Oxford 1976).

Granato, J.J.; Cross, P.M. and Stamey, T.A.: Trimethoprim diffusion into prostatic and salivary secretions of the dog. Investigative Urology 11: 205 (1973).

Hanley, H.G.: Cavernotomy and partial nephrectomy in renal tuberculosis. British Journal of Urology 42: 661 (1970).

Hatch, S. and Cockett, T.K.: Xanthogranulomatous pyelonephritis. Journal of Urology 92: 585 (1974).

Hodson, C.J.: Discussion on pyelonephritis. The radiological diagnosis of pyelonephritis. Proceedings of the Royal Society of Medicine 52: 669 (1959).

Kass, E.H.: Asymptomatic infection of the urinary tract. Transactions of the Association of American Physicians 69: 56 (1956).

Kass, E.H.: The role of asymptomatic bacteriuria in the pathogenesis of pyelonephritis; in Quinn and Kass (Eds) Biology of Pyelonephritis, p. 399 (Little Brown, Boston 1960).

Kaufman, D.B.: Katz, R. and McIntosh, R.M.: Secretory IgA in urinary tract infections. British Medical Journal 4: 463 (1970).

Kincaid-Smith, P. and Bullen, M.: Bacteriuria in pregnancy. Lancet 1: 395 (1965).

Kunin, C.M.: Asymptomatic bacteriuria. American Review of Medicine 17: 383 (1966).

Kunin, C.M. and Paquin, A.J.: Frequency and natural history of urinary tract infection in schoolchildren; in Kass (Ed) Progress in Pyelonephritis, p.33 (Davis, Philadelphia 1965).

Letcher, H.G. and Matheson, N.M.: Encrustation of the bladder as a result of alkaline cystitis. British Journal of Surgery 23: 716 (1935).

Marsh, F.P.; Murray, M. and Panchamia, P.: The relationship between bacterial cultures of the vaginal introitus and urinary infection. British Journal of Urology 44: 368 (1972).

Mayo, M.E. and Hinman, F.: Role of midurethral high pressure zone in spontaneous bacterial ascent. Journal of Urology 109: 268 (1973).

Medlar, E.M.; Spain, D.M. and Holliday, R.W.: Post mortem compared with clinical diagnosis of genitourinary tuberculosis in adult males. Journal of Urology 61: 1078 (1949).

Melicow, M.M.: Malakoplakia: report of a case, review of the literature. Journal of Urology 78: 33 (1957).

Moore, T.: Sterile pyuria. Proceedings of the Royal Society of Medicine 33: 593 (1940).

Norden, C.W.; Green, G.C. and Kass, E.H.: Antibacterial mechanisms of the urinary bladder. Journal of Clinical Investigation 47: 2689 (1968).

Norden, C.W. and Kass, E.H.: Bacteriuria of pregnancy: a critical appraisal. Annual Review of Medicine 19: 431 (1968).

North, J.D.K. and Miller, T.E.: Effect of protein intake on bacterial growth in the kidney. Abstracts of the Third International Congress of Nephrology 2: 248 (1966).

O'Flynn, J.D. and Mullaney, J.: Leukoplakia of the bladder — a report on 20 cases including 2 cases progressing to squamous cell carcinoma. British Journal of Urology 39: 461 (1967).

O'Grady, F.W. and Cattell, W.R.: Kinetics of urinary tract infection. I. Upper urinary tract. British Journal of Urology 38: 149 (1966).

O'Grady, F.W.; Gauci, C.L.; Watson, B.W. and Hammond, B.: In vitro models simulating conditions of growth in the urinary tract; in O'Grady and Brumfitt (Eds) Urinary Tract Infections, p.80 (Oxford, London 1968).

O'Grady, F.; Kelsey Fry, I.; McSherry, and A. Cattell, W.R.: Long-term treatment of persistent or recurrent urinary tract infections with trimethoprim-sulfamethoxazole. Journal of Infectious Disease (Suppl.): 128: 652 (1973).

Pengelly, A.W.; Stephenson, T.P.; Milroy, E.J.G.; Whiteside, C.G. and Turner-Warwick, R.T.: Results of prolonged bladder distension as treatment for detrusor instability. British Journal of Urology 50: 243 (1978).

Polk, B.F.: Urinary tract infections in pregnancy. Clinical Obstetrics and Gynaecology 22: 285 (1979).

Roberts, J.H.: Bubble bath cystitis. Journal of the American Medical Association 201: 207 (167).

Shand, D.G.; Nimmon, C.C. and O'Grady, F.: Relation between residural urine volume and response to treatment. Lancet 2: 1305 (1970).

Shirley, S.W. and Mirelman, S.: Experience with colocystoplasties, ceocystoplasties and ileocystoplasties in urologic surgery: 40 patients. Journal of Urology 120: 165 (1978).

Stamey, T.A.: Fair, W.R.; Timothy, M.M. and Chung, H.K.: Antibacterial nature of prostatic fluid. Nature 218: 444 (1968).

Stamey, T.A.; Govan, D.E. and Palmer, J.M.: The localisation and treatment of urinary tract infection. Medicine 44: 1 (1965).

Stamey, T.A.; Timothy, M.M.; Millar, M. and Mihara, G.: Recurrent urinary infection in adult women. California Medicine 115: 1 (1971).

Stephens, F.D.; Whitaker, J. and Hewstone, A.S.: True, false and sham urinary tract infection in children. Medical Journal of Australia 2: 840 (1966).

Wolin, L.H.: Voiding patterns in young healthy women. Journal of Urology 106: 923 (1971).

Chapter VI

Haematuria

The genitourinary system must be either visualised directly or outlined radiologically in all patients of all ages who present with macroscopic haematuria, or heavy recurrent microscopic haematuria, to determine the cause of the bleeding. Thus neoplasms, calculi, inflammatory and infectious diseases can be detected and treated before further tissue damage or death occurs.

Macroscopic haematuria, because of its possibly sinister significance, always requires urological investigation. Asymptomatic microscopic haematuria does not require further investigation unless there is a recurrent finding of more than 20,000 red blood cells per ml of urine.

Haematuria may result from local pathological changes within the genitourinary system or it may result from more widespread general causes. Haematuria is therefore classified as being due to local or general causes.

Local Causes of Haematuria

Bleeding may occur from one or both kidneys or ureters or the bladder, prostate or urethra. There may be more than one bleeding site. Haematuria may be initial, total or terminal. Initial or terminal haematuria suggests bleeding from the bladder outlet or posterior urethra respectively, whilst haematuria throughout the stream suggests a bladder or upper tract aetiology.

Neoplasm or Tumours

Neoplasm is the most important local cause (see chapter VII).

Kidney and Ureter: *Nephroblastoma* is an uncommon cause of haematuria in children. The prognosis has changed dramatically (90% 10-year survival for stages I and II) since the advent of combined surgery, radiotherapy and cytotoxic drug regimens (p. 166).

Adenocarcinoma of the kidney is an uncommon neoplasm, usually occurring in males over the age of 45 years, with a poor prognosis.

Transitional cell calyceal, pelvic and ureteric neoplasms are uncommon and must be differentiated from other non-opaque radiographic filling defects such as uric acid calculi.

Bladder: All transitional cell tumours of the bladder become malignant and are treated as such. Bladder transitional cell carcinomas are common causes of painless haematuria in men and women over the age of 50 years.

Prostate: Benign prostatomegaly is the most common cause of haematuria in older males. Carcinomatous changes occur in two thirds of men over the age of 70 but only 2% of sufferers die from the disease and this greatly influences the management.

Urethra: Urethral caruncles are uncommon distal mucosal granuloma tumours occurring in elderly females, while carcinomas of the urethra in males and females are very rare tumours, with a poor prognosis because of their usually late presentation.

Calculi

Renal and ureteric calculi usually have a primary aetiology while bladder calculi are usually secondary to obstruction. They may cause painful haematuria (see chapter IX).

Infection

Urethro-trigonitis is the most common cause of haematuria in the female. *Posterior urethritis* and *prostatitis* are common causes of haematuria in the male. *Pyelonephritis* is an uncommon cause of haematuria.

Tuberculosis is an uncommon cause but it is the author's experience that the incidence of genitourinary tuberculosis is increasing because of immigration although that of pulmonary tuberculosis is decreasing. *Bilharziasis* is a very rare cause of haematuria outside endemic areas such as the Middle East. See chapter V.

Glomerulonephritis and Papillary Necrosis

Glomerulonephritis may cause haematuria, particularly in children and young adults (p. 318). Papillary necrosis is discussed in chapter XII page 274.

Trauma

Genitourinary trauma is uncommon and the diagnosis is not usually difficult. Approximately 15% of kidneys which bleed following trauma are pathological. Considerable force is needed to damage a non-pathological kidney or bladder (see chapter XIII).

Physical Exercise

Physical stress haematuria may occur, either from the congested bladder outlet or from one or both kidneys, and is common now that jogging is popular. Rarely, renal angiography and venography may disclose the presence of vascular abnormalities such as aneurysms, arterio-venous fistulae or large sub-mucosal veins. Nephroscopy may enable diathermy destruction of some sub-mucosal vascular abnormalities but, because of their intra-renal situation, local excision is often difficult and a partial or complete nephrectomy may be necessary in selected patients.

General Causes of Haematuria

General or pre-renal causes of haematuria are uncommon.

Haemorrhagic Diseases

Diseases arising from platelet, capillary or coagulation defects may give rise to haematuria.

Cardiovascular Disease

Haematuria may be found in patients with:

  a) Congestive cardiac failure
  b) Hypertension
  c) Sub-acute bacterial endocarditis, embolus or infarction
  d) Polyarteritis nodosa or related diseases
  e) Inferior vena caval thrombosis.

Haemolytic Agents

Although the patient passes red urine the colour change is due to the presence of haemoglobinuria following haemolysis due to:

a) Anticoagulant drugs such as heparin or warfarin
b) Malaria or, more rarely, other infectious fevers
c) Incompatible blood transfusion
d) Paroxysmal nocturnal (cold) haemoglobinuria, which occasionally results from syphilis
e) Ingested chemical agents, such as detergents and carbolic acid.

Essential Haematuria

This term is used when no local or general cause for the haematuria can be found. Despite more refined methods of diagnosis, such as angiography, there still remains a small percentage of people, usually males, in whom the bleeding site and pathology cannot be identified.

Diagnosis and Investigation

In most cases the cause of haematuria can be diagnosed provided a full history, is taken, and a thorough general examination and appropriate special investigations are carried out.

History

Local Factors: The presence or absence of pain and/or dysuria associated with the haematuria is important, both in attempting to identify whether the bleeding is upper or lower tract in origin and also in suggesting whether the bleeding is due to infection, inflammation, calculi or neoplasia. The duration and extent of the bleeding, together with the precise colour and its position in the urinary steam, may indicate a possible anatomical site and aetiology.

General Factors: A history of haemorrhagic disease, cardiovascular abnormalities, or the ingestion of drugs or poisons, may suggest generalised reasons for the haematuria.

Examination

The general appearance of the patient may suggest the aetiology. The child with generalised oedema and a history of haematuria may have glomerulonephritis whilst the elderly man with recent weight loss and haematuria may well have a genitourinary malignancy. Fever associated with haematuria usually indicates an infective or renal neoplastic aetiology.

A renal mass may be detectable but it may not move downwards on respiration if it is fixed to the surroundings. A renal mass in a young child is more likely to be a congenital hydronephrosis than a neoplasm (p. 340).

Rectal examination may confirm a clinical impression of inflammation or neoplasia in the prostate gland.

Microscopic examination of the mid-stream urine specimen may fail to disclose the presence of red blood cells and this may be the first suggestion that the red urine is due to haemoglobinuria and suggest a generalised cause. Red blood cells, together with casts (blood cell, hyaline, granular), may suggest a nephritic cause for the haematuria whilst red blood cells, in the presence of organisms and pus cells, are indicative of a urinary tract infection. Red blood cells alone are suggestive of neoplasms or calculi, and a sterile pyuria of tuberculosis.

The requirement that the genitourinary system must either be visualised or outlined radiologically in all patients of all ages who present with macroscopic haematuria implies at least an initial intravenous pyelogram, followed by a panendoscopy, with or without retrograde pyelo-ureterogram studies, dependent upon the intravenous pyelogram findings.

The increasing sophistication and number of these and other special investigations, such as urinary cytology, angiography, venography, ultrasound, computerised tomography, radio-isotopic scan studies, lymphangiography and renal cyst puncture, has been one of the great advances in urology over the past 20 years (p. 100); they now enable an accurate preoperative diagnosis of benign and malignant space occupying lesions, or filling defects in the system, in almost all cases, together with an assessment of any involved metastatic lymph nodes or other metastases. This not only greatly assists the surgeon in planning an operation but may enable him to decide whether attempted radical curative, or lesser palliative surgery, is necessary.

Chapter VII

Neoplasms and Tumours

The prognosis for a patient with a genitourinary neoplasm differs according to tumour cell activity and invasion, delay in diagnosis and adequacy of treatment. All patients presenting with haematuria, whether painful or not, unexplained dysuria, a loin mass, a prostatic hard area or a testicular lump should be assumed to have a neoplasm until proven otherwise.

Renal, prostatic and testicular neoplasms are usually solid adenocarcinomas, whilst those arising from the calyceal-pelvi-ureteric collecting ducts, bladder and posterior urethra are usually transitional cell growths of varying grades of activity. The rare anterior urethral neoplasms are squamous or columnar cell in character.

Kidney Neoplasms

These may be classified by site into renal parenchymal neoplasms:

a) childhood nephroblastoma (Wilm's tumour)
b) adult adenocarcinoma (Grawitz tumour) and adenomas
c) secondary metastatic neoplasms
d) rare neoplasms such as benign connective tissue tumours, haemangiomas, oncocytomas, hamartomas and various sarcomas.

and renal collecting duct neoplasms — adult calyceal and pelvic transitional cell or, rarely, squamous cell tumours.

Childhood Nephroblastoma (Wilm's Tumour)

The cause of this tumour is unknown. It is the most common genitourinary neoplasm in childhood and is discussed further in chapter XIV. The neoplasm usually presents as a large, asymptomatic mass, occasionally with related weight loss, haematuria and abdominal pain.

The clinical differential diagnosis lies between a nephroblastoma, pelvi-ureteric hydronephrosis, multi-cystic kidney, neuroblastoma, mesenchymal hamartoma and a renal vein thrombosis, but the special investigations establish the diagnosis.

Modern surgery and associated irradiation and cytotoxic drug therapy enable an overall 70% 2-year survival and a 90% 2-year survival for stage I and II lesions.

*Adult
Adenocarcinoma
(Grawitz Tumour)*

The aetiology of the tumour is unknown. Renal adenocarcinoma occurs in all age groups and is the most common kidney neoplasm usually developing between the ages of 45 and 70 years and occurring more often in males (fig. 128a-d).

Pathology. *Macroscopic:* A golden yellow neoplasm which initially appears to be encapsulated. Rapid growth may produce areas of necrosis with occasional calcification. Cystic spaces are common. An oncocytoma (see below) neoplasm is brown coloured.

Microscopic: The neoplasm consists of large clear cells containing cholesterol, which is responsible for the yellow colour. Three microscopic types of cell arrangement are recognised:

    a) papillary
    b) glandular
    c) solid

Renal parenchymal neoplasms

128a A 50-year-old man presented with painless haematuria. An intravenous pyelogram revealed a left renal space occupying lesion with irregular distortion of the pelvi-calyceal system.

128b A left renal selective angiogram revealed a neoplastic blood supply to the space occupying lesion. Note the pooling of the medium within the primitive vessels.

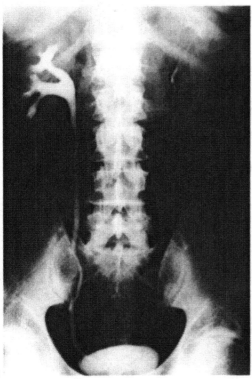

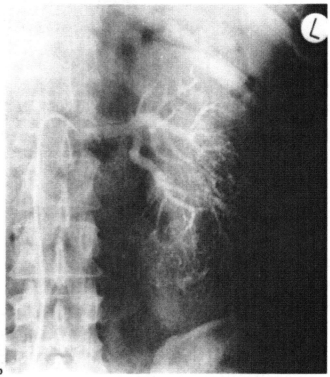

128a   128b

Renal parenchymal neoplasms (continued)
128c Computerised tomography displays the solid white neoplasm and also reveals metastatic para-aortic lymph nodes.

128d The neoplasm seen on radical removal of the kidney.

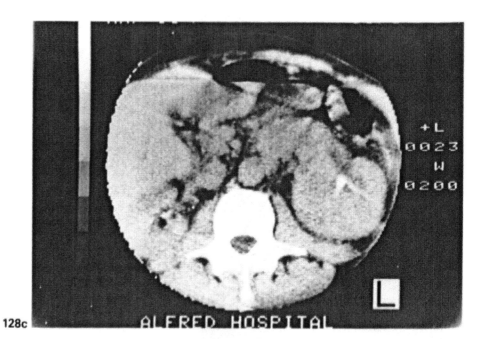

128c

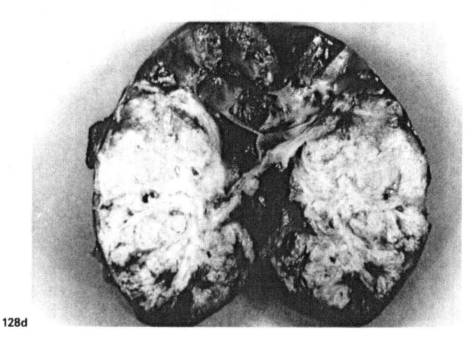

128d

The neoplasm may be well differentiated but is usually far more active and may be extremely anaplastic. Spread occurs by direct invasion of the surrounding tissues and lymphatic and vascular entrance. Lymphatic invasion of the para-aortic nodes and blood, spreading metastases to the lungs, liver, bones and adrenal glands, is common. Obstruction of the left renal vein may result in a left-sided varicocele (p. 72).

Presentation: Haematuria occurs in most cases whilst a mass associated with an aching pain in the loin is common.

Uncommon presentations include:

1) Lung, liver, bone and/or adrenal metastases, resulting in a persistent cough, pain and/or dysfunction
2) Fever (due to necrosis within the neoplasm)
3) Left-sided varicocele
4) Polycythaemia (p. 45, 365)
5) Ureteric clot colic
6) Rupture of the kidney due to haemorrhage
7) Inferior vena cava obstruction, which may be acute.

Diagnosis. See chapter III p. 94.

Treatment. *Primary neoplasm:* If possible, a thoraco-abdominal (for large upper pole neoplasms) or a trans-abdominal (so that the main renal artery and vein can be ligated quickly, with minimal handling of the neoplasm and a consequent reduction in haematogenous cell dissemination) radical nephrectomy (removal of the kidney, extra-renal fat and Gerota's fascia) is performed (Mimms et al., 1966; Robson et al., 1969). The removal of neoplastic extension into the inferior vena cava is possible (Schefft et al., 1978).

Metastases: Solitary metastases in the lung or brain can often be surgically excised or irradiated but for widespread metastases surgery is contraindicated.

Prognosis: The overall 5-year survival rate is only 33%.

Secondary Metastatic Neoplasms

Because of its large blood supply the kidney may be the site for many secondary metastases.

Other Renal Neoplasms

Adenoma: Renal adenomas are commonly found at post-mortem examination. They may develop into a renal adenocarcinoma.

Haemangioma: This may result in massive renal bleeding.

Oncocytomas: This rare neoplasm has a characteristic, relatively avascular angiographic appearance and a good prognosis after nephrectomy. The neoplasm is brown in appearance and the swollen cells, termed oncocytes, are packed with mitochondria.

Hamartoma: This relatively benign tumour (fig. 129) is composed of blood vessels, smooth muscle and fat and is therefore described as an angiomyolipoma. The neoplasm may be associated with tuberose sclerosis and may grow to a very large size. The angiographic appearance is usually diagnostic (Palmisano, 1967).

Sarcoma: This is a rare renal neoplasm.

Renal Collecting Duct, Bladder and Posterior Urethral Neoplasms

The calyces, pelvis, ureters, bladder and the posterior portion of the urethra are lined with transitional epithelium (chapter II) and neoplasms in these areas are classified into:

1) Various stages and grades of transitional neoplasia
2) The, fortunately rare, fatal squamous cell carcinoma; the even rarer adenocarcinoma, which only occurs at the bladder trigone, fundus or persistent urachus (p. 332); and the extremely rare rhabdomyosarcomas occurring in children.

Staging and Grading of Transitional Cell and Squamous Cell Neoplasms

The *staging* of transitional cell and squamous cell neoplasms (illustrated in figure 130) follows the International classification for bladder growths (T) but is modified here for simplicity:

Stage 0 (TIS)	Carcinoma *in situ*
Stage I (T1)	Infiltrating and non-infiltrating papillary neoplasms
Stage IIA (T2)	Invasion of superficial muscle
Stage IIB (T3a)	Invasion of deep muscle
Stage III (T3b)	Infiltration beyond the wall but with the neoplasm still mobile
Stage III-IV (T4a)	Involvement of adjacent organs
Stage IV (T4b)	Fixed or a squamous cell carcinoma

As indicated in figure 130, this classification particularly applies to the thicker walled bladder and is less clinically significant in the thinner walled pelvis and urethra. Stage IIb and III neoplasms usually require similar treatment and in the author's opinion should be treated as a single group.

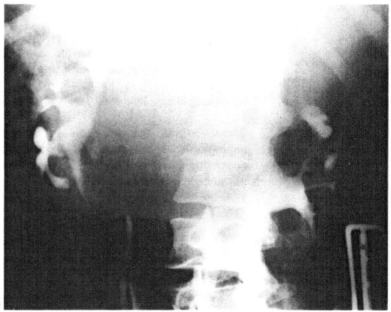

129

129 A 50-year-old woman presented with right-sided aching lumbar pain. An intra-venous pyelogram disclosed a large retroperitoneal mass distorting and involving the right kidney. Open surgical exploration revealed a hamartoma.

130 Transitional cell neoplasms. The sites and staging classifications. Pathological staging is often found to be worse than clinical staging, particularly with stage II and III growths.

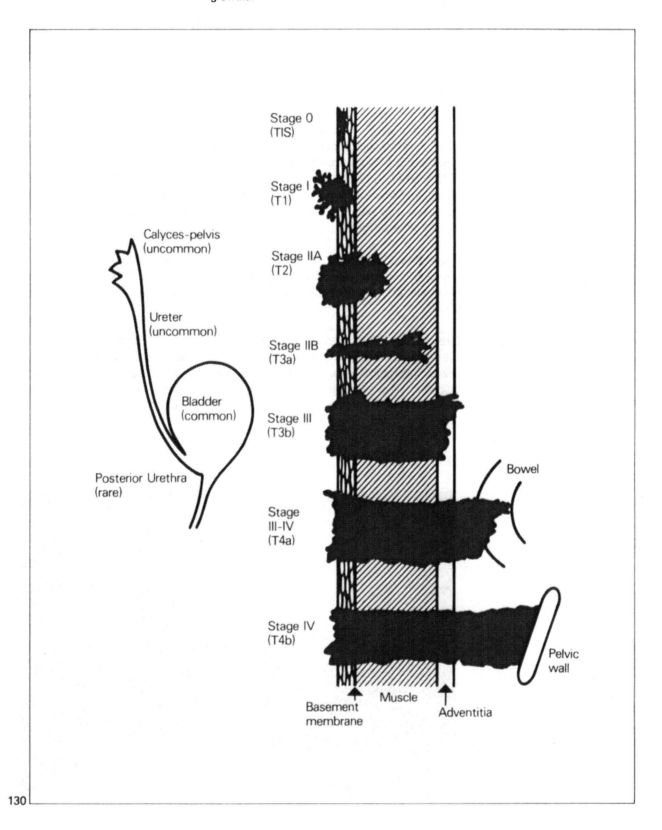

130

Squamous cell carcinoma arising from the urothelium is a death sentence and is graded as stage IV or T4b for this reason.

Grading relates to the histological cell structure:

Grade I	Papillary and well differentiated
Grade II	Papillary and moderately differentiated
Grade III	Solid or papillary and poorly differentiated
Grade IV	Solid and often ulcerated and anaplastic (includes all squamous cell carcinomas).

It should be appreciated that:

1) The prognosis for patients with these neoplasms is generally favourable for treated stage I to II, grade I to II neoplasms, but generally unfavourable for treated stage III to IV, grade III to IV neoplasms.

2) Attempted clinical staging is not necessarily pathologically accurate. The situation is often worse than the clinical assessment indicates.

3) Spread of the neoplasm occurs by direct extension, lymphatic and blood vessel invasion and the prognosis is dependent upon the length of time the neoplasm has been present, the site, the particular cell grade and the adequacy of treatment.

Renal Calyceal and Pelvic Neoplasms

These neoplasms (fig. 131-132) are uncommon and there is strong evidence to suggest that both analgesic nephropathy and 'Balkans' interstitial nephritis are pre-malignant precursors (Angerwall et al., 1969; Taylor, 1973).

Diagnosis: The intravenous pyelogram and/or retrograde pyelo-ureterogram reveals a *constant* filling defect or defects. Urine cytology may reveal malignant cells. The differential diagnosis lies between a uric acid calculus, when uric acid crystals may be identified in the urine and the serum uric acid level is often raised, and an impacted renal papilla (p. 274).

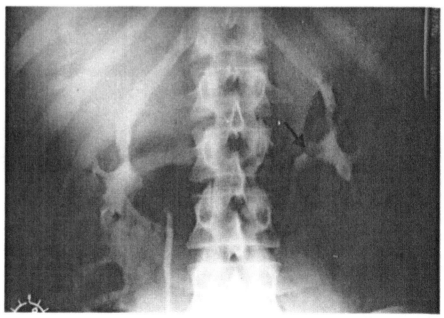

131

Renal calyceal neoplasms

131 A 60-year-old woman presented with painless haematuria. A constant filling defect in the left renal pelvis (arrow), highly suggestive of a neoplasm, is displayed in the intravenous pyelogram. Urine cytology revealed numerous malignant transitional cells and resulted in a left nephro-ureterectomy and cuff partial cystectomy operation, after panendoscopy had revealed no lower tract abnormality.

132 A 55-year-old woman presented with painless haematuria and gave a past history of heavy analgesic intake for headaches. An intravenous pyelogram revealed 2, constant, non-opaque filling defects in the right kidney which, despite normal urine cytology reports, were shown at operation to be neoplastic.

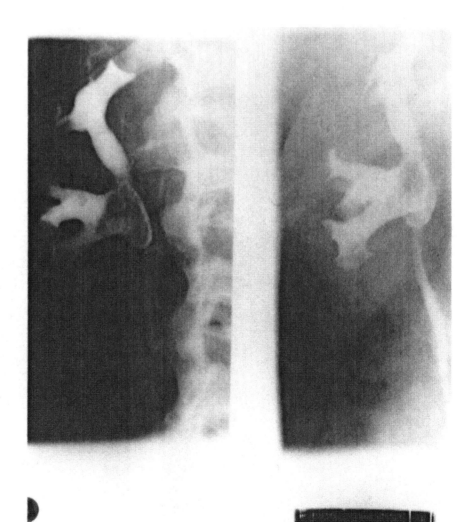

132

Ureteric Neoplasms

Treatment: If possible a nephro-ureterectomy and an associated partial cuff cystectomy around the ureteric orifice is performed through a loin and a second lower abdominal extraperitoneal incision. Following removal of the neoplasm the patient must undergo regular intravenous pyelogram and cysto-urethroscopic follow-ups for life.

Prognosis: Because of the usually late presentation, and the thin pelvic wall, the overall 5-year survival rate is only 30% for transitional cell neoplasm and 0% for squamous cell neoplasm.

These uncommon neoplasms are diagnosed, treated and followed as indicated for calyceal and pelvic neoplasms, with the exception that some patients with well differentiated superficial neoplasms require only local excision and oblique end-to-end anastomosis of the healthy ureter, rather than a nephro-ureterectomy-cuff cystectomy operation (fig. 133). Benign ureteric polyps are rare tumours (Williams and Mitchell, 1973; Petkovic, 1971).

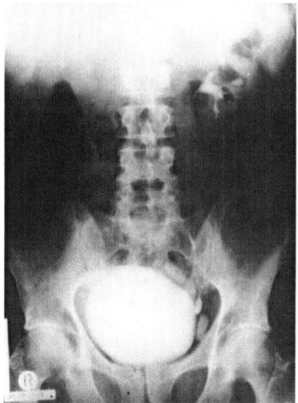

133a

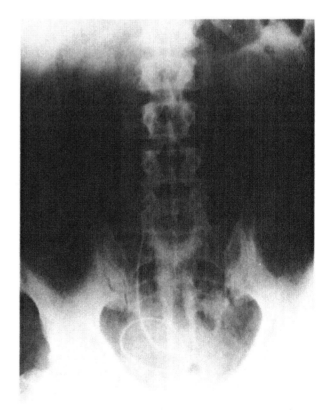

133b

Ureteric neoplasm

133a A 65-year-old man presented with painless haematuria. An intravenous pyelogram revealed a normal left system and a very poorly functioning right system.

133b,c A retrograde ureterogram disclosed an irregular filling defect in the mid ureter, suggestive of a ureteric neoplasm because of its irregular edge. Urine cytology revealed numerous malignant transitional cells.

133d A wide local excision of the neoplasm was performed.

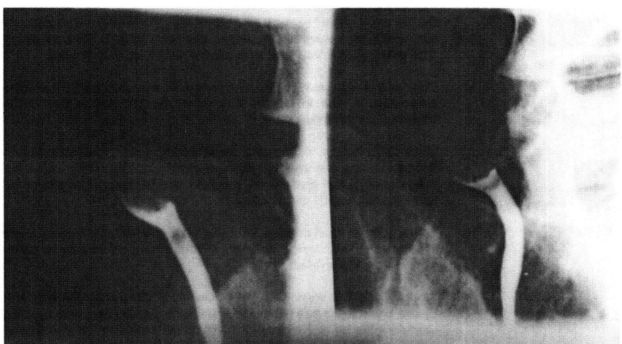

133c

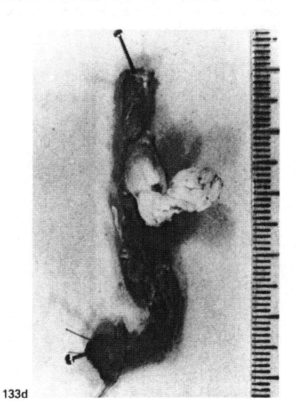

133d

Bladder Neoplasms

Most patients with bladder neoplasms (figs. 134-137) present with haematuria but some present with frequency-urgency of micturition (p. 77) without haematuria. An aniline dye intermediate, 2-naphthylamine and xenylamine have been proven (Heuper, 1934) to cause bladder carcinoma and are banned in the United States of America and the United Kingdom. Cigarette smoking is also a proven aetiological agent (Anthony and Thomas, 1970) as is schistosomiasis (Gelfand et al., 1967). Leukoplakia (O'Flynn and Mullaney, 1967) may result in the development of squamous cell carcinoma of the bladder (Pugh, 1973).

Bladder and urethral neoplasms are very rare in children but rhabdomyosarcomas of these tissues and the vagina may occur (p. 342). Their previously fatal prognosis has improved with modern cytotoxic drug therapy.

Diagnosis and Investigation: Malignant cells may be identified on urine examination. A constant bladder filling defect (fig. 136) may be found at intravenous pyelography.

Cysto-urethroscopy, excisional or incisional biopsy and bimanual examination confirm the diagnosis and enable the urologist to clinically assess the size, site, stage and grade of the neoplasm and to resect all or part of the lesion for histological examination.

Treatment: An initial decision, based on the above findings, must be made as to whether the planned treatment is to be attempted curative or palliative (Prout, 1976; Wallace, 1976).

Stage O (TIS): This uncommon flat carcinoma *in situ* usually presents with dysuria and appears as a red mucosal area or areas. The neoplasm must be carefully watched and treated by transurethral excision with a diathermy cutting loop but, should the histology indicate invasion of the basement membrane, then a total cysto-prostato-urethrectomy should be performed (Stams et al., 1977).

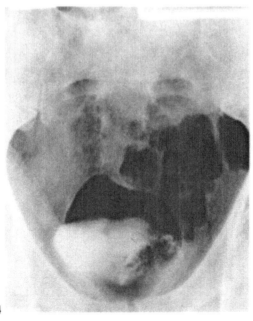

134

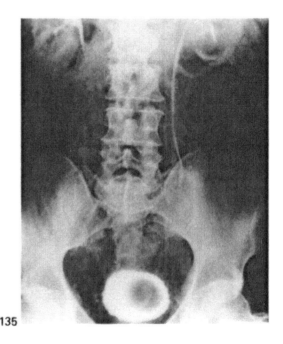

135

Bladder Neoplasm

134 57-year-old man, who had been a heavy cigarette smoker, presented with painless haematuria. A large constant bladder filling defect was seen on the intravenous pyelogram and confirmed by panendoscopy. Fortunately the neoplasm was superficial and papillary and could be treated by endoscopic resection.

135 This apparent constant bladder filling defect, in a 48-year-old man who presented with painless haematuria, is not a neoplasm but a large bowel gas shadow. Panendoscopy revealed no abnormality other than a vascular benign prostatomegaly.

136 This 80-year-old man presented with painless haematuria. An intravenous pyelogram revealed a large constant filling defect, occupying the left half of the bladder, infiltrating the left ureter and producing a left hydroureter and hydronephrosis. A total cysto-prostato-urethrectomy operation was performed in view of the well differentiated grade of the neoplasm and its site but the patient died of metastases 12 months later.

137 This multiple, superficial, rapidly recurrent bladder neoplasm was removed by cysto-prostatectomy operation and an ileal conduit urinary diversion performed. The urethra was removed separately.

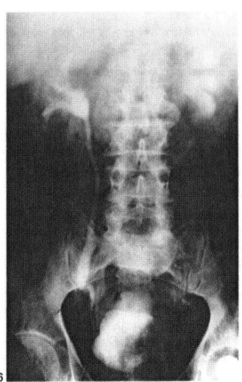

136

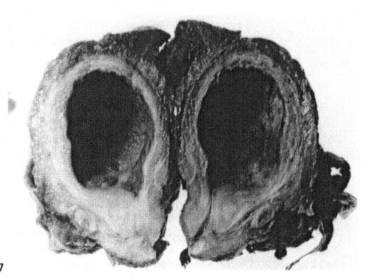

137

Stage I (T1) neoplasms: Most stage I neoplasms can be transurethrally excised with a diathermy cutting loop, unless they are very large or numerous, when they may be necrosed by the intravesical use of the Helmstein distension balloon (England et al., 1973) or excised by open surgical cystostomy.

A 10-year follow-up, by cysto-urethroscopy and occasional intravenous pyelography, at progressively increasing intervals of time, is essential in order to detect asymptomatic or symptomatic recurrent growth. Multiple and/or rapidly recurrent stage I neoplasms may require regular intra-vesical thiotepa or ethoglucid therapy (Riddle and Wallace, 1973); if this, combined with the above methods, is unsuccessful a total cysto-prostato-urethrectomy may be necessary, particularly in younger patients.

Stage IIA (T2) neoplasms: Treatment is as for stage I (T1).

Stage IIB and III (T3a and T3b) neoplasms: Total cysto-prostatectomy or cysto-prostato-urethrectomy, with or without pre- and/or post-deep x-ray therapy, provides the only hope for cure in this group but the morbidity and mortality of the operation is high, and it is often difficult to be certain, even at laparotomy, that the staging is correct.

There is increasing evidence that deep x-ray therapy alone, or local irradiation from surgically implanted radioactive metals, produces similar results, with less morbidity and mortality, to radical surgery in this group.

Palliative deep x-ray therapy, Helmstein balloon distension (Helmstein, 1972) and intra-vesical formalin therapy (Brown, 1969) may benefit the distressing bleeding and strangury of advanced bladder malignancy. A palliative total cystectomy has a high mortality (15%), because of the generally poor health of this group of patients but, in selected cases, may provide the best short term solution. Transcatheter arterial embolisation may also reduce bladder haemorrhage (Lang et al., 1979). The cytotoxic drug platinum diamminodichloride (cis-platinum) is at present undergoing clinical trials with very promising palliative results.

Stage IV (T4a and T4b) neoplasms: Palliative therapy is all that can be offered.

The place of cysto-prostatectomy: There are only three indications for the performance of this operation, with its associated urinary diversion (chapter VIII). The operation has a morbidity rate of 60 to 70% and a mortality of at least 5% when performed by experts (Whitmore and Marshall, 1962; Prout, 1976; Whitmore et al., 1977) for attempted cure, but these complication rates rise to a mortality of up to 15% when performed for attempted palliation.

Attempted curative cysto-prostatectomy is indicated in:

1) Extensive, recurrent, superficial grade I to II, stage I to II, multiple bladder carcinoma, in relatively young patients, in whom endoscopic surgery and/or intra-vesical cytotoxics have been shown to be ineffective. Prior irradiation of the bladder and lymph node drainage areas may improve the survival of some patients (Whitmore et al., 1977).
2) Stage II to III, grade II to III, transitional cell carcinoma of the bladder, where endoscopic surgery will not be curative and radical surgery alone may offer a cure. Pre-operative investigations and an initial laparotomy, with related lymph node dissection and biopsy, are carried out in order to ensure that the procedure is being performed for potentially curative and not palliative reasons (figs. 136-137).

The urethra should also be removed in those potentially curable patients with associated urethral neoplasia and all other potentially curable patients with neoplasia in the lower half of the bladder.

Attempted palliative cysto-prostatectomy has a place in palliation provided that:

1) The bladder is not fixed to the surrounding tissues.
2) The patient is in reasonable general and mental health and accepts the operation after a thorough explanation.
These circumstances are not always present and have undoubtedly resulted in the high mortality rate this operation has when attempted for palliation.

Prognosis: The prognosis of stage I to II and grade I to II bladder neoplasm is good (55% 5-year survival) but the prognosis of stage III to IV and grade III to IV neoplasm is poor (8% 5-year survival).

Carcinoma of the Urethra

As discussed in chapter II the urethra is lined with proximal transitional epithelium, mid and distal pseudostratified columnar ciliated cells, with stratified squamous epithelium lining the fossa navicularis and the external meatal area. This results in posterior urethral neoplasms being transitional in origin and anterior urethral neoplasms exhibiting pseudo-columnar or stratified squamous elements.

Urethral neoplasms are rare and have a poor prognosis, because of their usually late presentation with mechanical dysuria and/or a blood-stained urethral discharge. The vascular corpora spongiosum is rapidly invaded (fig. 138). Lymphatic metastases may spread to the inguinal nodes.

138 Carcinoma of the urethra. Note the infiltration of the corpora and the urethral stricture.

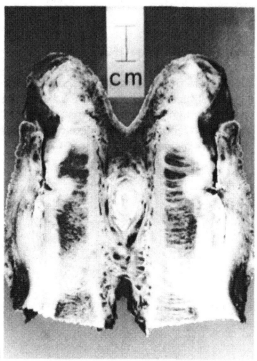

138

Treatment: Wide amputation of the urethral neoplasm, with a resultant urethroplasty, is performed for small anterior urethral neoplasms, whilst radioactive implant therapy is preferred for posterior urethral neoplasms, although cyst-prostato-urethrectomy, with urinary diversion, is still favoured in some centres. Large anterior urethral neoplasms have a poor prognosis, as previously indicated, but are usually best managed by a palliative urethrectomy operation and the creation of a perineal ureth-rostomy.

Palpable inguinal glands should be proven by biopsy to contain neoplasm and, if there is no evidence of further metastases, treated by irradiation or block dissection removal (Grabstald, 1973; Pointon and Poole-Wilson, 1968). A superficial inguinal lymph node block dissection usually results in a distressing, permanent, lower limb lymphoedema.

Prognosis: The overall 5-year survival figures average 40%, whether surgery or radioactive implant is used, but the prognosis for proximal growths is worse.

Benign Urethral Tumours

Condylomata Acuminata: These warts are common and usually arise at the external urinary meatus although, rarely, they may develop within the urethra. Perineal and peri-anal condylomata are not uncommon. The lesions tend to be more profuse in females.

Small external warts can be treated by applying a 25% suspension of podophyllin resin in liquid paraffin for 10 days, directly onto the lesion. Failure of this treatment, or the presence of a larger wart, requires scalpel or diathermy excision of both the wart and its base.

A *giant condyloma* of the penis is termed a Buschke-Loewenstein tumour and may be so large that partial penile amputation is required.

Urethral Polyps: These occur rarely in young boys and arise within the posterior urethra (Williams, 1969). Transurethral resection removes the lesion.

Caruncle: See page 155.

Carcinoma of the Prostate

Carcinoma of the prostate gland is found in 70% of Australians over the age of 70 years, although only 2% will die from it, and this natural history greatly influences urological management (Franks, 1973). Similar incidences have been recorded in other countries, except in Japan, where it is rare. The cause is unknown.

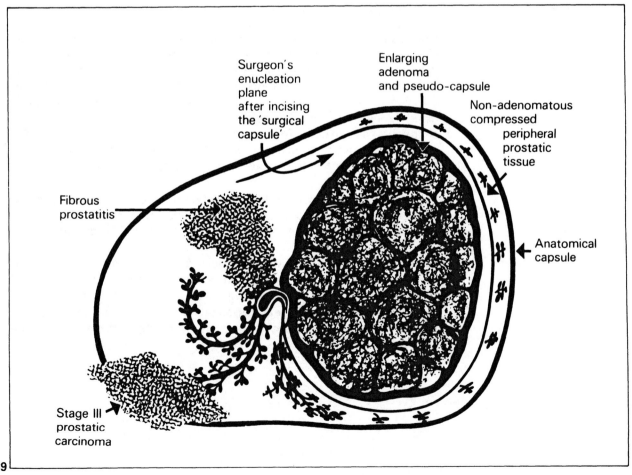

Pathology

As shown in figure 139 cancer of the prostate begins in the peripheral glands, usually as an adenocarcinoma with varying grades of activity. Rarely a squamous or transitional cell neoplasm is found and, very rarely, a sarcoma.

The neoplasm may remain at or about the same size, without metastasising, for 10 to 15 years, or it may rapidly spread (particularly when it occurs in men under the age of 55 years), both directly to surround the rectum, usually without breaching Denonvillier's fascia (p. 59), and through the lymphatic and blood channels. Urologists could be much more dogmatic about the treatment of prostatic carcinoma if we knew which neoplasms were going to progress and what the rate of progression was to be. This difficulty, compared with other genitourinary neoplasms and combined with the usual late presentation of the disease, means that palliative treatment is all that can be offered for most patients (Shuttleworth and Blandy, 1976).

139 Tumours of the prostate. Sites of prostatic tumours.

Staging

The staging of prostatic carcinoma is as follows:

Stage I	The carcinoma is not palpable and is within the anatomical capsule
Stage II	The carcinoma is palpable but is still within the anatomical capsule
Stage III	The carcinoma has breached the anatomical capsule
Stage IV	The carcinoma has invaded other structures or has distally metastasised (fig. 140)

It should be stressed again that clinical staging does not always correspond to pathological staging.

Presentation

Carcinoma of the prostate may present with the following:

1) *Symptoms and signs of prostatism:* (p. 248) and/or
2) *Symptoms and signs of metastases* — bone pain and/or pathological fracture and/or
3) *Uraemia* — due to distal ureteric infiltration (p. 284) and/or
4) *Local haemorrhage* — due to necrosis of the neoplasm and/or to prostatic fibrinolysin activity and, rarely,
5) *Rectal obstruction*
6) *General haemorrhage* — due to the release of large amounts of prostatic fibrinolysins.

As stressed in the chapter III all hard areas within the prostate gland are assumed to be malignant unless proved otherwise.

Diagnosis and Assessment

The majority of patients are diagnosed clinically but histological confirmation should be obtained before beginning treatment (Peck, 1960).

Serology: A high serum acid phosphatase level strongly suggests carcinoma of the prostate (p. 88). Despite the commonly given advice that a delay is essential between digitally examining the prostate gland and taking blood for enzyme determination this is not correct; there is no rise in the serum acid phosphatase concentration after examination of the benign gland (Christensen and Nielsen, 1972; Wiederhorn and Pickens, 1973) although a rise can occur following prostatic infarction (Stewart et al., 1950) or invasion procedures such as transrectal biopsy (Khan et al., 1976) or transurethral prostatectomy (Greene and Thompson, 1974).

Prostatic Biopsy: Prostatic tissue may be obtained from a perineal biopsy (p. 116) or following a prostatectomy operation performed for prostatism or lower urinary tract obstruction of urine (Barnes and Ninon, 1972).

Skeletal X-rays and Gamma Camera Scanning: Prostatic carcinoma metastases are usually sclerotic and occur most commonly in the pelvic girdle and the lumbar vertebrae (fig. 140) [p. 183], where the appearance may be confused with Paget's disease (O'Donoghue et al., 1978). Gamma camera scanning provides a more accurate method of diagnosing small metastases.

Intravenous Pyelogram: This may reveal obstructive infiltration of the lower ureters and/or lower urinary tract retention of urine.

Sternal Bone Marrow Biopsy: This is a necessary investigation before radical surgery is undertaken as it may reveal distal metastases.

Treatment

Stage I: This is a histological diagnosis and does not require any specific treatment other than regular urological examination throughout life.

Stage II: Treatment is the same as for stage I, apart from the under 55-year-old age group, who should undergo either a radical (removal of all the prostate gland, its anatomical capsule and a cuff of bladder outlet) open prostatectomy, local implantation or external irradiation of the lesion (Young, 1945; Whitmore, 1963; Flocks, 1969; Jewett, 1970; Alyea et al., 1977).

Stage III and IV: Palliative treatment is all that can be offered and includes bilateral orchidectomy, oestrogen hormone therapy, limited transurethral resection of the prostate gland, irradiation, or hypophysectomy. The discovery by Huggins (1944) that the growth of prostatic carcinoma was inhibited by performing a bilateral orchidectomy operation and/or by administering oestrogen has provided excellent palliation for many patients. A

140 Lumbar vertebrae and ileal osteosclerotic metastatic carcinoma of the prostate.

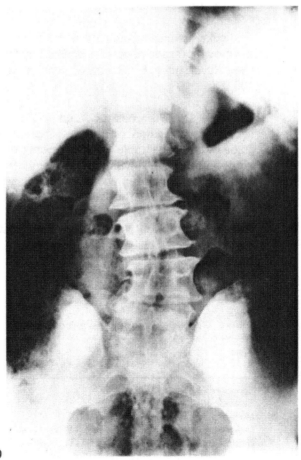

140

bilateral orchidectomy operation is often performed on diagnosis in this group of patients in view of its proven slowing of the growth of many prostatic carcinomas.

Oral stilboestrol, even at a therapeutically prostatic carcinoma cell cytotoxic level of only 1mg 3 times a day, may increase the incidence of coronary thrombosis, cerebrovascular accidents and nausea (Veterans Research Group, 1967).

Chlorotrianisene 25mg daily, may be better tolerated in particular patients, but also carries a risk of cardiovascular complications, as it also causes retention of sodium and water. Fosfestrol (diethylstilboestrol diphosphate) can be given intravenously, if rapid high dose treatment is required, as may be necessary in the patient presenting with retention of urine who is not considered fit enough to undergo a palliative transurethral prostatectomy. The oestrogen component of the posphorelated-oestrogen is liberated by the action of the enzyme acid phosphatase at the site or sites of neoplasia.

Hypophysectomy, by the implantation of radioactive yttrium, may provide instant pain relief from prostatic carcinoma bone metastases (Straffon et al., 1968).

Testicular Neoplasms

Testicular neoplasms represent a small group of genitourinary malignancies but they are extremely important because of the greatly improved prognosis now possible with modern investigations, surgery, irradiation and cytotoxic therapy (Javadpour, 1978). Any suspected testicular lump should be immediately explored by open surgery after lightly clamping the spermatic cord (see later).

Testicular neoplasms are almost unknown in American negroes but they are the most common neoplasm in white males between the ages of 20 and 35 years (average age 28 years), with a general male incidence of 2 per 100,000.

Classification

Germinal Cell Neoplasms: Pugh (1975) found that half of all germinal cell neoplasms consisted of pure seminomas whilst half contained a varying grade of teratoma (table I). Pathological classifications (figs. 141-142) suffer from the clinical disadvantage that they often depend upon the presence of the most differentiated elements found, rather than the most undifferentiated, although the latter (see later) cells greatly influence the prognosis.

Non-germinal Cell Neoplasms: Rare oestrogen secreting interstitial cell tumours, Sertoli cell tumours, lymphoid tumours and secondary metastases may also occur.

Table I. Classification of germinal cell neoplasms

Type	Incidence (%)
Seminoma	50
Seminoma-teratoma	10
Malignant teratoma intermediate (MTI)	24
Malignant teratoma undifferentiated (MTU)	14
Malignant teratoma trophoblastic (MTT)	2

Aetiology

The most popular theory is that seminomas develop from seminiferous epithelium whilst teratomas develop from multipotent embryonic cell rests.

Spread

Testicular neoplasms spread throughout the body of the testis and may invade the epididymis and cord. The tunica vaginalis acts as a very effective barrier to the penetration of the neoplasm until late in the process. Lymphatic spread occurs along the testicular lymphatics to the para-aortic lymph nodes, usually beginning at about the level of the second lumbar vertebrae, and from there to the mediastinal and supraclavicular nodes. There may be retrograde spread to para-aortic nodes below the level of this primary drainage and, extremely rarely, the inguinal nodes may become involved in this way. Haematogenous spread occurs more commonly in teratomas than in seminomas and may be responsible for the poorer prognosis of this group. The lung, liver, bones and central nervous system are common metastatic sites.

Diagnosis and Investigation

Any testis presenting with a solid swelling must be regarded as a neoplasm until proved otherwise. Sperm granuloma and granulomatous orchitis (p. 82) are not clinically distinguishable from a testicular neoplasm.

Testicular neoplasms

141 The homogeneous appearance of a testicular seminoma.

142 The mixed tissue appearance of a teratoma.

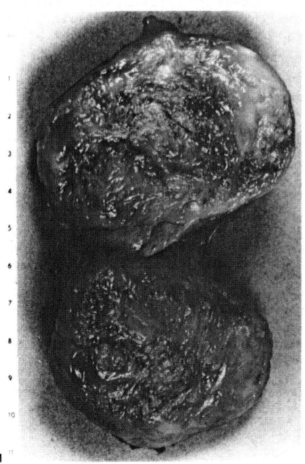

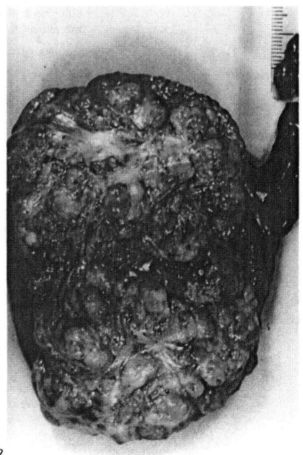

141   142

Although 50% of patients present with a painless, solid, non-transluminable enlargement of the testis, half present with a similar but painful enlargement. The pain may result from rapid neoplastic growth, stretching of the tunica vaginalis, haemorrhage or necrosis. The more rapidly growing neoplasms may be very painful and may be misdiagnosed as inflammatory epididymo-orchitis.

In order to avoid the increased risk of metastatic cell dissemination *it is essential that only gentle, infrequent palpation of the suspected neoplasm be performed.*

Special Investigations: These are performed in order to stage the neoplasm accurately and so aid the choice of specific therapy.

Radiology: Chest x-rays, intravenous pyelography, lymphangiography and inferior venacavagrams are performed in an endeavour to determine the presence of metastatic spread.

Serology: Over the past 5 years new and highly sensitive radioimmunoassays (RIA) for alpha-fetoprotein (AFP), follicle stimulating hormone (FSH) and human chorionic gonadotrophin (HCG), all of which may be produced by testicular teratomatous neoplasms, have significantly altered methods of diagnosis and treatment (Lange et al., 1976), although their accurate estimation (chapter III table II) requires considerable experience. Radioimmunoassay aids both the diagnosis and management of testicular tumours by:

1) Aiding the staging of the disease prior to possible lymphadenectomy
2) Enabling a more accurate follow-up of teratomatous neoplasms after the initial surgery.

Staging Testicular Neoplasms

Three stages of the spread of disease are recognised:

Stage I	Disease confined to the scrotum
Stage II	Lymph node involvement below the diaphragm
Stage III	More distant spread and/or bloodborne metastases.

Treatment

This consists first of an inguinal orchidectomy, to remove the primary neoplasm, secondly, treatment of the retroperitoneal lymph nodes (whether or not involvement can be demonstrated) and thirdly, treatment of more distant metastases.

Inguinal Orchidectomy: The spermatic cord is initially clamped at the internal inguinal ring with a light bulldog clamp and the testis is then mobilised and examined in detail. If malignancy is confirmed the testis, cord and coverings are removed. The peritoneum should be opened and palpation for possible lymph node metastases made. Should malignancy not be confirmed clinically the lump should be biopsied for immediate frozen section biopsy report. Dependent upon the biopsy findings, and the surgeon's clinical judgement, an inguinal orchidectomy is performed or the testis left *in situ* and the wound closed until the more accurate paraffin sections are available.

The excised neoplasm is examined histologically and the disease staged by a careful review of the clinical findings, pathology, radiology and serology results.

There is no place for an intra-scrotal biopsy of a suspected malignant testis, as this procedure may result in metastatic implantation of the neoplasm in skin and subsequent inguinal node involvement.

Retroperitoneal Lymph Nodes: *Seminomas* are amongst the most radio-sensitive neoplasms known and a course of 4,000 rads is always given to the retroperitoneal lymph nodes.

Teratomas are less radio-sensitive and, if potentially curable, require an open radical retroperitoneal lymph node excision, with or without supportive radiotherapy and/or cytotoxic drug therapy (see below). It is possible to remove all of the retroperitoneal lymph nodes completely (Kaswick et al., 1976) although there is some evidence that radiotherapy alone (Smithers et al., 1971) may be as effective as radical surgery with or without radiotherapy.

Radical retroperitoneal lymph node dissection results in ejaculatory impotence which does not occur with radiotherapy treatment.

Distal Metastases: X-ray therapy and triple drug therapy with bleomycin, vincristine and platinum diamminodichloride (cis-platinum), with the occasional excision of isolated metastases, as described by McGirr et al. (1977), may be of considerable value in individual cases.

Skinner (1976) has shown that improved survival rates have occurred with the use of such chemotherapy as an adjunct to both retroperitoneal node dissection and metastatic pulmonary excisions.

Follow-up

Three-monthly patient examinations, chest x-rays and serological testing are essential for the first 2 years, followed by 6-monthly examinations for the next 2 years and then yearly examinations for the next 10 years, in order to detect any metastatic spread and instigate appropriate therapy rapidly.

Prognosis

The prognosis depends largely on the most malignant element present within the removed specimen. Approximately 90% of patients with stage I or II seminomas are alive and have no detectable metastases 5 years after treatment, whilst 85% of all stage I and 70% of all stage II malignant teratoma intermediate (MTI) patients are alive and well 5 years after commencing treatment (Staubitz et al., 1974).

The detection of human chorionic gonadotrophin is a poor prognostic sign and few cases with malignant teratoma trophoblastic (MTT) elements survive for more than 2 years, whatever the therapy. Similarly, malignant teratoma undifferentiated (MTU) has a worse prognosis than malignant teratoma intermediate (MTI).

Penile Neoplasms

Carcinoma of the penis is almost unknown in those circumcised in infancy and is very rare in affluent countries. It is not uncommon in Latin America, Asia and Africa (Kayalwazi, 1966).

The age incidence varies widely, but averages 50 years in Africa and Asia and 60 years in Australia.

The neoplasm presents as an ulcer (fig. 143), a proliferative lesion, or an indurated area, usually well beneath the prepuce and associated with prepucial secretions and inflammation, producing an offensive smell and appearance (Frew et al., 1967).

Microscopically the neoplasm is usually well differentiated but 10% are anaplastic. Basal cell carcinomas are extremely rare.

Spread

Lymphatic spread occurs to the superficial inguinal nodes and/or to the deep inguinal nodes. Bloodborne metastases are uncommon although the corpora are often found to be invaded.

Differential Diagnosis

Ulcerative or indurated malignant penile lesions may resemble the following:

1) Syphilis, chancroid, or other venereal diseases, as discussed in the chapter on Venereal Disease (XIX), but the absence of spirochaetes, Ducrey's bacilli, etc. and tissue biopsy confirms the diagnosis.
2) Queyrat's erythroplasia produces a flat, red, moist, penile area and often requires biopsy differentiation, as does balanitis xerotica obliterans (p. 252). Occasionally erythroplasia of Queryat lesions progress to a squamous cell carcinoma (Payne, 1967).
3) Condylomata acuminata (Ogilvie, 1970).
4) Retention cysts, which are usually found in the region of the frenulum.
5) Rare cystadenomata and angioma.
6) Peyronie's disease. The site and character of this lesion usually enables an accurate clinical differential diagnosis to be made (p. 66).
7) Molluscum contagiosum. This viral dermatitis results in individual, pearl coloured, papular penile lesions, on the shaft of the penis and should present no difficulty in diagnosis. The lesions will remit spontaneously within a few months.

Treatment

1) If the neoplasm is small and confined to the prepuce then a circumcision is performed.
2) If the neoplasm has invaded the glans then local irradiation of the area is performed. If the growth recurs the penis is partially amputated.
3) If the neoplasm has invaded the shaft then a complete penile amputation is performed.
4) If the superficial inguinal nodes are still enlarged 2 weeks after removal of the primary neoplasm then they are biopsied and, if shown to contain metastases, removed by a block dissection or treated by irradiation. A superficial inguinal lymph block dissection usually produces marked lower limb lymphoedema and, as the results of surgery appear to be no better than irradiation, this latter method is usually preferred (Furlong and Uhle, 1953).

Prognosis

This varies from a 5-year survival of approximately 70% for lesions restricted to the glans penis to 30% for those with involved inguinal nodes (Hoppmann and Fraley, 1978).

Penile Sarcoma

This is an extremely rare neoplasm (Wheelock and Clark, 1943).

Scrotal Carcinoma

Since the demise of chimney sweeps and changes in the usage of oil in the cotton industry this neoplasm is rare (Kipling, 1968). The loose scrotal skin allows for wide excision of the squamous cell lesion which, if treated before inguinal lymph node involvement, has an excellent prognosis (fig. 144) [Dean, 1948; Ray and Whitmore, 1977].

143 Penile neoplasm. An ulcerative tumour which was treated by radical amputation of the penis.

144 Scrotal carcinoma. This tumour was treated by wide local excision.

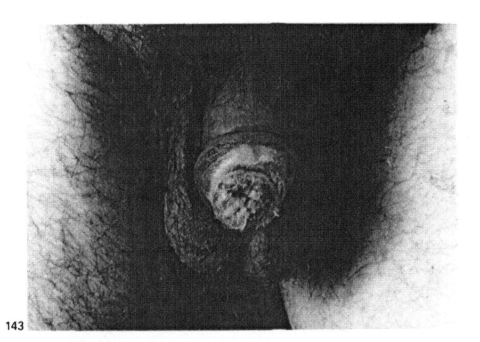

143

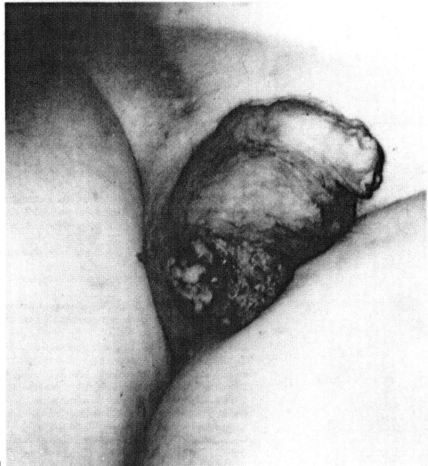

144

Differential Diagnosis   Sebaceous cysts of the scrotum are common and often multiple. Their non-ulcerated appearance and soft character enables a clinical differential diagnosis to be made. Large or multiple sebaceous cysts may require surgical excision. Extremely rarely a *melanoma* may develop in the scrotal skin.

Adrenal Neoplasms

Cushing's disease, phaeochromocytoma and hyperaldosteronism (Conn's syndrome) can all cause renal hypertension and are discussed in chapter XVII.

Adrenal neoplasms can be diagnosed by venogram or angiogram but there is a technical risk of producing adrenal infarction. Peri-renal air insufflation is also of value but carries a slight risk of producing an air embolus (p. 107). Adrenal scanning tests using ^{131}I, ultrasound and computerised tomography are safer and easier techniques and have now replaced venography and angiography as methods of diagnosis in most centres.

If there is doubt as to the location of the adrenal neoplasm both glands are explored via an extra-peritoneal incision, through the 11th or 12th rib-bed, with the patient in the prone position. Facilities for frozen section diagnosis must be available in order to diagnose small adenomata.

Large unilateral adenomata are best treated by excising all of the gland on that side, as the likelihood of multiple micro-adenomata being present in the residual tissue is high.

Aitchison et al. (1971) have indicated a preoperative method of distinguishing between adrenal hyperplasia and adenoma formation. Hyperplastic Cushing's disease is best treated with cortisone (p. 46) while hyperaldosteronism is best treated with spironolactone. Other types of adrenal hyperplasia are dealt with by selective surgical excision of varying portions of one or both glands.

References

Aitchison, J.; Brown, J.J.; Ferris, J.B.; Fraser, R.; Kaye, A.; Symington, T. and Robertson, J.L.S.: Quadric analysis in the preoperative distinction between patients with and without adrenocortical tumours in hypertension with aldosterone excess and low plasma renin. American Heart Journal 82: 660 (1971). 660 (1971).

Alyea, E.P.; Dees, J.E. and Glenn, J.F.: An aggressive approach to prostatic cancer. Journal of Urology 118: 211 (1977).

Angerwall, L.; Bengtsson, U.; Zetterlund, C.G. and Zsigmond, M.: Renal pelvic carcinoma in a Swedish district with abuse of a phenacitin-containing drug. British Journal of Urology 41: 401 (1969).

Anthony, H.H. and Thomas, G.M.: Bladder tumours and smoking. International Journal of Cancer 5: 266 (1970).

Barnes, R.W. and Ninon, C.A.: Carcinoma of the prostate: biopsy and conservative therapy. Journal of Urology 108: 897 (1972).

Brown, R.B.: A method of management of inoperable carcinoma of the bladder. Medical Journal of Australia 1: 23 (1969).

Christensen, P. and Nielsen, M.L.: Serum acid phosphatase; the influence of routine rectal examination with diagnostic palpitation of the prostate. Scandinavian Journal of Urology and Nephrology 6: 103 (1972).

Clemonson, J.: Statistical studies in the aetiology of malignant neoplasms. IV. Lung/bladder ratio. Acta Pathologica et Microbiologica Scandinavica (Suppl.) 247: 42 (1974).

Dean, A.L.: Epithelioma of scrotum. Journal of Urology 60: 508 (1948).

England, H.R.; Rigby, C.; Shepheard, B.G.F.; Tresidder, G.C. and Blandy, J.P.: Evaluation of Helmstein's distension method for carcinoma of the bladder. British Journal of Urology 45: 593 (1973).

Flocks, R.H.: Present status of interstitial irradiation in managing prostatic cancer. Journal of the American Medical Association 210: 338 (1969).

Franks, L.M.: Etiology, epidemiology and pathology of prostatic cancer. Cancer 32: 1092 (1973).

Frew, I.D.; Jeffries, J.D. and Swinney, J.: Carcinoma of the penis. British Journal of Urology 39: 398 (1967).

Furlong, J.H. and Uhle, C.H.: Cancer of the penis: a report of 88 cases. Journal of Urology 69: 550 (1953).

Gelfand, M.; Weinberg, R.W. and Castle, W.M.: Relations between carcinoma of the bladder and infestation with *Schistosoma haematobium* Lancet 1: 1249 (1967).

Grabstald, H.: Tumours of the urethra in men and women. Cancer 32: 1236 (1973).

Greene, F.T. and Thompson, I.M.: Effects of various manipulations on serum phosphatase levels in benign disease. Journal of Urology 112: 232 (1974).

Helmstein, K.: Treatment of bladder carcinoma by a hydrostatic pressure technique. British Journal of Urology 44: 434 (1972).

Heuper, W.C.: Cancer of the urinary bladder in workers of chemical dye factories and dyeing establishments. Journal of Industrial Hygiene 16: 225 (1934).

Hoppmann, H.J. and Fraley, E.E.: Squamous cell carcinoma of the penis. Journal of Urology 120: 393 (1978).

Huggins, C.: The treatment of cancer of the prostate Canadian Medical Association Journal 50: 301 (1944).

Javadpour, N.: National cancer institute experience with testicular cancer. Journal of Urology 120: 651 (1978).

Jewett, H.J.: The case for radical perineal prostatectomy. Journal of Urology 103: 195 (1970).

Kaswick, J.S.; Bloomberg, S.D. and Skinner, D.G.: Radical retroperitoneal lymph node dissection. How effective is removal of all retroperitoneal nodes? Journal of Urology 115: 70 (1976).

Kayalwazi, S.K.: Carcinoma of the penis: a review of 153 patients admitted to Mulago Hospital, Kampala. East Africa Medical Journal 43: 415 (1966).

Khan, R.M.; Cromie, W.J. and Edson, M.: Pre- and post-ejaculation serum acid phosphatase. Urology 8: 43 (1976).

Kipling, N.D.: Annual report by H.M. Chief Inspector of Factories 1967 (HMSO, London 1968).

Lang, E.K.; Deutsch, J.S.; Goodman, J.R.; Barnett, T.F.; Lanasa, J.A. Jr. and Duplessis, G.H.: Transcatheter embolisation of hypogastric branch arteries in management of intractable bladder haemorrhage. Journal of Urology 121: 30 (1979).

Lange, P.H.; McIntire, K.R.; Waldmann, T.A.; Hakala, T.R. and Fraley, E.E.: Serum alpha-fetoprotein and human chorionic gonadotrophin in the diagnosis and management of nonseminomatous germ-cell testicular cancer. New England Journal of Medicine 295: 1237 (1976).

McGirr, V.G.; Goldstein, A.M.; Thompson, D.M. and Utley, W.L.: Testicular tumours: treatment by surgery and radiotherapy. Australian and New Zealand Journal of Surgery 47: 491 (1977).

Mimms, N.M.; Christianson, B.; Schlumberger, F.C. and Goodwin, W.E.: A ten year evaluation of nephrectomy for extensive renal carcinoma. Journal of Urology 95: 10 (1966).

O'Donoghue, E.P.; Constable, A.R.; Sherwood, T.; Stevenson, J.J. and Chisholm, G.D.: Bone scanning and plasma phosphates in carcinoma of the prostate. British Journal of Urology 50: 172 (1978).

O'Flynn, J.D. and Mullaney, J.: Leukoplakia of the bladder — a report on 20 cases including 2 cases progressing to squamous cell carcinoma. British Journal of Urology 39: 461 (1967).

Ogilvie, M.M.: Virus in genital warts. British Medical Journal 1: 113 (1970).

Palmisano, P.J.: Renal hamartoma (angiomyolipoma): its angiographic appearance and response to intra-arterial epinephrine. Radiology 88: 249 (1967).

Payne, R.A.: Erythroplasia of Queyrat. British Journal of Urology 29: 163 (1967).

Peck, S.: Needle biopsy of the prostate. Journal of Urology 83: 176 (1960).

Petkovic, S.D.: A plea for conservative operations for ureteral tumours. Journal of Urology 107: 220 (1971).

Pointon, R.C. and Poole-Wilson, D.S.: Primary carcinoma of the urethra. British Journal of Urology 39: 240 (1968).

Prout, G.R.: The surgical management of bladder carcinoma. Urology Clinics of North America 3: 149 (1976).

Pugh, R.C.B.: The pathology of cancer of the bladder — an editorial overview. Cancer 32: 1267 (1973).

Pugh, R.C.B.: Pathology of the Testis, p.205 (Blackwell, Oxford 1975).

Ray, B. and Whitmore, W.F.: Experience with carcinoma of scrotum. Journal of Urology 117: 741 (1977).

Riddle, P.R. and Wallace, P.M.: Intracavity chemotherapy for multiple non-invasive bladder tumours. British Journal of Urology 45: 520 (1973).

Robson, C.J.; Churchill, M.B. and Anderson, W.: The results of radical nephrectomy for renal carcinoma. Journal of Urology 101: 297 (1969).

Schefft, P.; Novick, A.D.; Straffa, R.A. and Stewart, B.H.: Surgery for renal cell carcinoma extending into inferior vena cava. Journal of Urology 120: 28 (1978).

Shuttleworth, K. and Blandy, J.P.: Carcinoma of the prostate; in Blandy (Ed) Urology, p.926 (Blackwell, Oxford 1976).

Skinner, D.G.: Non-seminomatous testis tumours. Plan of management based on 96 patients to improve survival in all stages by combined therapeutic modalities. Journal of Urology 115: 65 (1976).

Smithers, D.W.; Wallace, E.N.K. and Wallace, D.M.: Radiotherapy for patients with tumours of the testicle. British Journal of Urology 43: 83 (1971).

Stams, U.K.; Gursel, E.O. and Veenema, R.J.: Prophylactic urethrectomy in male patients with bladder cancer. Journal of Urology 111: 177 (1977).

Staubitz, W.J.; Early, K.S.; Magoss, I.V. and Murphy, G.P.: Surgical management of testicular tumours. Journal of Urology 111: 205 (1974).

Straffon, R.A.; Kiser, W.S.; Robitaille, M. and Dohn, D.F.: Yttrium[90] hypophysectomy in the management of metastatic carcinoma of the prostate gland in 13 patients. Journal of Urology 99: 102 (1968).

Stewart, C.B.; Sweetser, J.H. Jnr, and Delory, G.E.: A case of benign prostatic hypertrophy with recent infarcts and associated high serum acid phosphatase. Journal of Urology 63: 128 (1950).

Taylor, J.S.: Carcinoma of the urinary tract and analgesic abuse. Medical Journal of Australia 1: 407 (1973).

Veterans Administration Co-operative Urological Research Group: Carcinoma of the prostate: treatment comparisons. Journal of Urology 98: 516 (1967).

Wallace, D.M.: Carcinoma of the urothelium; in Blandy (Ed) Urology, p.774 (Blackwell, Oxford 1976).

Wheelock, M.C. and Clark, P.J.: Sarcoma of the penis. Journal of Urology 49: 478 (1943).

Whitmore, W.F. Jr.: The rationale and results of ablative surgery for prostatic cancer. Cancer 16: 1119 (1963).

Whitmore, W.F. Jr.; Batata, M.A.; Gitoneim, M.A.; Grabstald, H. and Unal, A.: Radical cystectomy with or without prior irradiation in the treatment of bladder cancer. Journal of Urology 118: 184 (1977).

Whitmore, W.F. Jr. and Marshall, V.F.: Radical total cystectomy for carcinoma of the bladder: 230 consecutive cases five years later. Journal of Urology 87: 853 (1962).

Wiederhorn, A.R. and Pickens, R.L.: Serum acid phosphatase levels following prostatic massage: a re-evaluation. Journal of Urology 109: 855 (1973).

Williams, C.B. and Mitchell, J.P.: Carcinoma of the ureter — a review of 54 cases. British Journal of Urology 45: 377 (1973).

Williams, D.I.: Paediatric Urology, p.263-265 (Butterworths, London 1969).

Young, H.H.: The cure of carcinoma of the prostate by radical perineal prostatectomy (prostato-seminal vesiculectomy). History, literature and status of Young's operation. Journal of Urology 53: 188 (1945).

Discussion: in Transactions of the American Association of Genitourinary Surgeons: Preoperative irradiation of bladder carcinoma 70: 117 (1979).

Further Reading

Arduino, L.J. and Glucksman, M.A.: Lymph node metastases in early carcinoma of the prostate. Journal of Urology 88: 91 (1962).

Clark, P. and Anderson, K.: Tumours of the kidney and ureter; in Blandy (Ed) Urology, p.391 (Blackwell, Oxford 1976).

Holland, J.M.: Cancer of the kidney: natural history and staging. Cancer 32: 1030 (1973).

Marshall, F.F. and Walsh, P.C.: Extra-renal manifestations of renal cell carcinoma. Journal of Urology 117: 439 (1977).

Ray, B.: Condylomata acuminatum of scrotum. Journal of Urology 117: 739 (1977).

Rickham, P.P.: Malignant tumours involving the genitourinary system in childhood; in Johnston and Scholtmeijer (Eds) Problems in Paediatric Urology, p.180 (Excerpta Medica, Amsterdam 1972).

Van der Werf-Messing, B.: Carcinoma of the kidney. Cancer 32: 1056 (1973).

Chapter VIII

Urinary Diversion

Urinary diversion techniques have been devised mainly for patients in whom, for various reasons, there is a need to bypass the bladder. While these techniques were originally used for patients with ectopia vesicae (Simon, 1852) bladder malignancies are now the prime indication. Neurogenic bladder dysfunction, vesical decompensation from long standing obstruction, small capacity bladders and uncorrectable incontinence of urine are additional indications. Unfortunately, a perfect bladder substitute has yet to be devised.

The number of types of urinary diversion continues to grow, and those discussed here are listed in table I. Many factors need to be taken into consideration when selecting the best form of urinary diversion for an individual patient. Diversion operations are subdivided into upper and lower tract types and may be temporary or permanent. In patients with mechanical or

Table I. Urinary diversion procedures and their main complications and limitations

Procedure	Complications and limitations
Upper Urinary Tract Diversion — permanent	
1) Ileal conduit (Bricker diversion)	Chronic pyelonephritis, stone disease, reflux and loss of renal function, stomal stenosis
2) Non-refluxing colon conduit	Pyelonephritis < than with 1) above
3) Ureterosigmoidostomy	Pyelonephritis, hyperchloraemic acidosis, calculi, bowel obstruction, fistula
4) Rectal bladder with proximal colostomy	Infection, hyperchloraemic acidosis
5) Gersuny procedure	Pyelonephritis, enuresis, faecal soiling, stress incontinence
6) Initial sigmoid conduit + lateral ureterosigmoidostomy	Pyelonephritis less common than with 3) above hyperchloraemic acidosis (in theory)
7) Cutaneous ureterostomy	Of long term use in poor risk, short life-expectation patients only
Upper Urinary Tract Diversion — temporary	
1) Nephrostomy	Infection, calculi, difficult early postoperative replacement
2) Gibbons catheter	Calculi in some patients
3) Cutaneous pyelostomy	Infection, calculi < than in 1) above
4) Loop cutaneous ureterostomy	Risk of ureteral blood supply embarrassement
5) Silastic splint ureterostomy	Suitable only for temporary diversion
Lower Urinary Tract Diversion	
1) Urethral catheter	Infection, calculi, urethral diverticula
2) Suprapubic cystostomy	Leakage, fibrosis, infection, calculi
3) Cutaneous vesicostomy	Less infection and risk of calculus than in 1) above
4) Perineal urethrostomy	

functional obstructive disease both the cause and the site of obstruction must be considered, both to achieve the optimal method of diversion and to determine whether the diversion is to be temporary or permanent. It is essential to divert the urine above the highest functional level of obstruction. In patients requiring permanent diversion age and prognosis are the prime considerations in deciding the optimal form.

Upper Urinary Tract (Supravesical) Diversion

Permanent Diversion

Ileal Conduit. *Procedure:* This is also known as the Bricker urinary diversion (Bricker, 1950).

A 15cm segment of the ileum is isolated 15cm proximal to the ileocaecal valve. The continuity of the intestinal tract is restored by an ileo-ileostomy. The proximal end of the loop is closed and each ureter is anastomosed to the antimesenteric border of the proximal portion in an end-to-side manner (fig. 145). The distal end of the ileum is anastomosed to the anterior abdominal wall, usually in the right lower quadrant in a preselected location (fig. 146).

A stomal appliance is required for urine collection. Present day appliances can remain in place 5 to 7 days in between changes. Little compromise in the patient's life style is necessary. The ileal segment acts as a conduit rather than a reservoir, with the urine being propelled by peristalsis into the external collecting device. This lessens the likelihood of complications such as electrolyte imbalance, urinary calculi and infection which commonly occur in urinary diversions where the bowel has a reservoir function (see below).

Complications: Long term complications which are not unusual are acute and chronic pyelonephritis, stone disease and a progressive loss of renal function. There is a positive correlation between these complications and stomal stenosis, excess conduit length and uretero-ileal obstruction. Older patients, especially those with bladder cancer, rarely have difficulty, as these problems usually occur 10 to 15 years after diversion, but other methods of long term urinary diversion may be preferable in children. Stomal problems, especially stenosis, are more common in children.

Progressive renal deterioration has been noted in 30% of patients, with previously normal upper urinary tracts, when followed for up to 10 years (Magnus, 1977). In many of these patients obstruction or excess length was not present. Reflux, with or without infection, has been blamed for much of this deterioration. It is now thought by many that a non-refluxing colon conduit is indicated in patients with excellent long term prognosis, such as children with non-malignant disease.

Ileal conduit technique

145 Ileal conduit (Bricker) urinary diversion. Note the isolated segment of ileum with bilateral uretero-ileal anastomosis. The isolated segment of ileum should be taken at least 10cm from the ileocaecal valve in order to preserve the ileocolic artery and the vascular supply of the caecum and right colon and should be approximately 15cm in length.

146 Everted ileal stoma located in the right lower quadrant in a preselected site. A stomal appliance fits over the stoma for urinary collection.

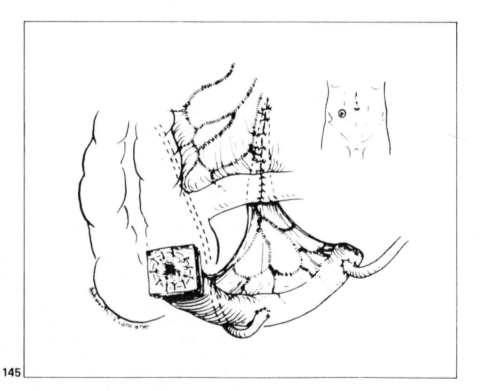

145

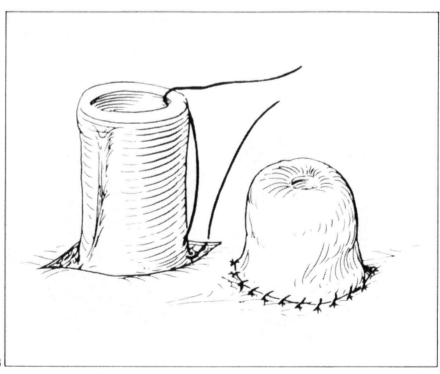

146

Non-refluxing Colon Conduit. *Procedure:* The non-refluxing sigmoid conduit has been used with increasing frequency since attention was redirected to this procedure by Mogg in 1965. This conduit system has two particular advantages over ileal diversion: the thicker muscular wall of the colon allows for an anti-refluxing anastomosis of the ureter to the colon and stomal problems are less common than with ileal conduits.

These beneficial effects have been confirmed in the laboratory where non-refluxing colon conduits were created on one side whilst refluxing ileal conduits were created on the contralateral system of dogs (Ritchie et al., 1974). After 3 months the incidence of pyelonephritis, confirmed histologically, was 7% in the non-refluxing renal units compared to 83% in the refluxing systems.

A 10 to 15cm segment of sigmoid colon is isolated, as in the ileal conduit, with a re-anastomosis of the colon in a standard fashion (figs. 147). The vascular supply is derived from the distal most sigmoid artery or the superior haemorrhoidal artery. A sigmoid conduit may be contraindicated in patients undergoing radical cystectomy for cancer, as the distal colon obtains its blood supply from the middle and inferior haemorrhoidals, which arise from the internal iliac artery, and which is usually sacrificed during cystectomy, thus jeopardising the integrity of the colonic anastomosis. The colon conduit does not have to be isoperistaltic although this is necessary in the ileal conduit diversion. The proximal end of the conduit is closed in two layers, making sure that the outer layer of non-absorbable suture material is not intraluminal, lest calculi form on these sutures. The ureter is then placed in a submucosal trough extraluminally created in the taenia (fig. 148). This trough should measure 3cm in length and should be wide enough not to obstruct the ureter. The trough for each ureter should be separated, to prevent narrowing of the bowel lumen when the tunnels are closed. Each ureter is laid in the trough and a small mucosal incision is made at the distal end of the trough and an end-to-side anastomosis of the ureter to the colonic mucosa is made with fine, absorbable sutures. The sides of the trough are then approximated to make a roof for the new anti-refluxing tunnel, making sure the ureter lies freely within the tunnel. This technique is identical to that used in the Leadbetter technique, for the intact uretero-sigmoidostomy, discussed below.

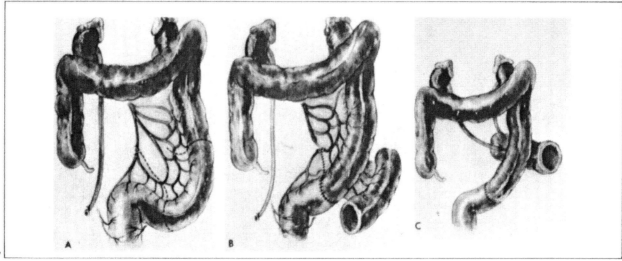

147

147 Sigmoid conduit diversion. Isolation of a segment of sigmoid colon (a). Note sacrifice of superior haemorrhoidal artery. Re-anastomosis of sigmoid colon and closure of proximal end of sigmoid conduit (b). Ureterocolonic anastomosis has been completed (c) — non-refluxing anastomosis (see fig. 148).

148 Ureterosigmoidostomy; technique of Leadbetter. a) Muscularis has been incised. b) Submucosal trough has been created. c) Anastomosis of the end of the ureter to the mucosa of the colon. d) Closure of muscular trough creating submucosal tunnel. e) Completed anastomosis. Note the staggered anastomosis of the ureter which prevents narrowing of the sigmoid colon.

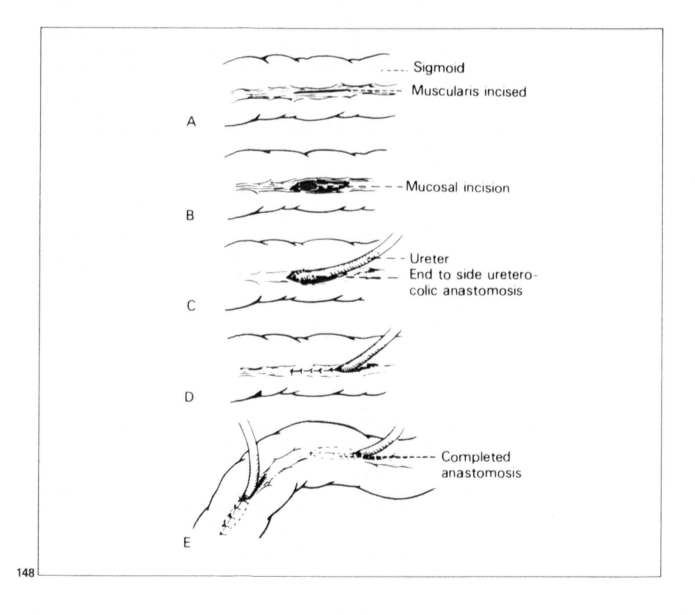

148

Complications: Although few series with colon conduits have been followed 10 years' allowing proper comparison with long term follow-up for ileal conduits, early clinical reports confirm the experimental evidence of a reduced incidence of pyelonephritis with the colon conduit. Other colon segments have been described, such as the ileocaecal segment, which may have an advantage in the patient who is later to be 'undiverted', especially in those patients requiring bladder augmentation (fig. 149).

Ureterosigmoidostomy: Transposition of the ureters into the intact sigmoid colon was the procedure of choice for supravesical urinary diversion for many years. Simon made the first attempt to divert the urine to the intact colon in 1852 and for the next 100 years this was the standard urinary diversion technique. The ileal conduit became popular in the 1950's. Stone disease and an extremely high incidence of acute pyelonephritis made ureterosigmoidostomy an extremely hazardous procedure until Coffey, in 1911, described the first attempt at an anti-refluxing anastomosis. The refinements of technique by Leadbetter in 1951 and Goodwin in 1953 further lessened these complications.

Transplantation of the ureters into the intact sigmoid colon has several possible advantages over conduit urinary diversion. The patient is able to maintain voluntary control over urination and has no appliance to wear (a distinct advantage in areas of the world where modern stomal appliances are not available). The absence of the stoma obviates all stomal problems, the most common complication of conduit diversion, and for this reason this type may be an ideal form of selected diversion for children. Because of these factors there is improved patient acceptance. The procedure is better tolerated in the older, poor risk patient, as it is quicker to perform than almost all forms of conduit diversion, with cutaneous ureterostomy being the obvious exception. It is especially useful as a palliative procedure in patients with a limited life span because of age or poor prognosis.

Disadvantages of ureterosigmoidostomy include the high incidence of pyelonephritis, renal deterioration and electrolyte imbalance. The normal colonic bacterial flora and the relatively high intraluminal colonic pressure have been implicated as the cause of the common resultant pyelonephritis. In addition, patients have essentially life-long watery diarrhoea, often with nocturnal enuresis and diurnal incontinence whilst passing flatus. It is necessary for them to evacuate the rectum every 2 to 3 hours, day and night. Definite *contraindications* to ureterosigmoidostomy include:

1) Incompetent anal sphincter mechanism
2) Creatinine clearance levels less than 40ml/minute
3) Two dilated ureters
4) Previous high dose pelvic irradiation
5) Severe inflammatory bowel disease.

Procedure: The extraluminal Leadbetter technique, or the open transcolonic technique of Goodwin, is used. In the Leadbetter technique (fig. 148) the ureters are anastomosed to the low sigmoid colon in the manner previously described for sigmoid conduits. This technique has the advantage that the colon is not opened, lessening the likelihood of abscess formation in the postoperative period. In the Goodwin technique the colon is opened and an anastomosis, similar to the Politano-Leadbetter technique to repair vesicouretero-reflux, is used (fig. 150). This operation has the advantage of creating the tunnel under direct vision making obstruction less likely. An adequate mechanical and chemical bowel preparation is required to minimise infective complications in the early postoperative period.

149 Ileocaecal cystoplasty.

150 **Open transcolonic technique of ureterosigmoidostomy.** [Adapted from Goodwin, W.E., Harris, A.P., Kaufman, J.J. and Beal, J.M.: Open Transcolonic Ureterointestinal Anastomosis. Surgery, Gynaecology and Obstetrics, 97: 295 (1953)].

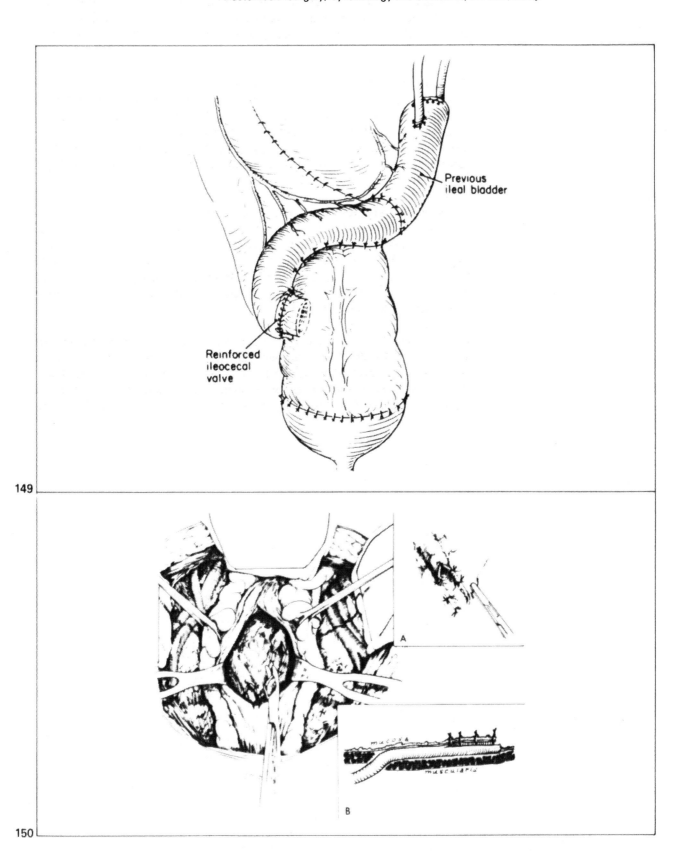

Complications: Pyelonephritis and hyperchloraemic acidosis are the most common problems following ureterosigmoidostomy and are the most common causes of failure of this procedure. Between 30 to 50% of patients will have to be converted to some other form of urinary diversion because of an inability to control these complications. Goodwin (1976) has stated that all intact ureterosigmoidoscopy patients will eventually develop episodes of pyelonephritis. Usually these episodes are mild and can be controlled by antibiotics.

Eventually 20 to 40% of these patients will show functional renal deterioration secondary to chronic pyelonephritis. Patients who can no longer be controlled with suppressive antibiotics should be immediately converted to a conduit form of diversion. An alternative is to convert the ureterosigmoidostomy into a rectal bladder, by performing a proximal diverting colostomy to separate the urine and faecal stream, the ureterocolonic anastomosis being left intact.

A low colonic anastomosis, sodium potassium citrate administration, frequent evacuation of the rectum every 2 to 3 hours, and a low chloride diet should decrease the incidence of hyperchloraemic acidosis. Zincke and Segura (1975), at the Mayo Clinic, reported only 4 of 173 cases with severe hyperchloraemic acidosis, but mild problems can appear in up to 70% of cases. Chronic acidosis is a cause of growth lag in children following a ureterosigmoidostomy.

When severe hyperchloraemic acidosis does occur a marked potassium loss may also result. Hyperchloraemic acidosis occurs as chloride and urea are selectively resorbed in the lower colon leading to a metabolic acidosis. Re-excretion of the chloride ion requires potassium, thus leading to potassium loss and a potentially severe hypokalaemia. Magnesium may also be lost, resulting in hypomagnesaemia. If severe hypokalaemia and hyperchloraemic acidosis occur care must be taken in correction: over zealous replacement of potassium may exacerbate an existing systemic acidosis by causing a shift in intracellular hydrogen ions to the extracellular fluid. Excessive bicarbonate administration may also cause difficulty as a rapid intracellular potassium shift may occur, increasing the hypokalaemia and the neuromuscular impairment. In such cases both potassium and bicarbonate must be replaced simultaneously, with careful acid base and electrolyte monitoring. Patients with a creatinine clearance of less than 40ml/minute may not be able to tolerate the hyperchloraemic acidosis and conversion to a conduit form of diversion may be required.

Other complications such as urinary tract calculi, bowel obstruction, urinary fistulae and sepsis occur more frequently with ureterosigmoidostomy than other forms of urinary diversion. Recently there has been an increasing number of reports of colon carcinoma occurring 5 to 30 years following ureterosigmoidostomy.

Rectal Bladder: An alternative to ureterosigmoidostomy is to use the rectum as a urine reservoir with a proximal diverting colostomy. Many patients and urologists feel that the colostomy is easier to manage than a urinary conduit, and often an appliance is not necessary. Since the faecal and urine channels are separated the incidence of pyelonephritis is less than that following ureterosigmoidostomy. A rectal bladder conversion is especially useful in patients with a ureterosigmoidostomy experiencing recurrent infections. An anti-reflux anastomosis should still be performed to lessen the possibility of infection. Because patients with rectal bladders have less colonic surface available for reabsorption, hyperchloraemic acidosis should not occur as readily; however, it has been reported in patients not evacuating their rectal reservoir frequently.

Gersuny Procedure: This technique involves the creation of a rectal bladder with a perineal colostomy, either anterior (Gersuny, 1898) or posterior to the rectum. The anal sphincter is utilised for control of the faecal stream. The urinary and faecal channels have been separated and this diminishes the incidence of pyelonephritis, but retraction of the septum between the anus and the perineal colostomy frequently causes a cloaca formation, with resultant pooling of faecal and urinary streams and pyelonephritis. Enuresis, faecal soiling and stress incontinence of urine are other common problems with the Gersuny and related procedures (fig. 151).

Sigmoid Conduit Combined with Ureterosigmoidostomy. *Procedure:* Hendren (1974) has described a staged approach to non-stomal urinary diversion in children, especially in ectopia vesicae. This has been applied even in patients with bilateral dilated ureters. A non-refluxing sigmoid conduit to the skin is created (see above) and continuity of the bowel is re-established. After a period of observation (at least 6-12 months) the conduit is assessed; if no reflux is seen the cutaneous anastomosis is taken down and an end-to-side anastomosis of the colon conduit to the intact sigmoid colon is performed. Some separation of the faecal and urinary channels results from this procedure.

Complications: In the early experiences of Hendren (1974) pyelonephritis has been less of a problem than when using a standard ureterosigmoidostomy operation. Long term follow-up, however, will be necessary before this procedure can be recommended as a method of choice. Problems with hyperchloraemic acidosis would theoretically, be just as likely to occur with this method as with ureterosigmoidostomy.

Cutaneous Ureterostomy: Cutaneous ureterostomy is the simplest form of supravesical urinary diversion. It is easy and quick to perform but problems with stricture at the skin level prevent its routine use. In order for this procedure to work satisfactorily the ureter should be sufficiently dilated to lessen the likelihood of stenosis. In patients with high ureteral obstruction there is often not enough ureteral length to allow a tension-free anastomosis with the skin. This procedure is suitable for palliation in patients with terminal malignant disease, or a solitary functioning kidney with a dilated ureter. Patients with one dilated ureter and a contralateral normal ureter can make use of this procedure by anastomosing the normal calibre ureter end-to-side to the dilated ureter (so called transureterostomy) and then anastomosing the dilated ureter to the skin. This procedure is applicable only to the poor risk patient with a short life expectancy.

Rectal urinary diversion
151a 'Rectogram' of a child with bladder extrophy. Note absence of reflux.

151b Intravenous pyelogram. Note small amount of post-micturition residual urine. Nocturnal enuresis was a minor problem with this patient.

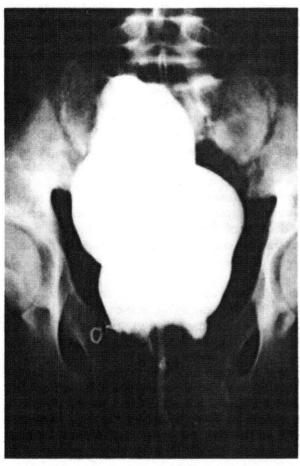

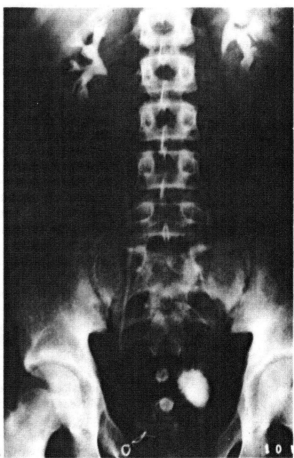

151a   151b

Temporary Diversion

Temporary supravesical diversion is utilised for 3 clinical indications:

1) As a rapid method of decompressing the obstructed upper urinary tract (see p. 269)
2) As part of a staged reconstruction of the urinary tract
3) For acute short term decompression of the upper urinary tract after reconstructive surgery.

Nephrostomy. *Procedure:* Nephrostomy is the most proximal form of urinary diversion and entails inserting a silastic tube from the renal pelvis to the flank, traversing the renal parenchyma. An external urinary collecting device is required. A nephrostomy tube may be inserted by open surgical exposure of the renal pelvis and lower renal pole and placing the nephrostomy tube through the lower pole cortex into the lower calyx and the renal pelvis. This procedure is often used in reconstructive operations on the upper tract to decompress the collecting system until the suture line becomes water tight (approximately 12-14 days). It is useful in patients with acute urinary obstruction and sepsis as well as in patients with chronic obstruction and uraemia from various causes. Recent popularisation of percutaneous nephrostomy has largely replaced open surgical nephrostomy in the acutely ill, poor risk patient. Modern angiographic technique and equipment can be modified to pass small catheters percutaneously accurately, under fluoroscopic control, into the renal pelvis, with low morbidity.

Complications: Nephrostomy tubes and operations have the advantages of being proximal and relatively easy to insert. Their disadvantages arise from the fact that they entail the introduction of a foreign body into the urinary tract with its almost certain sequela of infection. Tubes left indwelling for periods longer than a few weeks can act as a nidus for calculus formation. Because of these complications long term nephrostomy drainage is rarely indicated, except in those patients with a limited life expectancy. Technical problems also ensue in changing the tubes, especially if they should fall out in the early postoperative period.

Gibbons Catheter: Gibbons (1976) has described the use of a specially designed silicone catheter, which can be passed cystoscopically through the ureteral meatus into the obstructed ureter to the renal pelvis. This is self-retained and has been used in some patients for up to 3 years without significant calculus encrustation, although this remains a problem in others. Its advantages include the ease of introduction and its easy reversibility. It is especially useful in patients suffering from ureteral obstruction from a malignant or benign retroperitoneal obstruction (p. 282). Technical difficulties involving introduction of the catheter may occur, but its attempted insertion remains the first choice for supravesical urinary diversion in the obstructed, acutely ill, uraemic patient.

Cutaneous Pyelostomy: Cutaneous pyelostomy implies a direct anastomosis of the renal pelvis to the skin. Its application is useful in the infant with a large hydronephrosis secondary to lower tract obstruction (p. 274, p. 326) as the first step in a staged urinary tract reconstruction.

The procedure is simple, safe and rapid and reduces the risks of infection and calculus formation resulting from nephrostomy tubes. Since the infant will wear diapers in the neonatal period it is no problem for the parents to simply place the diapers around the flank, to collect the urine from each cutaneous pyelostomy site, rather than the more usual perineal location. Staged reconstruction can then be delayed until the child's general health has improved and age has improved the reconstruction technical success rate. The procedure is easily reversible.

Loop Cutaneous Ureterostomy: If the renal pelvis is not large enough to reach the skin without tension then the most proximal loop of ureter can be brought to the skin and anastomosed in an elliptical fashion leaving the medial border of the ureter intact. One must be certain that a pelvi-ureteric junction obstruction is not present. The operation has the same advantages as a cutaneous pyelostomy but has the disadvantage that the ureteral blood supply can be embarrassed. Modification of this technique with a Y-ureterostomy, or circle ureterostomy techniques, have been enjoying increasing popularity because of their easy reversibility and lessened risk to the ureteral blood supply. Occasionally it is preferable to insert a proximal *in situ* diverting silastic tube temporarily if the ureter is considerably dilated and operative speed is essential.

Lower Urinary Tract Diversion

Temporary forms of lower urinary tract diversion are commonly used (p. 233) but, in frail elderly patients, the catheter may need to be permanent.

Urethral Catheters

The development of silicone Foley urethral catheters (p. 234) has reduced the complications of infection, stricture and diverticular formation but urethral damage is an inevitable complication of long term implacement (p. 252). Frequent changes of appropriate sized catheters and twice-daily 1 in 400 aqueous hibitane cleansing of the external urinary meatus reduces the risks of such complications.

Recent experiences with intermittent self-catheterisation, especially by female patients, makes this an attractive alternative to either a permanent indwelling Foley catheter or a suprapubic tube. The writer has patients who have practised intermittent self-catheterisation for years, with stable upper tracts and negative urine cultures. This procedure requires a cooperative, dexterous patient, as the bladder must be emptied a minimum of 3 times a day.

Suprapubic Cystostomy

This involves inserting a small Supracath (p. 240) catheter for temporary drainage or a large gauge catheter, for long term drainage, directly into the bladder, extraperitoneally, through a small incision in the lower abdomen. Long term suprapubic cystostomy avoids the risk of urethral stricture formation but is not free from the complications of infection and calculus formation. Leakage of urine can occur around the catheter and there is an eventual progression towards a fibrosed small capacity bladder. Weekly irrigation with 0.25% acetic acid or 10% 'Renacidin'[1] may decrease the likelihood of calculus formation, whilst long term suppressive oral antibiotics such as co-trimoxazole and nitrofurantoin can decrease infective complications.

1 'Renacidin' (Guardian)

Cutaneous Vesicostomy

In patients where intermittent catheterisation is not possible and where the diversion is likely to be permanent a tubeless form is advisable. As discussed earlier a cutaneous vesicostomy may be the procedure of choice (Lapides et al., 1960) in children or adults with very large bladders and relatively normal upper tracts. The bladder is sewn directly to the lower abdominal wall, utilising various flap techniques to prevent stenosis. An external urinary collecting device or diapers are placed over the 'stoma'.

The incidence of infection and calculus formation is much lower than that resulting from tubed forms of lower tract diversion. Whilst this method is used primarily as a temporary form of diversion in patients being considered for later reconstruction, it may act as a permanent form of diversion, particularly in selected cases of neurogenic bladder.

Perineal Urethrostomy

Suturing the perineal urethra to the skin may be an ideal operation for patients with gross urethral stricture disease (p. 253) or in those patients who have experienced multiple failed urethroplasty operations. It is often used as a temporary diversion for staged urethral reconstruction.

All attempted permanent methods of lower urinary tract diversion may be unsuccessful and require conversion to one of the previously described upper tract methods.

References

Bricker, E.M.: Bladder substitution after pelvic evisceration. Surgical Clinics of North America 30: 1511 (1950).

Coffey, R.C.: Physiologic implantation of the severed ureter or common bile duct into the intestine. Journal of the American Medical Association 56: 397 (1911).

Gersuny, R.: Case Reports. Royal Society of Physicians of Vienna. Zentralblatt fur Chirurgie 26: 497 (1889).

Gibbons, R.P.; Correa, R.J.; Cummings, K.B. and Mason, J.T.: Experience with indwelling ureteral stent catheters. Journal of Urology 115: 22 (1976).

Goodwin, W.E.: Complications of ureterosigmoidostomy; in Smith and Skinner (Eds) Complications of Urologic Surgery: Prevention and Management, p.229 (Saunders, Philadelphia 1976).

Goodwin, W.E.; Harris, A.P.; Kaufman, J.J. and Beal, J.M.: Open transcolonic ureteral intestinal anastomosis. Surgery, Gynecology and Obstetrics 97: 295 (1953).

Hendren, W.H.: Urinary tract refunctionalisation after prior diversion in children. Annals of Surgery 180: 494 (1974).

Lapides, J.; Agemian, E.P. and Lichtwardt, J.R.: Cutaneous vesicostomy. Journal of Urology 84: 609 (1960).

Leadbetter, W.F.: Consideration of problems incidence to the performance of ureteroenterostomy: report of a technique. Journal of Urology 65: 818 (1951).

Magnus, R.V.: Pressure studies and dynamics of ileal conduits in children. Journal of Urology 118: 406 (1977).

Mogg, R.A.: Treatment of neurogenic urinary incontinence using the colonic conduit. British Journal of Urology 37: 681 (1965).

Ritchie, J.P.; Skinner, D.G. and Waisman, J.: The effect of reflux in the development of pyelonephritis in urinary diversion; an experimental study. Journal of Surgical Research 16: 256 (1974).

Simon, J.: Ectopia vesicae: operation for directing the orifices of the ureter into the rectum. Lancet 2: 568 (1852).

Further Reading

Zincke, H. and Segura, J.W.: Ureterosigmoidostomy: critical review of 173 cases. Journal of Urology 113: 324 (1975).

Chapter IX

Urinary Calculi

Almost all calculi are composed of urinary waste products such as calcium oxalate, ammonium magnesium phosphate or uric acid; less than 0.1% contain, in addition, constituents such as haematin, fibrin, bilirubin and sulphonamide. As the vast majority of calculi contain calcium they are radio-opaque, to a degree dependent upon the percentage of calcium present.

Many urinary waste products are poorly soluble in water but some are present in urinary concentrations which double or quadruple their water solubility product. This enhanced solubility is due to the presence of 'solubility factors' secreted by the kidney. Minor changes in the concentrations of these waste products and/or a reduction of the solubility factors may result in crystal precipitation. It is therefore not surprising that calculi are very common. Unfortunately drug addiction is increasing and must always be suspected if a history of renal colic is not supported by accompanying radiological evidence.

Clinical Types of Calculus

Primary Metabolic Calculi

Primary metabolic calculi are very common and are usually less than 1cm in diameter. They consist of the normal urinary waste products and are usually not infected. They develop in the kidney, but in less affluent countries possibly because of an inadequate diet, may develop in the bladder (Valyasevi et al., 1967).

Very large primary renal calculi, occupying all of the renal pelvis and most of the calyces, are termed staghorn calculi, and consist mostly of calcium and ammonium magnesium phosphate. They are always infected, usually with proteus organisms.

Secondary Calculi

Secondary calculi result from mechanical or functional distal obstruction and are commonly found in the bladder (p. 245).

Composition

The composition and appearance of the types of calculus are shown in table I.

Table I. Major composition and appearance of commonly found calculi. Cystine and xanthine calculi are extremely rare

Composition	Appearance	Incidence (%)
Calcium oxalate	Hard, sharp, irregular	78
Calcium ammonium magnesium phosphate	Crumbling, rough, irregular	15
Uric acid	Hard, smooth or irregular	7

Aetiology of Renal Calculi

Urinary crystallisation may occur idiopathically or, because of greater saturation, damaged or abnormal urothelium and/or alteration in the urinary pH levels (Hodgkinson and Nordin, 1969).

Greater Saturation

Conditions of greater saturation, leading to urinary crystallisation, can arise from an increase in metabolic waste products (Harrison and Rose, 1974), dehydration or stasis.

Increased Metabolic Waste Products: Types of metabolic waste product increase liable to lead to calculus formation are shown in table II.

Dehydration: By altering urinary saturation characteristics dehydration increases the risk of calculus formation.

Stasis: Congenital abnormalities of the kidney, such as medullary sponge kidney and pelvi-ureteric mechanical or functional obstruction, together with acquired causes, such as prostatomegaly, urethral strictures, and fibrosis resulting from pyelonephritis, papillary necrosis or trauma, may create stasis and consequent infection which will aid crystallisation.

Table II. Types of increase in metabolic waste products leading to greater urinary saturation with an increased risk of calculus formation

1. Hypercalcaemia
   Idiopathic (30 % of cases)
   Primary hyperparathyroidism (2 % of cases)
   Dietary excess — particularly milk
   Prolonged immobilisation
   Secondary carcinomatosis
   Multiple myeloma
   Hypervitaminosis D
   Sarcoidosis
   Renal tubular acidosis — bone demineralisation

2. Hyperuricaemia (7 % of cases)

3. pH changes — infective alkalosis, generalised acidosis or hyperchloraemic acidosis resulting idiopathically, from urinary diversion operation, or congenital renal tubular acidosis

4. Oxaluria — rare

5. Cystinuria — rarely severe enough to form calculi

6. Xanthinuria — extremely rare

Renal lymphatic obstruction: Randall (1937) and Carr (1969) described various plaques and concentrations occurring within the calyceal region of many kidneys routinely examined both radiologically and at post-mortem. They postulated that (fig. 152):

1) The lymphatics of the kidney ended in a direct relationship with the calyceal fornices.
2) A considerable amount of calcified material was removed from this area by the lymphatics
3) Obstruction of these lymphatics due to congenital, inflammatory or excessive overload conditions could result in the formation of a calcified nucleus which could grow by progressive precipitation.

152 The formation of urinary calculi. A diagrammatic illustration of Randal and Carr's lymphatic obstruction theory (see text) of the formation of primary renal calculi.

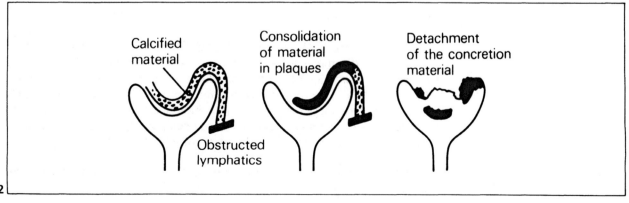

152

Damaged or Abnormal Epithelium

The following epithelial-related changes may lead to calculus formation:
1) Irregular areas of epithelium (from the abnormalities described on p. 208), may encourage precipitation.
2) Loss of solubility factor secretion, which may be related to vitamin A deficiency.
3) All calculi have an organic matrix and extensive research is at present being conducted into the formation of this matrix, as it undoubtedly plays some role in calculus formation, perhaps by providing a suitable primary nucleus which encourages peripheral crystallisation and calculus growth. Certain epithelia may produce excessive amounts of such matrix (Boyce et al., 1962).

Urinary pH

As can be seen in figure 153 the solubility of various urinary waste products, other than oxalate, is influenced by the urinary pH. Organisms, such as Proteus, which can split urea and so produce an alkaline urine, greatly aid the desposition of calcium ammonium magnesium phosphate, while renal tubular acidosis (p. 45), by preventing renal distal tubular cells from exchanging hydrogen for sodium and potassium ions, also creates a similar situation by preventing the urinary pH from falling below 6. The resultant acidosis causes bone demineralisation and an excessive release of bone calcium, which often results in the formation of a very large urinary calculus. By contrast, uric acid, cystine and xanthine calculi precipitate much more readily in an acidic urine.

Diagnosis of Urinary Calculi

Although symptoms and signs are common, 25% of patients with urinary calculi are asymptomatic. Bilateral calculi occur in 15% of patients and males form calculi slightly more commonly than females.

Signs and Symptoms

Renal and Ureteric Signs and Symptoms: Renal and ureteric pain, haematuria and fever are common, with frequent urgent micturition occurring as the calculus approaches the uretero-vesical junction (fig. 154). Acute renal and ureteric colic produces an agonising, gripping pain, intermittently radiating from the loin to the groin, testicle or labia, with a constant, lesser, background colic. Smaller calculi, which can be gripped more firmly by the smooth muscle contraction, usually produce greater pain than larger calculi. Severe colic is associated with nausea, vomiting and shock, and may be difficult to separate clinically from acute abdominal, myocardial or pulmonary disasters.

Renal calculi can also produce an intermittent or constant aching pain in the lumbar region. The pain is usually exacerbated by renal palpation but is often difficult to distinguish from non-renal, musculo-skeletal back pain which usually does not radiate anteriorly. Musculo-skeletal pain is usually exacerbated by physical exercise and/or postural movements.

Bladder and Urethral Symptoms and Signs: Aching supra-pubic or perineal pain, often exacerbated by movement or voiding, with associated frequency and urgency of micturition, due to a secondary infected or non-infected cystitis, are common symptoms. Large calculi can often be palpated during a rectal or bimanual examination and pain may be experienced in these areas during such a procedure. Calculi passing through the urethra may cause retention of urine if they are sufficiently large.

Investigation

Urine Microscopy: Mid-stream urine specimen microscopy and culture may reveal red and white cells, crystals and infection.

153 The influence of the urinary pH on the solubility of various urinary waste products.

154 Renal and ureteric colic symptoms and signs.

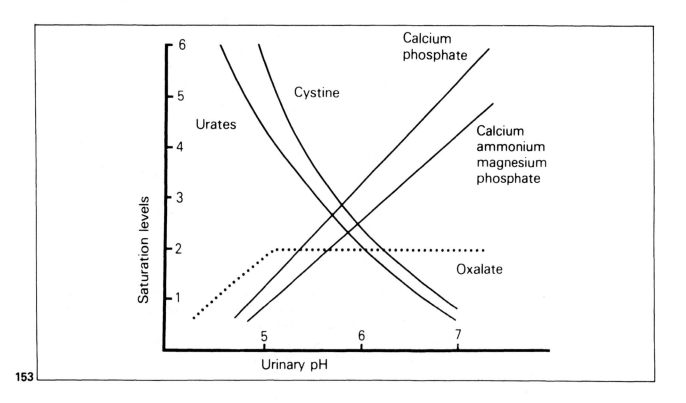

Calcium phosphate

Cystine

Urates

Saturation levels

Calcium ammonium magnesium phosphate

Oxalate

Urinary pH

153

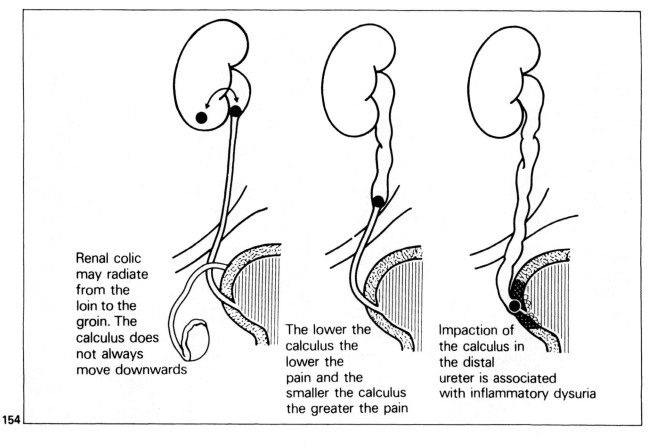

Renal colic may radiate from the loin to the groin. The calculus does not always move downwards

The lower the calculus the lower the pain and the smaller the calculus the greater the pain

Impaction of the calculus in the distal ureter is associated with inflammatory dysuria

154

Radiological: An intravenous pyelogram usually confirms the diagnosis of a calculus (figs. 155-157). As 95% of urinary calculi contain some calcium they are commonly detected in the initial plain abdominal and pelvic x-ray, unless they are superimposed upon bone shadows, obscured by bowel gas, very small, faintly calcified, or the x-ray is of poor quality. Pelvic vessel wall calcifications (phleboliths) are usually multiple, outside the line of the ureter, and have a translucent centre. Should a calcified density suggestive of a calculus be seen in a straight abdominal and pelvic x-ray then it must be distinguished from other calcified elements, such as mesenteric glands in the abdomen and phleboliths in the pelvis, either by:

1) Taking a lateral x-ray and proving that the calculus is anatomically in the line of the kidney or ureter, or
2) Displaying it, in the injection phase of the pyelogram, as being within the lumen of the system, or
3) Displaying it as a constant filling defect in the case of a non-opaque calculus.

A renal pelvic, ureteric or bladder neoplasm may also appear as a constant, non-opaque filling defect and, despite estimates of serum uric acid levels and urinary cytology examinations, the true diagnosis may only be made by surgical exploration.

Cysto-urethroscopy: Not all bladder and urethral calculi are radio-opaque, nor are they revealed as a filling defect in the cystogram phase of the intravenous pyelogram. Cysto-urethroscopy occasionally results in the detection of such calculi during the investigation of patients presenting with haematuria, urinary tract infection and/or dysuria.

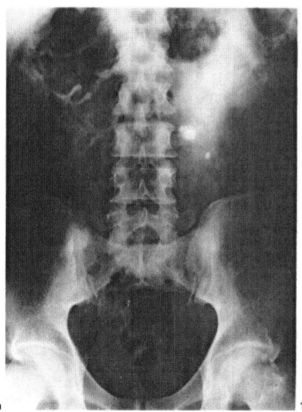

155a

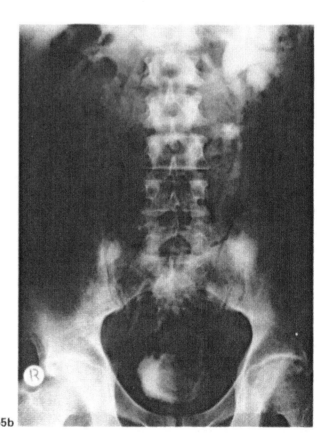

155b

**Further
Investigation of
Primary Renal
Calculi**

Despite proven aetiological factors it is not possible to determine a precise cause of renal calculus formation in at least 85% of patients. Further investigations should however be carried out on all patients with recurrent or multiple calculi and all patients initially presenting with a calculus larger than 1cm as this group has a higher percentage of detectable, and sometimes curable aetiological factors. In addition to a thorough history (it is surprising how many patients drink very large quantities of milk) and physical examination (rarely a parathyroid tumour may be found) these further special investigations include:

1) Mid-stream urine specimen microscopy, chemistry, pH and culture
2) Serum creatinine, urea and electrolyte levels (fasting venous blood specimen)
3) Serum calcium, phosphate, alkaline phosphatase, uric acid and protein levels (fasting venous blood specimen)
4) 24-hour urinary calcium and creatinine excretion and pH
5) Analysis of all calculi passed or surgically removed.

Diagnosis of opaque renal or ureteric calculi by intravenous pyelography.
155a A 50-year-old man presented with left renal colic. A straight abdominal and pelvic x-ray reveals 2 calcifications in this area.

155b An intravenous pyelogram demonstrates that the lateral calcification is within the lumen of the upper ureter whilst the medial calcification, a mesenteric lymph node, is not.

156a A 45-year-old woman presented with right renal colic. The straight abdominal and pelvic x-ray discloses a faint calcification in the line of the right pelvic ureter.

156b An intravenous pyelogram demonstrates a ureteric calculus.

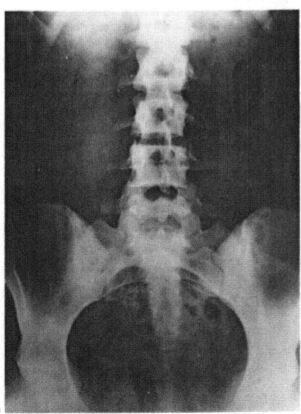
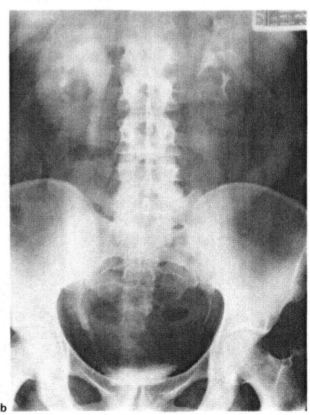

156a   156b

Expensive and detailed investigations, such as urinary oxalate and cystine excretion levels, cannot be routinely justified and are only performed in selected cases.

The findings in 212 patients with primary recurrent renal calculi from the author's practice are shown in table III.

Fate of a Formed Urinary Calculus

The possible fates of formed primary renal calculi are shown in figure 158.

Table III. Findings on further investigation of 212 patients with primary recurrent renal calculi

Finding	Number of patients
No abnormality	90
Idiopathic hypercalciuria	75
Urinary tract infection	22
Hyperuricaemia	12
Medullary sponge kidney	5
Urinary diversion operation	4
Primary hyperparathyroidism	2
Congenital oxalura	1
Cystinuria	1

Intravenous pyelography (continued)

157a A 30-year-old woman presented with left renal colic. A straight abdominal and pelvic x-ray reveals a dilated loop of bowel in the region of the left kidney but no other abnormality.

157b An intravenous pyelogram discloses 2 filling defects within the left pelvi-calyceal system, which appear to be uric acid calculi, but could be neoplasms.

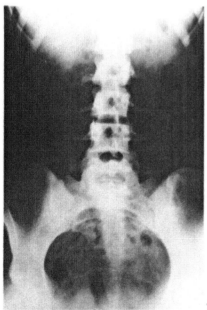

157a

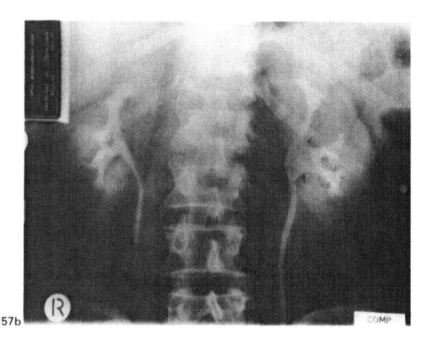

157b

158 Possible fates of a formed primary renal calculus.

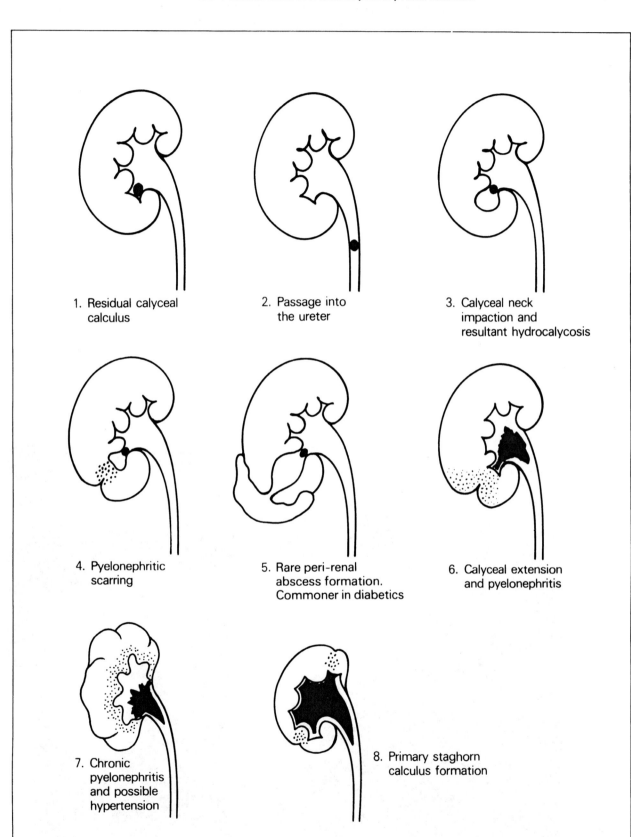

1. Residual calyceal calculus

2. Passage into the ureter

3. Calyceal neck impaction and resultant hydrocalycosis

4. Pyelonephritic scarring

5. Rare peri-renal abscess formation. Commoner in diabetics

6. Calyceal extension and pyelonephritis

7. Chronic pyelonephritis and possible hypertension

8. Primary staghorn calculus formation

Renal Calculi

Parenchymal calculi: (figs. 159-160) or more commonly, calcification, may result from acquired infection, congenital medullary sponge kidney, or renal tubular acidosis, as previously described.

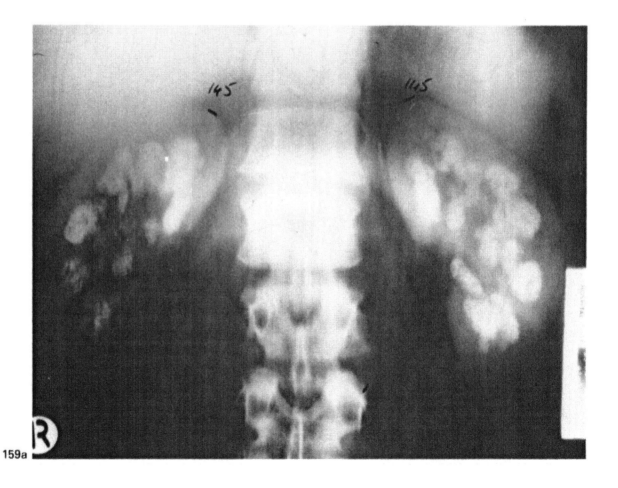

159a

Renal parenchymal calculi

159a This 40-year-old man presented with a 2-year history of aching lumbar pain and one episode of right renal colic. The straight renal x-ray tomogram reveals multiple parenchymal calcification due to medullary sponge kidneys.

159b An intravenous pyelogram reveals good renal function.

160 Multiple parenchymal and calyceal calculi resulting from primary hyperparathyroidism.

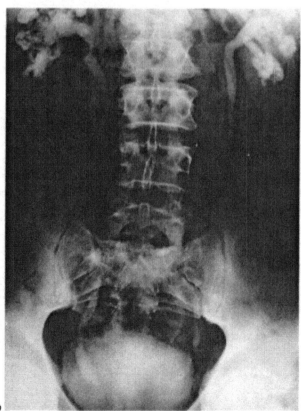

159b

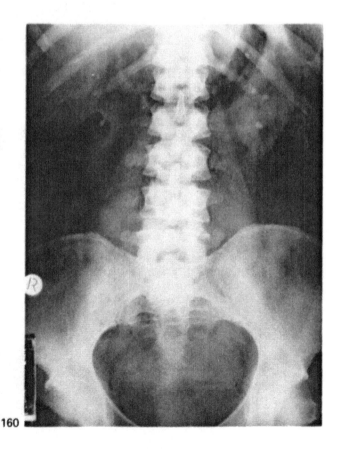

160

Calyceal calculi: (figs. 161-162) are very common. They may:

1) Remain *in situ* without increasing in size
2) Pass into the renal pelvis or ureter and then either spontaneously pass or remain in the new position (fig. 162)
3) Increase in size and extend into the pelvis (fig. 163).
   Obstruction or infection may result in progressive renal destruction and, rarely, hypertension (chap. XVII)
4) Obstruct the calyceal neck, resulting in a hydrocalycosis or pyocalycosis with associated renal cortical scarring (fig. 163)
5) Cause extreme calyceal neck obstruction and associated infection, resulting in the formation of a peri-renal abscess or, extremely rarely, a granulomatous inflammatory renal reaction described as xantho-granulomatous pyelonephritis (Hatch and Cockett, 1964). Xantho-granulomatous pyelonephritis is discussed further on page 136.

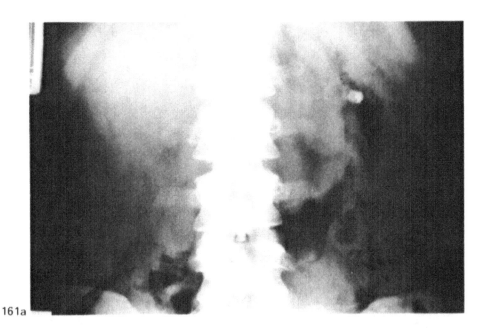

161a

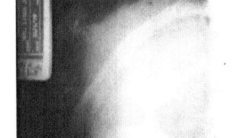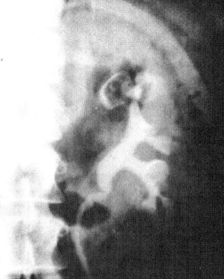

161b

Calyceal calculi

161a A 35-year-old woman presented with left renal colic. A straight renal x-ray indicates a possible left calyceal calculus.

161b The intravenous pyelogram reveals that the calculus is impacted at the neck of an upper major calyx, obstructing 2 minor calyces. The calculus was removed through a cortical scar.

162 Calyceal calculi may pass into the renal pelvis and continue to grow. Open surgical extraction of all the calculi, and sterilisation of the kidney, is necessary in order to prevent recurrence. A rounded pelvic calculus may indicate a primary pelvi-ureteric hydronephrosis.

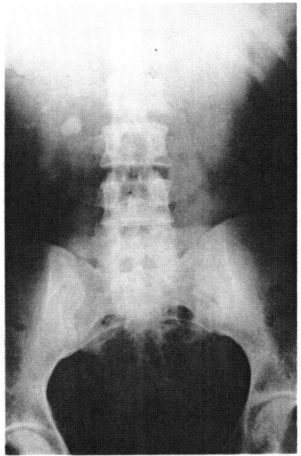

162

Ureteric Calculi

Almost all ureteric calculi (fig. 164) are derived from the kidney, except those resulting from gross ureteric obstruction such as a megaureter (p. 10, 328).

Most calculi which enter the ureter are of sufficiently small size to pass spontaneously into the bladder without resultant renal damage (Brown, 1979) but surgical removal may be necessary if they remain impacted and cause continued pain (Williams, 1963).

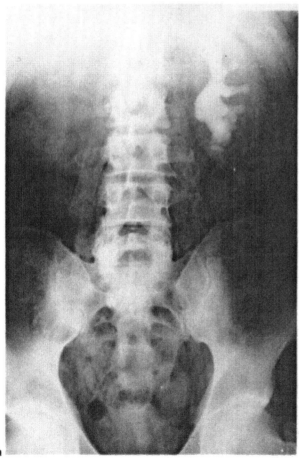
163a

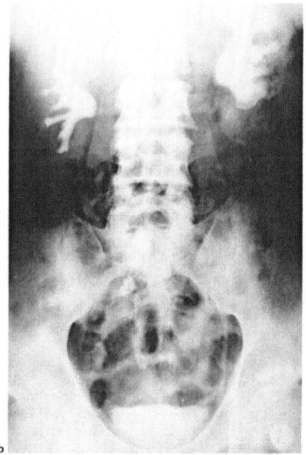
163b

Staghorn calculus

163a A proteus infected staghorn calculus occupying all of the renal pelvis and most of the calyces.

163b An intravenous pyelogram study reveals a poorly functioning left kidney and a normal right system. An uneventful removal of the staghorn calculus was performed.

Small ureteric calculus

164a A 30-year-old man presented with severe right renal colic. A straight abdominal and pelvic x-ray discloses some calcifications in the pelvis but no other abnormality.

164b An intravenous pyelogram confirms the diagnosis of an impacted renal calculus in the lower aspect of the right ureter and also indicates which of the pelvic calcifications is the calculus.

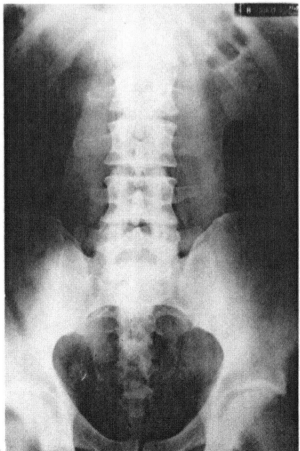

164a

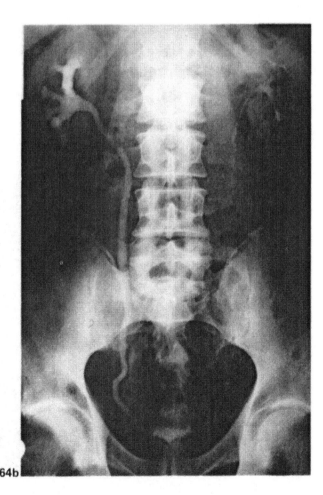

164b

Bladder Calculi

Because most bladder calculi are secondary to mechanical or functional obstruction they will increase in size or number unless surgically removed (fig. 165). The primary obstructive cause must be corrected at the same time.

Prostatic Calculi

Prostatic calculi are asymptomatic and do not require specific treatment. They result from recurrent prostatitis which may require treatment (p. 140). Because of their digital movement, multiplicity and x-ray appearance (fig. 166) they should not be confused with areas of prostatic carcinoma.

Urethral Calculi

Most urethral calculi have formed elsewhere and are passing through the urethra (fig. 167) but true urethral calculi can result from urethral stricturing and associated inflammation-infection.

Management of Urinary Calculi

Small, single, non-infected calcium oxalate renal calyceal calculi are very common. They do not usually cause sufficient symptoms to justify attempted surgical removal unless, as previously indicated, they pass into the calyceal neck, pelvis or ureter and remain impacted (fig. 161b). Bladder and urethral calculi require surgical removal but prostatic calculi do not require any specific treatment.

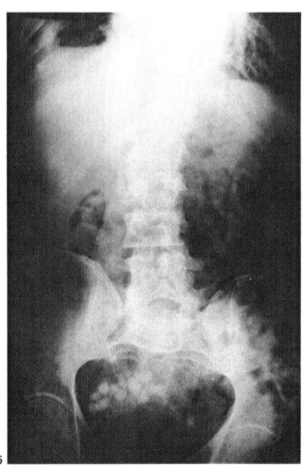

165

165 Secondary multiple bladder calculi. Note the elevation of the bladder base due to the primary prostatic enlargement.

166 Infective prostatic calculi. Note the congenital sacral agenesis.

167 A secondary bladder calculus impacted in the urethra. Open surgical extraction was necessary.

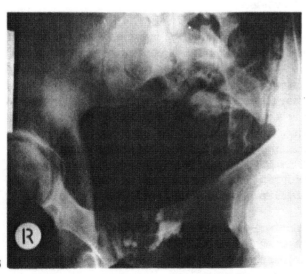

166

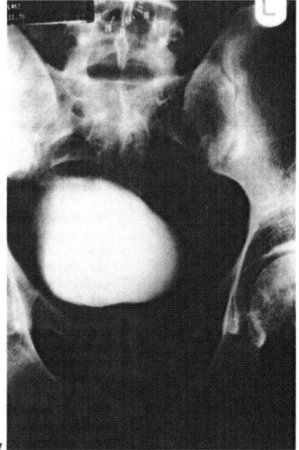

167

Non-surgical
Management

Relief of Pain: Severe renal colic may require 10 to 20mg of omnopon or 50 to 100mg of pethidine intravenously or intramuscularly every 1 to 6 hours, dependent upon the severity of the pain and the patient's body build and temperament. Such high dose analgesic therapy should only be given after excluding the possibility of an acute abdomen and drug addiction. A patient suffering from acute renal colic never has a completely normal intravenous pyelogram, and this investigation, in a limited form, may be necessary to establish the diagnosis.

Preventing Calculi from Increasing in Size or Recurring. *General measures:* Should the previous investigations indicate that a specific aetiological factor is present then, if possible, it should be corrected. This particularly applies to mechanical and functional obstructive causes, excessive milk in the diet, hyperparathyroidism and a fluid intake of less than 3,500ml/day. A high bland fluid intake may be the only therapy necessary for many patients with recurrent uric acid or cystine calculi.

Specific measures require careful medical supervision and full patient cooperation.

Calcium: A calcium diet of less than 260mg/day does reduce urinary calcium levels but increases urinary oxalate levels. This situation can be managed by controlling the dietary oxalate and avoiding grapefruit, orange and cranberry juice, tea and beer. A low calcium-low oxalate diet is well tolerated by most patients. A high phosphate intake (1.5g of phosphorous per 24 hours) is often of value as it reduces hypercalciuria, decreases intestinal absorption of calcium and enhances the urinary excretion of 'solubility factors' (Cordonnier and Talbot, 1948) provided that the dose is kept at a level at which vascular and tissue calcification will not occur. A starting dose of 500mg of orthophosphate sodium 3 times a day is usually sufficient but may be increased in selected patients. Diarrhoea and dyspepsia may necessitate dose reduction. A low phosphate diet is of little value. It may reduce the urinary phosphate but it usually increases the urinary calcium. Hydrochlorothiazide, 50mg twice daily, reduces calcium excretion but increases magnesium and potassium excretion. It is of value in some patients but potassium replacement tablets may be necessary. Hyperuricaemia and an increased resistance to insulin may also occur.

Oxalate: Chocolate, beer, rhubarb, berries, prunes and spinach are high in oxalate content and best avoided.

Phosphate: Any urinary tract infection must be vigorously treated and the urine regularly examined for asymptomatic infection. In patients without idiopathic hypercalciuria a low phosphate diet (no milk, cheese or ice-cream and minimal bread, chocolate and nuts) together with aluminium hydroxide gel (45ml 4 times daily) may reduce the urinary phosphate excretion level to less than 250mg per day and thereby assist in reducing the chances of recurrent calculus formation. Acidification of the urine (aluminium chloride in doses resulting in a urinary pH below 5.4) may also be of value (fig. 153). Methylene blue, 65mg 3 times a day, which may interfere with the matrix-crystallisation process (Boyce, 1962) is occasionally of value in preventing the recurrence of both calcium phosphate and calcium oxalate calculi.

Uric acid: Allopurinol, a xanthine oxidase inhibitor, reduces the urinary urate excretion level and, in doses of 200 to 600mg/day, has been proven to be most effective in reducing recurrent uric acid calculus formation. Urinary alkalinisation (5-15g/day of sodium bicarbonate and the avoidance of conditions conducive to a low urinary pH, such as dehydration) is of considerable value in those who form recurrent uric acid calculi, as is the avoidance of a high protein (producing an acid urine) and a high purine (producing an increased urinary urate) diet, although a low purine diet is usually not acceptable to patients. The intense use of allopurinol, a high fluid intake and heavy alkalinisation may be sufficient to dissolve formed calculi.

Cystine: These extremely rare calculi are effectively dissolved by D-penicillamine (2-4g/day) which combines with cystine to form a disulphide which is 50 times more soluble than cystine itself. The precise dose of D-penicillamine can be titrated against the urinary cystine levels. Alkalinisation of the urine, together with a high fluid intake is also essential.

Xanthine: These extremely rare calculi result from heritable absence of the enzyme xanthine oxidase. Xanthine is the least soluble of all the purines. The calculi are treated by a combination of low purine diet, high fluid intake and alkalinisation.

Many calculi pass spontaneously and cause no harm other than temporary pain. The probable and possible indications for surgical removal of a calculus are discussed below.

Surgical Management

Severe constant pain provides the common indication for most operations but, in many situations, several factors must be considered before advising operative or conservative management.

Indications for Surgery. *Symptoms:* Severe continuing pain is the most usual reason for advising attempted operative removal.

Total renal function: The total renal function greatly influences the decision to operate. Most staghorn calculi destroy kidneys and should be removed on diagnosis (Brown, 1978).

Infection: The presence of infection in an obstructed system is an indication for early corrective surgery.

Site: Large calculi, particularly those situated in the renal pelvis or upper ureter, are usually not difficult to remove by open surgery but small calculi, situated deep within a calyx, provide a technical challenge. Small calculi in the lower ureter usually pass spontaneously, as indicated earlier, but should the patient's symptoms dictate removal then an attempted endoscopic extraction is performed.

Related abnormalities: A pelvi-ureteric obstruction may require a pyeloplasty, in addition to a pyelolithotomy, whilst a prostatic obstruction requires a prostatectomy in addition to open or closed removal of any associated bladder calculi.

Degree of obstruction: A gross hydroureter or hydronephrosis requires early surgical relief.

Past history: There is less indication to perform an early operation on a patient with a past history of a previous spontaneous calculus expulsion providing the calculus is small.

Pregnancy: Almost all surgery is inadvisable in the first 3 months of pregnancy and open pelvic surgery is extremely difficult in the last 3 months of pregnancy.

Socio-economic: It is often preferable to surgically remove relatively asymptomatic, non-infected, moderately obstructive calculi, from patients who live hundreds of miles from medical assistance or in whom persistent symptoms are preventing them from financially supporting their families.

Age: Endoscopic calculus extractions in children are rarely necessary.

Sex: Females spontaneously extrude calculi more easily than males.

Surgical Considerations: *Renal calculus surgery:* Pyrah (1979) has written on the special considerations applicable to renal calculus surgery. These include an immediate preoperative x-ray to check that the calculus has not moved, complete removal of the calculus and grossly diseased renal tissue, intra-renal and calculus swab cultures, and adequate operative and postoperative chemotherapy. In addition postoperative chemical analysis of the calculus should be done so that the patient can be given appropriate advice on diet, drugs and fluid intake.

Staghorn calculi: Staghorn calculi (fig. 163a) present a particular problem but, unless the patient is grossly uraemic or unfit for surgery, attempted open removal of the calculus should be undertaken as the mortality and morbidity of non-surgical intervention are high (Singh et al., 1971) and the results of surgery are good (Maddern, 1967; Boyce and Elkins, 1974).

Brown (1978), using Gil-Vernet's (1965) technique, has shown that, provided no stone fragments greater than 1cm in area are left *in situ* and that postoperative sterilisation of the urine is achieved, the recurrence rate is very low.

In highly selected situations it is possible to dissolve staghorn calculi with fluid introduced via a percutaneous nephrostomy tube (Dretler, 1979).

Ureteric calculus surgery: Calculi impacted in the ureter can be removed by an open, extra-peritoneal, ureterolithotomy operation or, if they are less than 0.6cm in size and situated in the lower third of the ureter, removed with an endoscopic stone basket (fig. 168).

In addition to respecting the relevant technical surgical requirements necessary for renal calculus surgery ureterolithotomy operations also require early, gentle and adequate proximal and distal ureteric control, prior to removal of the calculus, so that it is not dislodged back into the kidney or further down the ureter.

168 A Dormier stone basket, with a filiform tip. The basket is gently passed beyond the calculus, the wires opened as shown, and the instrument withdrawn, entrapping and removing the calculus.

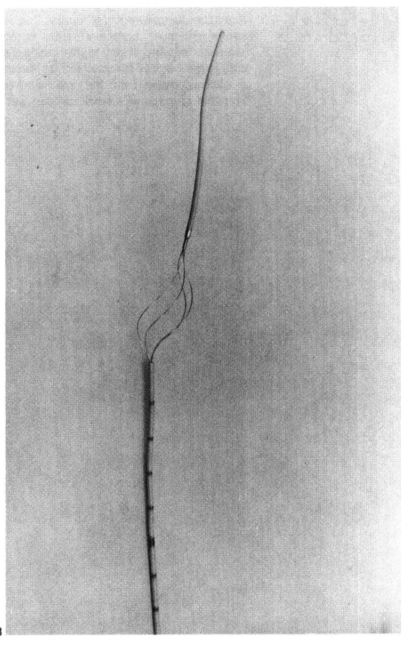

168

Bladder and urethral calculus surgery: As indicated almost all bladder and urethral calculi are secondary to obstruction in this area and therefore usually require open or closed surgical removal in association with open or closed correction of the primary obstructive cause (fig. 167).

Vesical calculi can be crushed, using a visualising lithotrite, and the fragments washed from the bladder or, if very large and very hard, removed by open suprapubic cystostomy. Cysto-urethroscopic extraction and/or irrigation removal is commonly used for multiple small calculi. Ultrasonic litholapaxy has recently been employed.

Parathyroid surgery: This may be required if hyperparathyroidism has been proven. Such surgery requires identification of all 4 parathyroid glands, by dissection along the superior and inferior thyroid arteries, and identification of all suspected adenoma tissue by frozen section histology. Rarely parathyroid adenoma are located infrasternally.

Spontaneous rupture of the kidney: This is rare (fig. 169) and presents with severe renal colic, combined with a higher than usual level of background loin pain, requiring heavy regular analgesic therapy. The renal 'rupture' occurs at the calyceal fornices and, as illustrated in figure 169b, extravasation of contrast media from the renal hilum is seen. The condition may result from the passage of a small calculus but usually this is not proven.

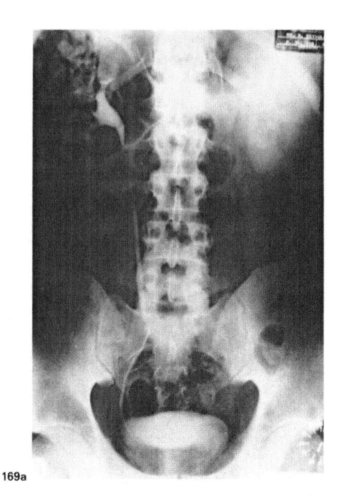

169a

Spontaneous rupture of the kidney

169a A 28-year-old man presented with severe left renal colic and a high level of persistent background loin pain. No calculus was seen on a straight x-ray but the intravenous pyelogram displayed a grossly obstructed left nephrogram with urinary extravasation.

169b A later film shows the extravasation appearing from the renal hilum. No detectable calculus was passed or identified. High dose analgesic therapy was necessary for 48 hours before the pain resolved.

169c Two months later the patient had a normal pyelogram.

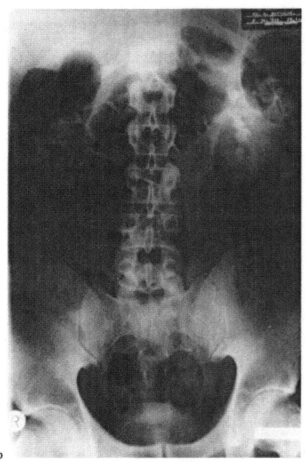

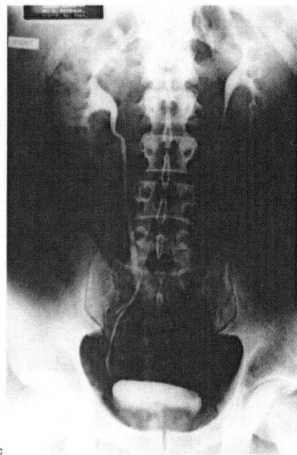

169b

169c

References

Boyce, W.H. and Elkins, I.B.: Reconstructive renal surgery following anatrophic nephrolithotomy: follow-up of 100 consecutive cases. Journal of Urology 111: 307 (1974).

Boyce, W.H.; King, J.S. and Fielden, M.C.: Total non-dialysable solids in human urine, XIII. Immunological detection of a component peculiar to renal calculus matrix and to the urine of calculus patients. Journal of Clinical Investigation 41: 1180 (1962).

Brown, R.B.: The 5-year fate of 57 attempted conservative staghorn calculus operations. British Journal of Urology 51: 61 (1978).

Brown, R.B.: A cost analysis study of the management of lower ureteric calculi. British Journal of Urology 51: 420 (1979).

Carr, R.J.: Aetiology of renal calculi: micro-radiographic studies. Renal stone research symposium (Churchill, London 1969).

Cordonnier, J.J. and Talbot, B.S.: The effect of the ingestion of sodium and phosphate on urinary calcium in recumbency. Journal of Urology 60: 316 (1948).

Dretler, S.P.: Renal stone dissolution via percutaneous nephrostomy. New England Journal of Medicine 300: 341 (1979).

Gil-Vernet, J.M. Jr.: New surgical concepts in removing renal calculi. Urologia Internationalis 20: 255 (1965).

Harrison, A.R. and Rose, G.A.: The incidence, investigation and treatment of idiopathic hypercalciuria. British Journal of Urology 46: 261 (1974).

Hatch, L.S. and Cockett, T.K.: Xanthogranulomatous pyelonephritis. Journal of Urology 92: 585 (1964).

Maddern, J.P.: Surgery of the staghorn calculus. British Journal of Urology 39: 237 (1967).

Randall, A.: The origin and growth or renal calculi. Annals of Surgery 105: 1009 (1937).

Singh, M.; Tresidder, G.C. and Blandy, J.P.: Long-term results of removal of staghorn calculi by extended pyelolithotomy without cooling or renal artery occlusion. British Journal of Urology 43: 658 (1971).

Valyaseri, A.; Halstead, S.B. and Pantuwatana, S.: Studies of bladder stone disease in Thailand. American Journal of Clinical Nutrition 20: 1340 (1967).

Williams, R.E.: Long-term survey of 538 patients with upper urinary tract stone. British Journal of Urology 35: 416 (1963).

Further Reading

Blandy, J.P.: The management of renal calculi. Annals of the Royal College of Surgeons of England 48: 159 (1971).

Hodgkinson, A. and Nordin, B.E.C.: Renal Stone Research Symposium (Churchill Livingstone, London 1969).

Pyrah, L.N.: Renal Calculus (Springer-Verlag, Berlin 1979).

Wickham, J.E.A.: Urinary Calculus Disease, (Churchill Livingstone, London 1979).

Chapter X

Lower Urinary Tract Obstruction

Mechanical causes are responsible for the vast majority of patients developing lower urinary tract obstruction of urine, but neurological, parasympathetic drug-induced, infective or functional causes should always be suspected in a person presenting under the age of 50 years. The diagnosis and management of the neurogenic bladder is discussed in chapter XI. Because of the preponderance of prostatic, bladder outlet and urethral stricture pathology males commonly develop retention of urine, or mechanical voiding difficulty, while this is rare in females.

Obstruction of urine at or below the bladder outlet may produce varying degrees of dysuria or 1 of 4 types of retention:

1) Acute
2) Subacute
3) Chronic
4) Chronic with overflow.

Chronic retention of urine with overflow is a potentially reversible condition and must not be confused with senility.

Because of serious renal back pressure, and occasionally infective damage, patients presenting with non-neoplastic uraemic chronic retention have a 6-fold increase in morbidity and mortality compared with those presenting with non-uraemic acute and subacute retention of urine.

Aetiology

The causes of lower urinary tract obstruction of urine are listed in table I.

Obstruction in Males

Babies and Young Children: These may be born with mechanical obstructions such as phimosis, meatal stenosis, urethral stricture or diverticula, Marion's bladder neck stenosis or posterior urethral valves; acquired obstruction may arise from balanitis, with or without phimosis or paraphimosis, urethral polyps, a foreign body or, very rarely, neoplasm. Meatal ulceration, constipation, infection and neurological causes, such as spina bifida occulta, may also result in obstruction to voiding or retention of urine. These causes, and the role of distal external meatal stenosis are discussed more fully in the chapter on Paediatric Urology.

Young Males: In young males obstruction may be due to a progression of the previously discussed causes or to acquired acute prostatitis, with or without the very rare development of a prostatic abscess, or a urethral stricture. Occasionally foreign bodies are inserted into the urethra. Neurological, drug-induced and, rarely anxiety-induced obstructions may also occur in this group.

Older Males: Benign and malignant prostatomegaly and urethral strictures are the commonest cause of urinary obstruction in older males although drug-induced or neurological causes are not uncommon.

Elderly Males: In addition to the previous causes this age group may develop progressive bladder muscle and nerve degeneration with a resultant atonic bladder. Faecal impaction may also cause or precipitate urinary obstruction (p. 320).

Table I. The causes of lower urinary tract obstruction of urine

Lower urinary tract obstruction

mechanical causes	neurological causes	other causes
Phimosis	Congenital	Infection
Meatal stenosis	Spina bifida	Acute prostato-urethritis
Urethral stricture	Vascular malformations	Prostatic abscess
Posterior urethral valves	Sacral agenesis	Urethral abscess
Balantitis xerotica obliterans	Spinal cord neoplasm	Drugs
Urethral polyps	Quadri/paraplegia	Many drugs may
Foreign bodies	Non-surgical	interfere with normal
Urethral neoplasms	Surgical	nerve, nerve-muscle
Marion's disease	Metastasis	junction, and muscle
Calculi	Abscess	action
Prostatic hyperplasia	Prolapsed intervertebral disc	
Fibrous prostatitis	Subacute cord degeneration	
Prostatic neoplasm	Multiple sclerosis	Anxiety
Bladder neoplasm	Diabetes mellitus	Atonia
Retroverted gravid uterus	Tabes dorsalis	Faecal impaction
Post-obstetric trauma	Arteriosclerosis	
Postoperational trauma		

Obstruction in Females

Babies and Young Children: Rarely, females are born with severe distal external meatal stenosis or may have acquired severe vulvo-vaginitis and/or a urethral prolapse. These problems are discussed in more detail in the chapter on Paediatric Urology.

Adult Women: Obstruction of urine is uncommon but may occur through such causes as anxiety, post-obstetric or postoperative trauma, multiple sclerosis, retroverted gravid uterus or atonia.

Immediate Management

Acute or subacute retention of urine is a painful state and requires temporary bladder drainage, while the patient is investigated to determine the cause of retention and the appropriate therapy.

Chronic and chronic-overflow retention of urine represent advanced stages of obstruction and both obstructive, and often infective, damage have developed in the bladder, ureters and kidneys. Chronic over-stretching of the detrusor muscles and nerves results in a lack of pain sensation, although the bladder may contain one or more litres of urine. Bladder drainage may be required therefore, not for pain relief, but to allow the over-stretched bladder and the obstructed kidneys to recover their optimal function. It is stressed that bladder drainage is only required for gross uraemic chronic retention of urine and many patients with chronic non-uraemic retention or moderately uraemic chronic retention of urine, who are otherwise well, do not require such pre-operative drainage, which always carries the risk of introducing infections.

If bladder drainage be necessary it is continued until the renal function improves to below 20mmol of urea per litre. Such optimal renal function may necessitate many weeks of drainage, in addition to other measures designed to improve the patient's general health. Once urinary drainage is undertaken the patient may undergo a massive diuresis and careful fluid and electrolyte management during this stage is essential. Should the renal function not improve to a satisfactory level after long term bladder drainage surgical relief of the obstruction may have to be undertaken; alternatively the patient may be best advised to remain with a permanent indwelling 'tissue inert' bladder catheter (see below).

Bladder Drainage

Urethral Catheterisation

Types of Catheter: Urethral catheters are of 3 basic types (fig. 170a):
1) Non self-retaining Jaques or Nelaton catheters, originally made of metal, gum elastic or rubber, and now of soft plastic or semi-rigid silastic, which are less 'tissue irritant'. The head of the catheter contains one or more openings and was traditionally shaped (spike, coude, bi-coude) to negotiate the bend of the urethra but is now commonly rounded and blunt as this shape and consistency passes less traumatically along the urethra and is not sharp or rigid enough to create false passages. A curved tip Tiemann catheter is occasionally used if difficulty is experienced in negotiating the bend (see below). Non-self retaining catheters are used to obtain bladder urine specimens, estimate residual bladder urine, and occasionally for longer term bladder drainage (see below).

2) Self-retaining 2- and 3-way balloon Foley catheters (fig. 170b), which are used for longer term continuous bladder drainage, are also made of soft or more rigid silastic coated latex or of pure silastic. A 3-way Foley catheter

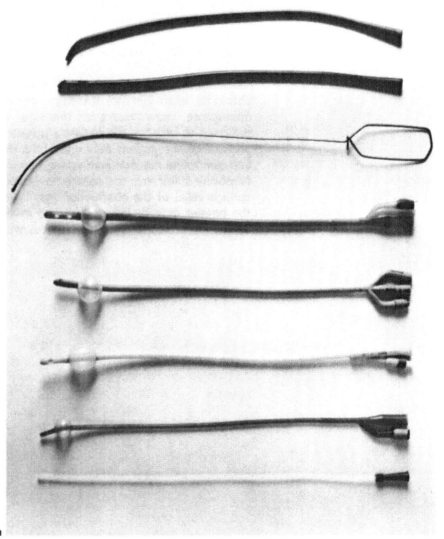

170a

Urethral catheters.

170a From below upwards: 1. Jaques or Nelaton non self-retaining catheter. 2. Self-retaining 2-way Foley silicone coated latex catheter. 3. Self-retaining 2-way Foley pure silicone coated latex catheter. 4. Self-retaining 3-way Foley silicone coated latex catheter. 5. Self-retaining 3-way Foley haematuria catheter. 6. Catheter introducer. 7. Plastic whistle tip catheter. 8. Tiemann catheter.

170b Foley and Jaques catheters. From above downwards: 1. A pure silastic 2-way Foley catheter is used for long term bladder drainage. 2. A 3-way Foley haematuria catheter is used to drain and irrigate blood and urine. 3. A 2-way silicone coated latex catheter is used to drain clear urine for a short period of time. 4. A non self-retaining Jaques or Nelaton catheter is used to obtain a bladder urine specimen and/or to estimate the bladder residual urine.

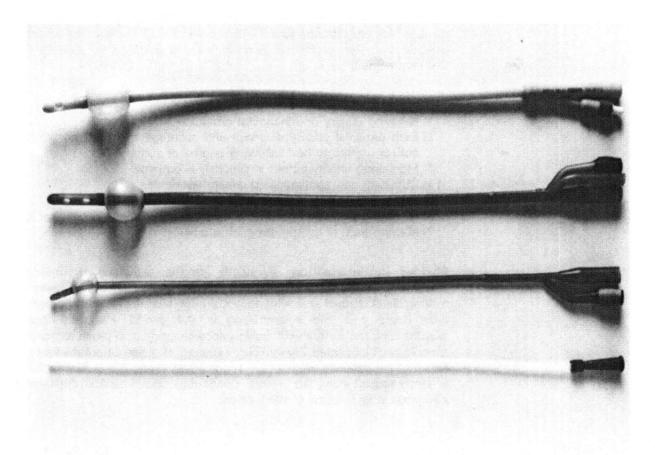

170b

has a small balloon inflator tube, incorporated in the wall, together with a second tube through which saline, or other fluid, can be introduced into the bladder, and a third tube through which the fluid and urine can be drained from the bladder. 2- and 3-way Foley catheters made completely from silicone are expensive but are the most suitable for long term bladder drainage as urine encrustation is minimal and the catheters can remain *in situ* for up to 2 months before needing replacement.

3) Postoperative prostatic or bladder surgery catheters, such as the more rigid walled 3-way catheter, which is used because of its ability to drain urine and blood and withstand intermittent manual bladder washouts (see later) until the area heals. It is important to appreciate that the drainage efficiency of these catheters depends more on the flow rate than the output tube lumen (Whitaker, 1975). A haematuria Foley catheter, with walls made rigid by the incorporation of a spiral metal thread (fig. 170c) is expensive but ideally suited for postoperative drainage, as the firmer walls permit very efficient syringe evacuation of any clot obstruction. Non self-retaining, firm walled, plastic whistle-tip wide lumen catheters, like haematuria Foley catheters, also allow blood clots to be syringed and irrigated from the bladder. (Bladder drainage should always be into a closed-system bag containing a 'bacterial trap' sufficiently large for the passage of blood stained irrigation.)

Catheter Sizes: There are 3 different size systems used. In Australia and America the Charriere or French scale is used; this is double the size of the Benique scale used in France. In England a third scale is used.

The normal adult male urethra accepts a 22 Charriere catheter or instrument, which corresponds to a 44 Benique and a 13 English. The external catheter diameter, expressed in millimetres, is obtained by dividing the Charriere number by 3.

Uses: Catheters are used for:

1) Relieving urinary or urinary clot retention
2) Both proximal urinary diversion and splintage to allow the bladder and/or urethra to heal following trauma or surgery
3) Monitoring urinary output in seriously ill patients
4) Obtaining non-contaminated urinary specimens
5) Estimating bladder residual urine
6) Managing surgically untreatable incontinence of urine (see chapter XV)
7) In cystogram or cystometrogram studies.

Bladder Catheterisation: A strictly aseptic technique is observed (Headlund, 1976). After sterilisation of the glans penis and external meatal/distal urethral area with aqueous 1:400 hibitane (alcoholic preparations cause pain and inflammation in the genital area) and locally anaethetising the urethra with sterile xylocaine, using a no touch technique, a sterile, well lubricated 2-way Foley catheter, of a size determined by the lumen of the patient's urethra (10F at age seven years, 22F in most adults), is gently passed along the urethra. Continuous closed bladder drainage is instigated after inflation of the balloon.

Urethral catheters (continued)
170c A haematuria catheter incorporates a firm metal thread in its wall, enabling efficient suction irrigation of blood clots. Note the balloon inflation tube running in the wall but not narrowing the catheter lumen.

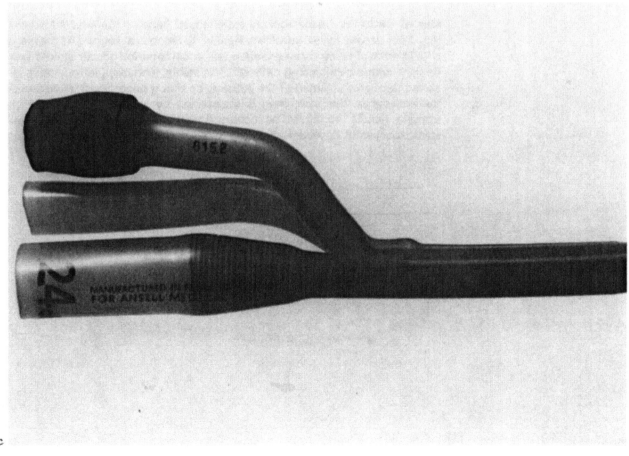

170c

In addition to using the smallest suitable catheter, to reduce the degree of initially sterile and later secondarily infected urethritis, care should be taken to avoid bacterial contamination of the now continuous drainage system by:

1) Never distrupting the drainage system. Urinary bags are emptied by draining and not by changing the bags
2) Twice daily 1 in 400 aqueous hibitane swabbing of the external urinary meatus and surrounding areas, including the catheter
3) Maintaining the adult patient's fluid intake a minimum of 4 litres per 24 hours.

If the urine is infected at the time of catheterisation prophylactic broad spectrum chemotherapy is given by injection (IV or IM) for 48 hours to minimise the dangers of a possible instrumentation-induced bacteraemia (p. 249).

While the catheter remains *in situ* any urinary tract infection will persist and chemotherapy given for the infection will be largely ineffective; in addition its administration may aid the formation of drug-resistant organisms and produce other undesirable antibiotic side effects.

For these reasons prophylactic chemotherapy is best avoided for long term catheter drainage but must be given at the times of greatest bacteraemic risk (surgical correction of the obstruction, replacement of a catheter, postoperative bladder washouts, etc.) and must be given intravenously to achieve a rapid satisfactory serum level. Such intermittent chemotherapy may also be necessary should a patient with catheter drainage develop systemic signs or symptoms of infection.

Use of Catheter Introducer: In experienced hands a catheter introducer (fig. 171) usually gives sufficient rigidity to enable a successful passage should manual Foley catheterisation fail. A catheter introducer should only be used with a blind ending catheter. The sterile, lubricated introducer is inserted through the lumen of the catheter so that it becomes stretched over the introducer; this stretching is maintained by locking the catheter introducer handle (fig. 172). The increased rigidity of the system usually enables successful catheterisation but it also increases the risk of trauma

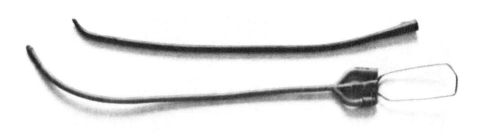

171

Difficult urethral catheterisation

171 Difficult bladder catheterisation can usually be achieved, in the absence of a severe urethral stricture, by the use of either an upgoing tip Tiemann catheter or a catheter introducer.

172 When using a catheter introducer the handle must be locked so that the introducer tip is maintained within the head of the catheter (a) and does not protrude through an opening (b).

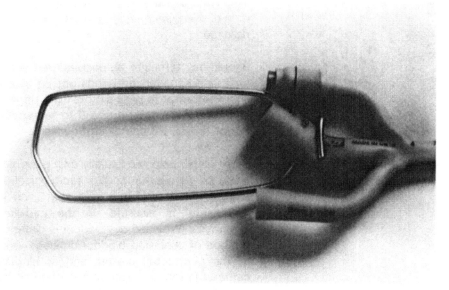

172a

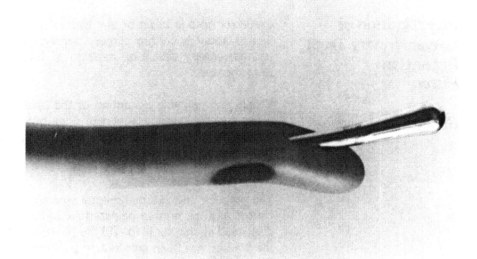

172b

and false passage formation; for this reason, gentle passage is essential. Urethral strictures may require the use of urethral sounds or filiform bougies with catheter followers (see later). Even experienced hands cannot always negotiate a grossly obstructed urethra (fig. 173).

Failed Bladder Catheterisation: The 3 most common reasons for failure to introduce the catheter are:

1) Failure through inexperience to negotiate the posterior urethra
2) The presence of a urethral stricture
3) The presence of an unsuspected urethral calculus or foreign body. (An oblique x-ray of the extended urethra usually indicates such calculi or foreign bodies).

Persistent forceful urethral catheterisation and its associated trauma and false passage formation are common causes of either bacteraemia (and it must be remembered that despite the advances in resuscitation and chemotherapy Gram-negative septicaemia has a 20% mortality rate [Altemeier et al., 1967]) or lifelong stricture formation. Another, less common consequence, may be urinary incontinence, due to external sphincteric damage.

Should any difficulty be encountered in a patient with painful retention of urine and experienced hands not be available, the inexperienced operator should attempt to pass a more rigid, upgoing tip Tiemann catheter (fig. 171) and then, if this fails, proceed to suprapubic catheterisation rather than attempt to use a catheter introducer.

Suprapubic Catheterisation

After visual, palpable (usually only possible in acute and subacute retention of urine), percussion and/or radiological evidence of a distended bladder, and preparation of the skin area with local anaesthetic, a suprapubic 'Supracath' is inserted, in the mid-line, one inch above the pubic symphysis. Provided the bladder is distended this is a safe and satisfactory method of achieving bladder drainage whilst investigations and correction of the obstructed urethra and/or bladder outlet continues. Suprapubic catheterisation is a desirable method of bladder drainage in females, particularly following vaginal trauma or surgery, where the tissues have become contaminated.

Investigation of Lower Urinary Tract Retention
History

Particular note is taken of any history of haematuria (see chapter VI), previous bladder or urethral surgery, venereal disease, lower genitourinary tract trauma, urinary calculi or insertion of foreign bodies, anxiety states and drug therapy.

General Examination

Visible and palpable distention of the bladder is present in most cases of acute and subacute retention of urine but, because of the previously discussed bladder muscle changes, this is not always so in patients presenting with chronic retention of urine, although their large, insensitive, elastic, bladders can usually be percussed.

The prepuce and external meatal area should be examined for obstructive causes and the urethra palpated for stricture, foreign bodies or calculi. As discussed in chapter III (p. 79) the prostate gland should be examined after the bladder has been emptied. In patients who present with chronic retention of urine and who do not require preoperative bladder drainage accurate

173 Severe filarial elephantiasis and a urethral stricture prevented temporary urethral relief of an acute urinary retention and a supra-pubic cystostomy was performed. Excision of the elephantiasis tissue was performed successfully (Courtesy of Mr H. Awang and Mr P. Bruce).

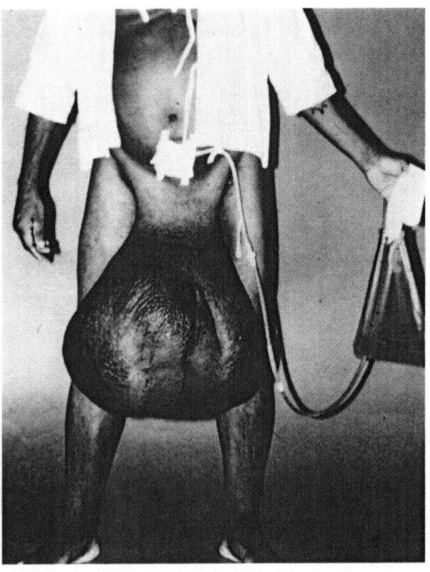

173

prostatic size and tissue assessment is made at the time of cysto-urethroscopy. Large (> 60g) benign glands are best removed by open enucleation while smaller benign glands and all carcinomatous glands are best treated by endoscopic surgery (see later).

A full neurological examination is mandatory.

Laboratory Tests: The non-urethrally contaminated catheter, supra-pubic or midstream urine specimen, is examined chemically and microscopically and cultured if indicated.

Special Investigations
Serology: Serum creatinine or urea and serum electrolyte estimations are usually normal in cases of acute or subacute retention of urine but are often abnormal in cases of chronic retention.

Intravenous Pyelogram: This is an essential investigation in all cases of urinary retention presenting with a history of haematuria but it is not essential in those patients presenting without haematuria and with normal serum creatinine and electrolyte findings. In this latter common situation a straight abdominal and pelvic x-ray, to determine the renal, bladder and other soft tissue outlines and the possible presence of urinary calculi or skeletal abnormalities, is all that is necessary. Figures 174-180 illustrate some of the abnormalities resulting from lower urinary tract obstruction of urine.

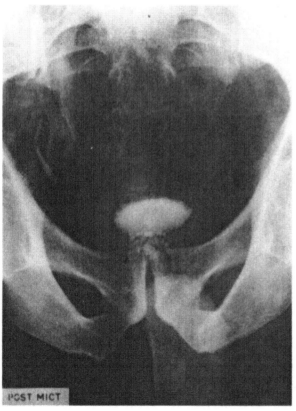

174 POST MICT

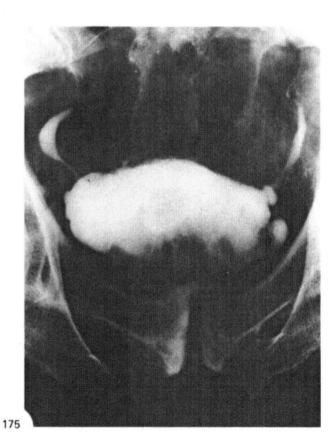

175

The complications of chronic retention of bladder urine

174 This man is unable to completely empty his bladder. Note the thick, trabeculated bladder wall and the prostatic calculi.

175 This man has a large residual bladder urine, multiple small pulsion diverticula, and some early dilatation and tortuosity of the lower ureters.

176 A large single pulsion diverticulum. Note the trabeculated bladder.

177 Non-uraemic chronic retention of urine. This man has a normal upper system but a large residual bladder urine.

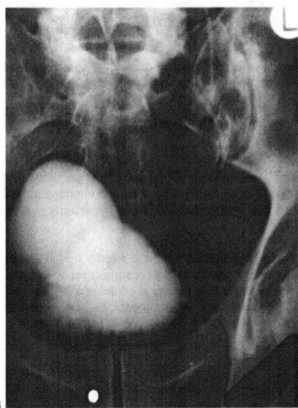

176

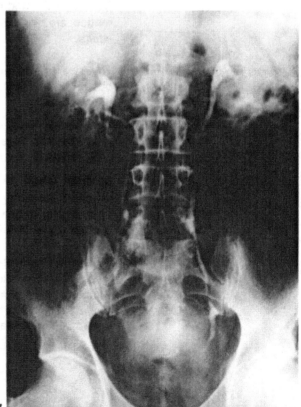

177

Micturating Cysto-urethrogram: This investigation is of value in diagnosing suspected posterior urethral valves and in investigating neurogenic retention.

Urodynamics: These investigations may also assist in distinguishing between mechanical and neurogenic causes of retention.

Cysto-urethroscopy: Cysto-urethroscopy enables a disagnostic assessment of the urethra, bladder outlet and bladder and, in addition, often enables the therapeutic correction of the cause of the retention.

Other Investigations: In view of the age of most patients presenting with retention of urine a chest x-ray, an electrocardiograph and a full blood examination are essential preoperative general screening tests.

Treatment of the Causes of Obstruction

In *children* balanitis with lower urinary tract obstruction from phimosis is treated by circumcision, as are meatal ulcers resistant to analgesic ointment. The uncommon distal external meatal stenosis is treated by dilatation, meatotomy and/or meatoplasty. Urethral polyps and posterior urethral valves are transurethrally resected and urethral diverticula excised. Urethral strictures are dilated, urethrotomised or excised. Large ureteroceles are removed via an open operation and both ureters re-implanted in an anti-reflux manner. Marion's disease is treated by dilatation of the bladder neck or, in very severe cases, by transurethral resection. Foreign bodies are removed by endoscopic or open surgery as are operable neoplasms. Infection and faecal impaction are treated with chemotherapy and disimpaction respectively, but both causes may also require temporary bladder drainage. See also chapter XIV.

Bladder outlet and prostatic pathology, together with urethral stricture formation, are responsible for most cases of lower tract obstruction of urine in *adults*.

Benign Prostatic and Bladder Outlet Obstruction

The size of the prostate gland is not always related to the degree of obstruction. There are 3 types of benign prostatic or bladder outlet obstruction:

1) Bladder neck hypertrophy (Marion's disease)
2) Prostatic hyperplasia
3) Prostatic fibrosis.

Bladder Neck Hypertrophy (Marion's Disease): This condition, of unknown aetiology, presents in boys and young men and is characterised by a varying degree of muscular and connective tissue hypertrophy at the bladder outlet (Marion, 1927).

Prostatic Hyperplasia: Benign hyperplasia begins in middle age. The submucosal and middle groups of the glands in the prostate form adenomas. Although these changes are multiple they usually predominate in one area, producing a disproportionate prostatic enlargement. As the adenoma develops it encourages the formation of a fibrous pseudo-capsule as indi-

Complications of chronic retention of bladder urine (continued)

178 Uraemic chronic retention of urine. Note the poorly functioning left kidney, the obstructed right kidney and the upward deviation of the terminal right ureter, highly suggestive of a large prostatic obstruction.

179 Gross uraemic chronic retention of urine. Note the very large bladder and the poor radiological renal function.

180 Multiple secondary bladder calculi resulting from urinary stasis and, occasionally, infection.

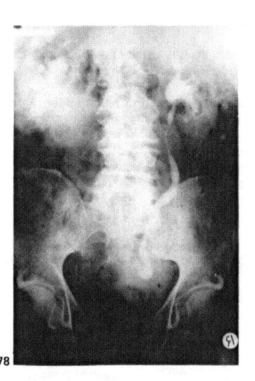

178

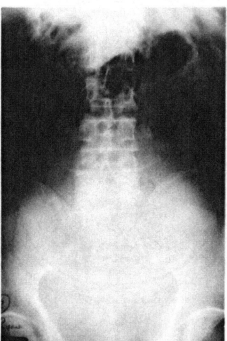

179

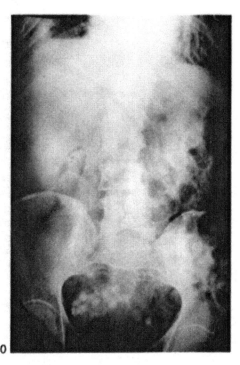

180

cated in figure 181. The plane between this pseudo-capsule and the compressed joint peripheral prostatic tissue and true anatomical capsule is the one the surgeon's finger must enter in order to enucleate the adenoma. This pathogenesis means that there is still prostatic tissue left after an 'adenomatous prostatectomy' although the amount is very small. Prostatic carcinoma can develop in later years from this small amount of residual prostatic tissue.

Prostatic Fibrosis: The prostate gland undergoes an infective or non-infective fibrosis of unknown aetiology which, although there has often been very little increase in size, can result in severe obstructive damage by narrowing both the bladder outlet and the prostatic urethra.

Complications

Prostatic, bladder outlet or urethral obstruction may give rise to the following complications.

Local tissue distortion and bladder hypertrophy. The prostatic urethra is compressed and the bladder neck occluded by the changes. This produces symptoms of hesitancy and a poor strength stream due to the difficulty in opening the bladder outlet (p. 54). The bladder muscle bundles hypertrophy in an endeavour to obtain stronger voiding power. This produces trabeculation of the bundles (fig. 174), with advanced cases showing

181 Prostatic pathology. The sites of development and the surgeon's adenoma enucleation plane. Note the obstruction and distortion of the prostatic urethra.

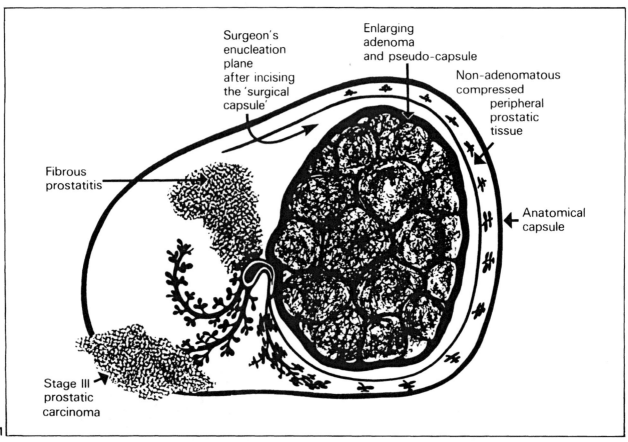

pulsion diverticula of the bladder mucosa where it is unsupported by muscle (figs. 175-176). Trabeculation can occur from neurological or infective causes and therefore does not necessarily imply mechanical obstruction (fig. 182).

Residual Bladder Urine. The unobstructed normal bladder is able to completely empty itself but prostatic obstruction impairs this ability (fig. 177) and thereby produces frequency of micturition with, in advanced cases, overflow incontinence of urine. As previously indicated infection and bladder calculi may develop because of the urinary stasis (Abrams and Griffith, 1979).

Hydro-ureter, hydronephrosis and uraemia. The hypertrophied bladder muscle and the residual urine combine to obstruct the lower ureters and, in advanced cases, this results in uraemia (figs. 178-179).

Infection and secondary calculus formation. Stasis of urine aids the development of infection and both may aid the development of urinary calculi (fig. 180) and uraemia.

Indications for Prostatectomy

Prostatic retention of urine. As previously indicated this condition calls for hospitalisation and investigation and, almost always, a prostatectomy operation performed as soon as the patient's general health and renal function permits.

182 Bladder trabeculation. This usually results from mechanical obstruction but can result, as illustrated here, from neurogenic or, in children, infective causes. Note the pulsion diverticula and the prostatic calculi, suggestive of chronic infection.

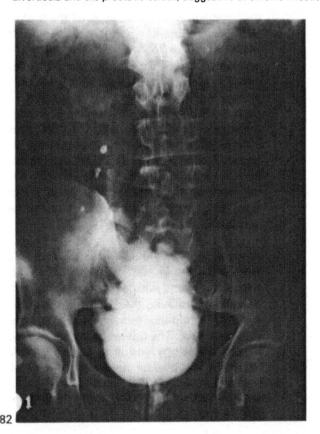

182

Severe or progressive prostatism. The most important symptom resulting from prostatic obstruction is hesitancy and this is usually associated with a poor strength stream. Frequency of micturition, both during the day and night, commonly occurs but in the absence of hesitancy and a poor strength urine stream it rarely, if ever, justifies a prostatectomy operation. Haematuria may occur from enlarged sub-mucosal prostatic veins but other causes, such as a bladder neoplasm or a vesical calculus, are found in 3% of all patients with benign prostatic obstruction. An intravenous pyelogram, together with the clinical findings, may assist in deciding whether to proceed with a prostatectomy operation or to continue to review the patient.

Patients unsuitable for prostatectomy. The elderly, senile, ill patient, with overflow uraemic retention of urine, will usually not benefit from a prostatectomy operation and is best treated with an indwelling silastic tissue inert urethral catheter; this should be changed, using a strictly aseptic technique, each month.

Types of Prostatectomy

Transurethral (Young's) prostatectomy. This is a traditional but inaccurate description as the operation is performed per-urethrally (Young, 1913). Over 90% of prostate gland obstructions are of a size (60g or less) that the operation can be performed within 60 minutes, thus minimising the complications of blood loss, bacteraemia and water intoxication associated with the procedure (see below). Isotonic irrigating solutions are used throughout the operation, also reducing the incidence of red blood cell lysis which, if excessive, can cause acute tubular necrosis. Prophylactic intravenous chemotherapy is given before, during and after the operation in view of the 26% incidence of bacteraemia (Gray and Scott, 1953; Creevy and Feeney, 1954).

The urethra must be able to accommodate at least a 24F resectoscope and the resection must remove all of the prostate gland from the bladder neck to the verumontanum, without damage to the external sphincter, unless the tissue is known to be malignant, when a sub-total palliative resection is performed in order to avoid the increased risk of postoperative incontinence in such patients. All major bleeding should be controlled before the patient leaves the operating theatre and a postoperative irrigating and drainage 3-way Foley catheter is left *in situ* for 1 or 2 days, until the urinary drainage is clear. The operation is safer, provided that it is done for the right indications, than open prostatectomy and only requires 3 or 4 days hospitalisation (Sing et al., 1973). Resection of the bladder neck only is performed on patients with severe Marion's disease, while incision of the bladder neck is on occasion all that is necessary to relieve obstruction in selected patients with minimal prostatic lateral lobe enlargement (Jenkins and Allen, 1978).

Open trans-vesical (McGill) prostatectomy. The first prostatectomy was performed in 1887 by McGill of Leeds via an extra-peritoneal, trans-vesical approach, with extraction of the prostatic adenoma by blind finger enucleation, utilising the previously described surgical plane. A postoperative bladder catheter remains *in situ* for at least 7 days, allowing the bladder incision to heal. The operation is always preceded by cystoscopy to exclude bladder pathology and is suitable for large benign prostate glands, particularly if the bladder needs to be opened (e.g. for the removal of large, hard secondary bladder calculus), but suffers from both this disadvantage and the fact that bleeding from the prostatic fossa is difficult to visualise and control.

Open retropubic (Millin) prostatectomy. This improved method of open prostatectomy (Millin, 1947) is now favoured by most urologists. After preliminary cystoscopy an extra-peritoneal, retro-pubic abdominal approach enables incision of the anterior prostatic capsule and subsequent adenoma enucleation. Direct visualisation of the bleeding prostatic fossa vessels greatly aids haemostasis during the operation and, as the bladder has not been opened, the postoperative drainage catheter can be removed within 1 to 3 days.

Complications of Prostate Gland Surgery

Death. Measured over a 3 months postoperative period, patients presenting with prostatism, acute or subacute retention of urine have a mortality rate of 0.5% but patients presenting with uraemic retention of urine, with overflow, have a mortality of 2% (Brown, unpublished data).

Excessive bleeding. *At operation:* A careful preoperative history-taking, to exclude a history of bleeding and coagulation defects, hypotensive anaesthesia and care in selection of the operative procedure have greatly reduced the incidence of severe operative bleeding. Fibrinolysins may be released from the prostatic cells and antifibrinolytic therapy may be required (Fearnley, 1965).

Secondary haemorrhage. This may occur up to 8 weeks after a prostatectomy. Evacuation of all clots from the bladder, using an air- and water-tight Toomey syringe and a whistle tip, or a haematuria catheter, is necessary should clot retention occur.

Infection Bacteraemia-septicaemia. As previously indicated bacteraemia occurs in 26% (Gray and Scott, 1953) of all transurethral prostatectomies and Marshall (1967) found an incidence of 60% in retropubic prostatectomies. Bacteraemia is potentially lethal (Altemeier et al., 1967) and aseptic, prophylactic precautions must be taken with any form of urological instrumentation (Mitchell and Gillespie, 1964). Appropriate prophylactic intravenous chemotherapy is given at the time of operation and for 48 hours afterwards, in an endeavour to destroy any circulating bacteria. Established septicaemic shock requires immediate expert resuscitation (Murdoch et al., 1968; Eremin and Marshall, 1969).

Urine. Infection usually resolves spontaneously after removal of the catheter, provided an adequate prostatectomy has been performed.

Wound. Infection of the wound is now uncommon.

Epididymitis. This is now very uncommon. Prophylactic preoperative vas deferens ligation is unnecessary (Sing et al., 1973).

Osteitis pubis. This is extremely rare now because of better control of urinary tract infection and the greatly reduced incidence of open prostatectomy and suprapubic fistulae. Vertebral osteomyelitis is a very rare complication and results from hospital-induced *Staphylococcal aureus* infection.

Irrigating fluid overload and gaemolysis. Suitable non-haemolytic isotonic irrigating solutions are advised (Creevy, 1947; Nesbit and Glickman, 1948). Many urologists continue to use non-isotonic sterile water and admit to few complications. Madsen (1979) has estimated that 600ml of water could be absorbed into the circulation during a transurethral prostatectomy before significant haemolysis would occur. Careful attention to surgical technique and the height of the irrigating solution minimises this serious complication.

Deep vein thrombosis. Careful positioning of the lower limbs on the operating table and early postoperative ambulation has greatly reduced the incidence of this potentially serious complication.

External sphincter damage incontinence or prostatic capsule perforation. These are extremely rare complications (p. 355, p. 310).

Post-prostatectomy urethral strictures. This is the most common post-prostatectomy complication. In the author's series (Brown, unpublished data) stricture occurred in 2.5% of all endoscopic prostatectomies and 1% of all open prostatectomies. Strictures occur mostly at the external meatal-pre-fossa navicularis area and, less commonly, in the bulbous (fig. 184) or more anterior urethra. The incidence of stricture formation is reduced by (Lentz et al., 1977):

1) Performing an adequate pre-prostatectomy meatotomy when necessary
2) Selecting a suitable sized sheath for the particular urethra (determined by initial urethral calibration)
3) Limiting the time of the operation
4) Performing a perineal urethrotomy introduction or an open prostatectomy, if indicated
5) Correct choice and hygienic management of a suitable sized and material postoperative catheter
6) Use of a postoperative meatal dilator in selected patients.

A preoperative internal urethrotomy (Emmett et al., 1963) is very occasionally indicated in those patients with an established operative bulbous or membranous urethral stricture or a uniformly tight urethra.

Postoperative failure to void satisfactorily. This is usually due to a chronically atonic bladder, which may require continuous catheter drainage for several months before its tone improves, or there may have been surgical failure to remove all of the obstructing prostate gland and bladder neck.

Infertility. Destruction of the bladder outlet ('internal sphincter') usually means that subsequent ejaculations enter the bladder rather than passing along the urethra.

Prostatic Abscess

A prostatic abscess is a rare cause of acute retention of urine in young or middle-aged patients. Treatment includes temporary bladder drainage, chemotherapy and rarely, endoscopic unroofing of the abscess.

Obstruction from Prostate Carcinoma

Carcinoma may still develop in residual prostatic tissue following open prostatectomy, as indicated on page 246, or may develop independently (fig. 181). Although radical prostatectomy, which implies removal of all of the prostate gland including its true anatomical capsule and the bladder neck, is carried out in a few highly selected cases in an attempt to cure, almost all patients present at a stage when only palliative treatment with oestrogen, bilateral orchidectomy, transurethral resection or radiotherapy can be offered (p. 183).

Urethral stricture
183a,b Urethrograms should always be done with the penis extended and separated from the bone shadows. Note the contrast medium injector. No urethral abnormality appears in either study but the external sphincter verumontanum and the internal sphicter are clearly outlined.

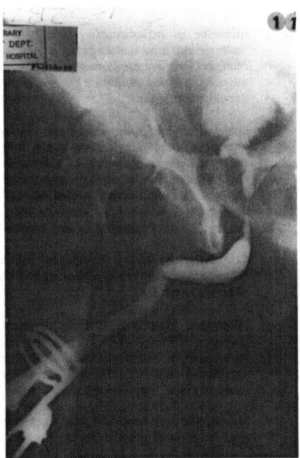

183a

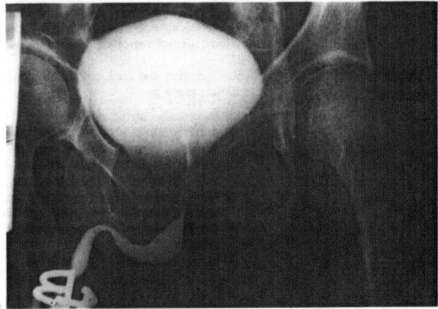

183b

Urethral Stricture

Aetiology

Traumatic stricture. Internal urethral trauma (p. 298) is common and usually occurs at or just inside the external urinary meatus or in the bulbous or prostatic urethra. As discussed in the chapter on Paediatric Urology (p. 348) external meatal stenosis resulting from a poorly executed circumcision is not uncommon. Severe external trauma commonly results in fibrosis in the anterior urethra or at the prostato-membranous junction (figs. 184-185).

Infective or inflammatory stricture. Gonorrhoeal and/or nonspecific urethritis strictures usually occur in the anterior urethra and may be single or multiple. They are not common in our community because of early adequate diagnosis and treatment. Tuberculosis, which commonly occurs in the posterior urethra, and bilharzial strictures are very rare.

Inflammatory strictures usually occur in the bulbous urethra or the external meatal area and occasionally result from an indwelling catheter. Using tissue inert silastic catheters, of a size such that urethral secretions can exit, and cleansing the external urinary meatal area twice daily with 1 in 400 aqueous hibitane, greatly minimises the chances of stricture formation. Foreign body insertion, or chemical irrigation of the urethra, are unusual causes of inflammatory strictures involving the anterior urethra.

Congenital stricture. Congenital strictures include posterior urethral valves, anterior urethral membranes and distal external meatal stenosis (see chapters I and XIV).

Idiopathic stricture. Balanitis xerotica obliterans is a condition of unknown aetiology which fibroses the external urinary meatus and a varying amount of the anterior urethra. Meatoplasty correction is required in the established case but sublesional cortisone injection therapy, performed at an early stage, may prevent such fibrosis (Poynter and Levy, 1967).

Neoplastic stricture. Urethral carcinoma is rare, but does occur more often in patients with severe benign urethral strictures.

Surgical Pathology

Congenital strictures have neat, sharp edges and are rarely extensive or infected, thus greatly aiding any attempted endoscopic or open surgical correction; however, many acquired strictures, except those at the external meatus, are inflamed and/or infected and extend well beyond the point of maximal urethral narrowing, making excisional surgery much more difficult.

Complications of Urethral Stricture

Local infection and back pressure obstructive complications are common and may result in:

1) Progression of the stricture
2) A peri-urethral abscess, which may aid the formation of a diverticulum and/or calculi, or may burst through the skin forming a urethral fistula. In grossly untreated cases multiple fistulae may result in the formation of a 'watering-can penis, scrotum and perineum'
3) Retrograde epididymo-orchitis is not uncommon (fig. 185). Prostatic abscess formation and pyelonephritis are rare
4) Bladder, ureteric and renal back pressure damage, with eventual uraemia
5) Rarely, carcinoma of the urethra.

Urethral stricture (continued)
184 A single urethral stricture due to external trauma.

185 Multiple urethral strictures due to surgical internal trauma. The dye is shown entering the prostatic ejaculatory ducts, which have enlarged openings caused by the long standing severe urethral obstructions.

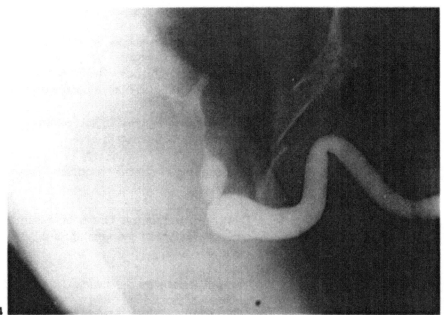

184

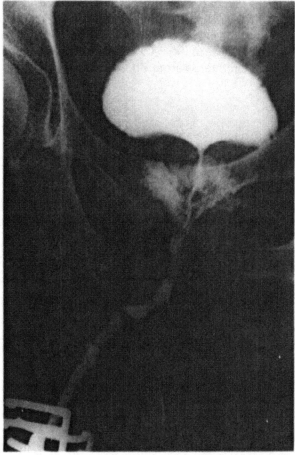

185

Clinical Presentation   Uncomplicated urethral strictures produce a thin stream with a progressively poorer strength, eventually leading to urinary retention. Inflammation and infection may present features ranging from a discharge, termed 'morning gleet', to haematuria, fever, epididymitis, abscess or fistula formation. Life threatening gross back pressure obstruction and infection may develop in untreated patients.

Diagnosis   **History.** Younger patients presenting with a mechanically poor strength stream should be suspected of having a urethral stricture.

Physical examination. This may reveal the induration of a stricture or one or more of the previously described complications.

Urethrogram. Figures 183a,b illustrate normal urethrograms and 184-185 severe urethral stricturing.

Micturating cysto-urethrogram. This may provide more detailed information.

Cysto-urethroscopy. This is an essential aid to both accurate diagnosis and assessment of the stricture and any associated lower tract complications.

Management of Urethral Stricture   **Benign Strictures.** *Intermittent dilatation:* Using local anaesthesia, plastic or steel dilators (fig. 186a,b) are passed through the stricture at progressively increasing intervals of time. This method of treatment is regarded as successful if the patient eventually requires only a maximum of 4 dilatations a year, which is the case in the majority. Urethral instrumentation fever, now known to be due to bacteraemia, has been known since the time of Hippocrates. Other complications such as bleeding, false urethral passages (fig 187) or retention of urine may also result from the passage of urethral dilators. In an endeavour to avoid these complications, urethral

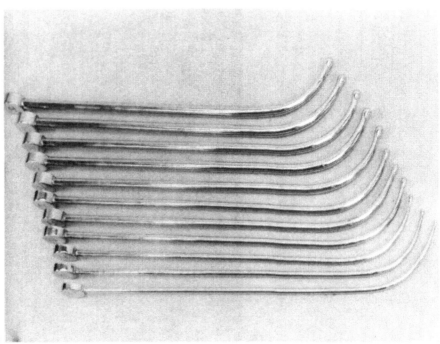

186a

186 Urethral stricture dilatation. Most benign urethral strictures can be satisfactorily managed by intermittent dilatation, using metal (a) or plastic (b) dilators.

187 A false passage in the urethral bulb resulting from the traumatic passage of a small metal dilator.

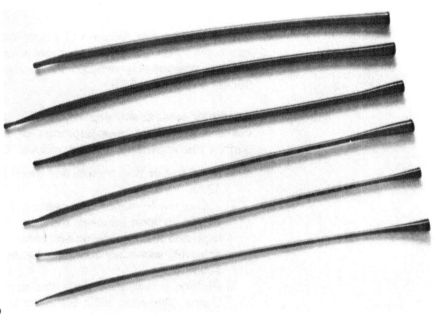

186b

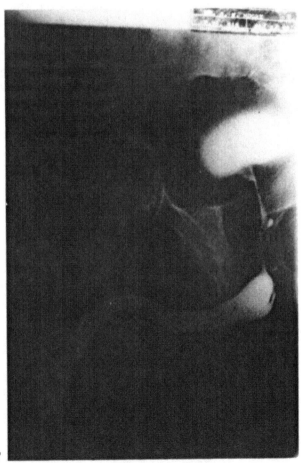

187

dilatation must be carried out gently with a careful aseptic technique (Mitchell and Gillespie, 1964) and the selected associated use of appropriate chemotherapy (Creevy and Feeney, 1954).

Continuous dilatation: This method is occasionally of value in softening a difficult urethral stricture and so enabling more efficient future intermittent dilatations.

Internal urethrotomy: Division of a tight stricture, or strictures, under direct telescopic vision, greatly assists more efficient future intermittent dilatation and has considerably reduced the incidence of urethroplasty operations (Kinder and Rous, 1979).

Attempted curative urethroplasty: Initial ventral excision of the stricture requires a secondary re-anastomosis of the proximal and distal healthy urethral openings. This may be achieved by:

1) Resection of the stricture and direct end-to-end anastomosis (Jesen, 1970)
2) Aiding the formation of a healthy, non-inflamed, non-pocketed strip of skin to form between the proximal and distal urethrotomy openings, and then mobilising and suturing this strip of skin, as a tube, so achieving secondary continuity between the urethrotomies (Johanson, 1953)
3) Grafting a skin tube from the scrotum or the shaft of the penis (Turner-Warwick, 1960; Blandy et al., 1968).

The results of urethroplasty operations are very good although the more posterior the stricture the more difficult the operation and less successful the result.

Relief of urinary retention in urethral stricture. Patients with urethral strictures who default from their planned intermittent dilatation programme may develop retention of urine if the stricture becomes extremely narrow. Retention of urine may also occur following a difficult urethral dilatation. The degree of stricturing is usually so severe that it is not possible to pass a urethral catheter initially. Filiform bougies (fig. 188a,b) are inserted into the

188 Filiform bougies in the relief of stricture. Retention of urine due to a urethral stricture often requires the passage of several fine filiform bougies (a) until one, directed by its fellows filling the obstructed space, passes through the stricture (b). A follower is screwed onto the successful filiform and then introduced into the bladder, so relieving the retention.

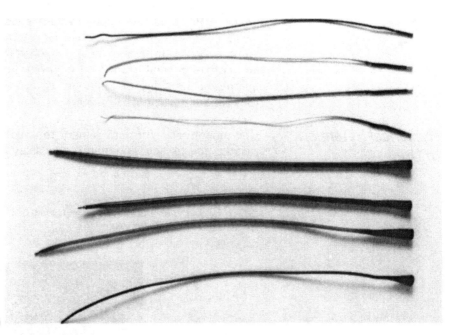

188a

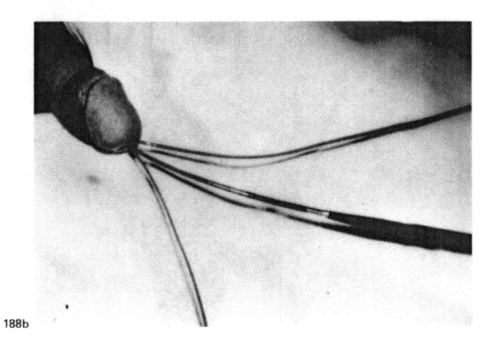

188b

urethra until one negotiates the stricture and enters the bladder. A hollow follower, with one or more distal openings, is then screwed onto the successful filiform bougie and passed through the stricture into the bladder (fig. 189). Should filiform bougies and followers and the necessary expertise not be available then suprapubic bladder drainage (p. 240) should be used and the patient transferred to a urological centre for further assessment and treatment.

Neoplastic strictures. See chapter VII.

Atonic Bladder

This is a common condition caused by primary muscle and/or nerve degeneration or by secondary bladder damage resulting from mechanical and/or functional bladder outlet or urethral obstruction. Many elderly patients with bladder atonia do not require specfiic treatment as they are relatively asymptomatic, non-infected, and not undergoing progressive or severe back pressure upper system changes. Patients who experience these complications may require long term continuous bladder drainage, using a silastic urethral catheter (which is replaced each month), measures to improve general health and intermittent chemotherapy if there are any symptoms or signs of infection. Drugs which contract bladder muscle (p. 268) are occasionally of value.

Hysterical Retention of Urine

This uncommon form of urinary retention should be treated with psychiatric advice, sedation, and if necessary intermittent bladder drainage.

189 A follower with a drainage opening (inset) being passed through the stricture, guided by the successful filiform.

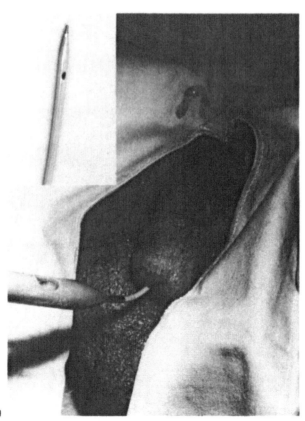

189

References

Abrams, P.H. and Griffith, D.J.: The assessment of prostatic obstruction from urodynamic measurements and from residual urine. British Journal of Urology 51: 129 (1979).

Altemeier, W.A.; Todd, J.C. and Inge, W.W.: Gram-negative septicaemia: a growing threat. Annals of Surgery 166: 530 (1967).

Blandy, J.P.; Sing, M. and Tresidder, G.D.: Urethroplasty by scrotal flap for long urethral strictures. British Journal of Urology 40: 261 (1968).

Brown, R.B.: The complications of prostatectomy. Australian Medical Journal (in press).

Creevy, C.D.: Hemolytic reactions during trans-urethral prostatic resection. Journal of Urology 58: 125 (1947).

Creevy, C.D. and Feeney, M.V.: Routine use of antibiotics in trans-urethral prostatic resection: a clinical investigation. Journal of Urology 71: 615 (1954).

Eremin, J. and Marshall, V.C.: The diagnosis and management of refractory shock. Medical Journal of Australia 1: 778 (1969).

Gray, D.N. and Scott, W.W.: The incidence and type of bacteraemia at the time of various prostatectomy procedures. Read at Clinical Society of Genito-urinary Surgeons (Feb. 3rd, 1953).

Jenkins, J.D. and Allen, N.H.: Bladder neck incision — A treatment for retention with overflow in the absence of adenoma. British Journal of Urology 50: 395 (1978).

Jesen, C.: Resection of urethral stricture end to end anastomosis. Scandinavian Journal of Urology and Nephrology 4: 87 (1970).

Johanson, B.: Reconstruction of the male urethra in strictures: Application of the buried intact epithelium technique. Acta Chirurgica Scandinavica (Suppl.) 176: 3 (1953).

Kinder, P.W. and Rous, S.N.: Treatment of urethral stricture disease by internal urethrotomy: clinical review. Journal of Urology 121: 45 (1979).

Lentz, C.H.; Mebust, W.K.; Foret, J.D. and Melchoir, J.: Urethral strictures following transurethral prostatectomy. Review of 2,223 resections. Journal of Urology 117: 194 (1977).

Madsen, P.O.: Induction of diuresis following transurethral resection of the prostate. Journal of Urology 23: 701 (1970).

Marion, G.: De l'hypertrophie congenitale du col vesical. Journal d'Urologie Medicale et Chirurgicale 23: 97 (1927).

Marshall, A.: Retropubic prostatectomy. A review with special reference to urinary infection. British Journal of Urology 39: 307 (1967).

McGill, A.F.: Suprapubic prostatectomy. British Medical Journal 2: 1104 (1887).

Mitchell, J.P. and Gillespie, W.A.: Bacteriological complications from the use of urethral instruments: principles of prevention. Journal of Clinical Pathology 17: 492 (1964).

Murdoch, J.C.M.; Speirs, C.F. and Pullen, H.: The bacteraemic shock syndrome. British Journal of Hospital Medicine 1: 345 (1968).

Nesbit, R.M. and Glickman, S.I.: The use of glycine as an irrigating medium during transurethral resection. British Journal of Hospital Medicine 59: 1212 (1948).

Poynter, J.H. and Levy, J.: Balanitis xerotica obliterans: effective treatment with topical and sublesional corticosteroids. British Journal of Urology 39: 420 (1967).

Sing, M.; Blandy, J.P. and Tressider, G.C.: The evaluation of transurethral resection for benign enlargement of the prostate. British Journal of Urology 45: 93 (1973).

Turner-Warwick, R.T.: A technique of posterior urethroplasty. Journal of Urology 83: 416 (1960).

Whitaker, R.H.: A look at the three-way catheter. British Journal of Urology 47: 103 (1975).

Young, H.H.: A new procedure (punch operation) for small prostatic bars and contracture of the prostatic orifice. Journal of the American Medical Association 60: 253 (1913).

Further Reading

Fearnley, G.R.: Fibrinolysis (Arnold, London 1965).

Hedlund, P.O.: Urinary Bladder Catheterisation. (Mockridge, Bulmer, Sydney 1967).

Millin, T.: Retropubic Urinary Surgery. (Livingstone, Edinburgh 1947).

Chapter XI

The Neurogenic Bladder

Nervous control of the bladder implies conscious control imposed on an intrinsic emptying mechanism by important centres in the cerebral cortex, hypothalamus, sacral spinal cord and the bladder wall, linked by excitatory and inhibitory pathways (p.55).

A neurogenic bladder may be defined as one whose function is disturbed by an abnormality affecting one or more of these centres, their interconnecting pathways or the neurotransmitter substances (Oyarsky, 1967).

Normal Bladder Function

The bladder functions as a urinary reservoir (Smith, 1976). There is a low resting pressure (5-10cm H_2O), which allows ease of filling by the ureter (normal peak pressure 10-20cm H_2O). Bladder resting pressure remains low, despite increased filling, until the volume reaches a capacity of approximately 400ml. A feeling of bladder fullness is then experienced, but may be inhibited or suppressed if micturition is not desired. Urgency is associated with rises in intravesical pressure and only normally occurs with considerable distension of the bladder.

The second function of the bladder is complete evacuation of urine at will. The inhibitory influences are removed and reflex contraction of the detrusor allowed to occur. This results in opening of the bladder neck and prostatic urethra, with associated synergistic relaxation of the external sphincter. Peak intra-vesical pressure during micturition is 30 to 60cm H_2O, peak flow is 15 to 30ml/second, and a normal micturition will void about 400ml in 20 to 30 seconds (Hinman, 1971). These parameters of normal function can be measured by means of:

1) Cystometrograms (CMG)
2) Voided flow rates (VFR)
3) Intra-vesical pressure measurements
4) Urethral pressure profiles (UPP)
5) Electromyography of the external sphincter.

Disturbances of Micturition

Tabes dorsalis due to tertiary syphilis affects the dorsal root ganglia and may thus deprive the bladder of sensation, breaking the reflex arc. Desire to void, awareness of fullness, urgency and pain are lost, with the result that the bladder overdistends. Overflow incontinence is the end result.

Sensory Denervation

Although this disease is very uncommon it is mentioned to emphasise the importance of bladder overdistension as an extremely damaging secondary (myogenic) factor affecting the neurogenic bladder. The overstretched detrusor loses tone and the ability to contract. The cystometrogram is flat and prolonged in the denervated, atonic, overstretched bladder (fig. 190).

190 **Normal and abnormal cystograms**

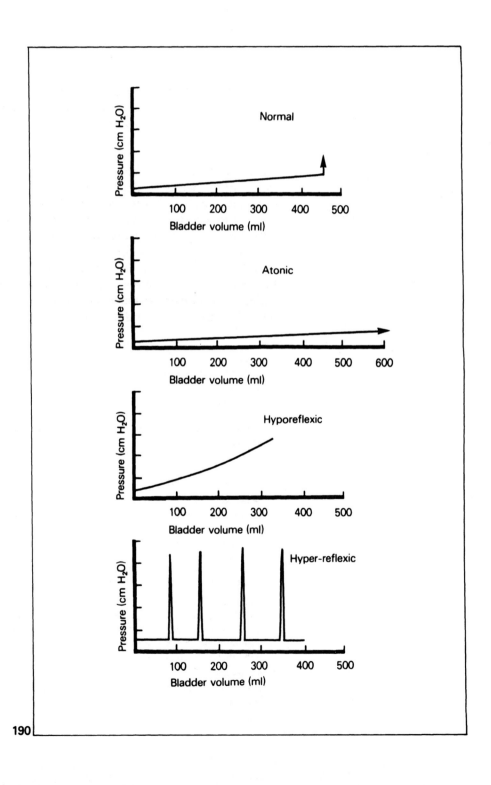

Hyper-reflexic (Upper Motor Neurone) Bladder

Division of or damage to the spinal cord above the sacral micturition centre produces a hyper-reflexic bladder. It is also called the upper motor neurone bladder because there is associated damage to the upper motor neurones of skeletal muscle and a resultant spastic paralysis below the level of spinal cord damage. The bladder sacral reflex is intact but disconnected from higher centres and the pelvic floor and somatic external sphincter are spastic. Although normal bladder sensation is lost, after a period of spinal shock varying from days to weeks, reflex activity returns to the bladder and contraction of the detrusor occurs purely as a result of stretch. These reflexes are not inhibited and a typical cystometrogram develops (fig. 190). These reflex contractions of the detrusor may be enhanced by various types stimulation (e.g. tapping of the lower abdomen, or pinching, stroking of skin). Although quite powerful bladder contractions may occur normal relaxation of the external sphincter does not. In fact, an active contraction of the external sphincter may be associated with detrusor contraction (detrusor-sphincter dysnergia), leading to very high intravesical pressures, incomplete emptying, and ultimately bladder trabeculation, diverticula, reflux and upper tract dilatation.

Areflexic (Lower Motor Neurone) Bladder

Damage to the sacral micturition centre, the cauda equina, or the pelvic nerves destroys the reflex arc and may result in an areflexic bladder. A lower motor neurone paralysis of the skeletal muscles is associated with nerve injury which affects the second, third or fourth sacral myotomes with sensory loss in the corresponding dermatomes. The bladder is without a reflex arc and contraction depends on local stretch responses in the bladder wall, which are most inefficient. Although the external sphincter is not overactive (in fact it may be paralysed and flaccid), passive tone inherent in the smooth muscle fibres and elastic tissue of the sphincter complex is sufficient to prevent effective urination. Voiding may be enhanced by abdominal straining, Valsalva and Crede manoeuvres, but is typically intermit-

Table I. The important causes of neurogenic bladder presenting as acute quadri/paraplegia

1. Spinal trauma
   Causing spinal fracture and/or dislocation most commonly due to:
   a) motor car accidents
   b) industrial accidents/falls
   c) surfing, diving, sporting accidents
   d) gunshot wounds

2. Spinal surgery
   For neoplasm, vascular malformation, prolapsed intervertebral disc. Cord compression may be due to:
   a) primary pathology
   b) operative damage
   c) postoperative haematoma
   d) postoperative cord infarction due to spinal artery thrombosis

3. Spinal metastasis
   Usually associated with prodromal symptoms such as paraesthesia, weakness, frequency and difficulty of micturition, which, if recognised and acted upon, may prevent complete spinal cord compression with dubious recovery. This is an acute surgical emergency

4. Spinal abscess
   Usually secondary to spinal osteomyelitis (tuberculosis or other pathogen) but occasionally primary

5. Spina bifida

tent. The cystometrogram shows a lack of reflex activity, pressure tending to rise linearly with volume (fig. 190); however, in the slowly developing situation, gradual bladder overdistension may lead to an atonic bladder with a flat cystometrogram. Associated weakness of the skeletal component of the anal sphincter may be found, and erectile function may be absent.

The Uninhibited Bladder

Here the nerve lesion involves the cerebral higher centres and inhibitory pathways leading to a loss of inhibitory control; bladder awareness is present but the bladder functions in a reflex fashion with normal relaxation of the external sphincter — thus voiding is not obstructive in character and bladder emptying is usually complete. This type of bladder activity is commonly seen in elderly people with cerebrovascular disease, Parkinson's disease and senile dementia (a group in which bladder outlet obstruction is also commonly present).

It must be emphasised that these classical descriptions are of complete lesions. Many neurogenic bladders present as incomplete lesions or develop slowly over many years so that the full characteristics may not be observed initially. Complicating factors such as overdistension, infection, anxiety, catheter drainage, drug treatment and surgery may intervene and modify the natural history of the condition.

Clinical Presentation
As Acute Quadri/Paraplegia

In this group there is a sudden or rapidly progressive onset of spinal cord dysfunction producing painless lower urinary tract retention of urine. Spinal cord lesions above T11 will produce a hyper-reflexic (upper motor neurone) bladder, whilst those occurring below L1 will produce an areflexic (lower motor neurone) bladder, with a variable response seen between these two levels.

A short phase of spinal shock occurs during which no reflex activity is present; this usually lasts a few days but may last weeks. These patients have paralysis and loss of sensation below the level of the lesion in the spinal cord. They are unable to void and must not be allowed to develop overdistension of the bladder as this will prolong the period of areflexic bladder activity and impair recovery. It is important to be aware of the possibility of concomitant spinal injury in the patient unconscious due to a head injury. The important causes of this presentation are listed in table I.

Known Neurological Disease with Bladder Symptoms

Patients with recognised neurological disease who develop bladder symptoms present with a combination of bladder irritability (due to uninhibited reflex activity) and mechanically difficult micturition. They complain of frequency, urgency, urge-incontinence and/or recurrent urinary infection. It is essential that those bladder symptoms due to the neurogenic abnormality are separated from those due to mechanical obstruction or some other complication such as infection (Summers, 1978). Table II lists some of the neurological disturbances which may present in this way.

Unsuspected Neurological Disease with Bladder Symptoms

This is the most important group because the diagnosis of a neurogenic bladder may easily be overlooked. Presentation occurs with either painless urinary retention, often as overflow incontinence, or as frequency, urgency and urge-incontinence. The former presentation is largely associated with unsuspected cauda equina or pelvic nerve plexus dysfunction, while the latter presentation is the result of partial uninhibited bladder activity of a hyper-reflexic type.

Table II. Neurological diseases from which patients developing bladder symptoms may be known to be suffering

1. Multiple sclerosis
   There is no distinct pattern of neurogenic bladder behaviour because of the patchy and variable nature of the spinal cord lesion

2. Tabes dorsalis

3. Subacute combined degeneration of the cord

4. Parkinson's disease
   It is not commonly recognised that this condition is associated with uninhibited bladder activity

5. Cerebral arteriosclerosis/senile dementia
   The classic cause of uninhibited bladder activity

6. Spinal cord tumour, vascular malformation

It is important to recognise these situations since some may be correctable (e.g. prolapsed intervertebral disc, spina bifida occulta). In others, early recognition of the neurogenic basis of the problem will help to prevent deterioration, due to overdistension, in what may be a temporary neurogenic disturbance (e.g. after pelvic surgery or in multiple sclerosis); again, in others it helps to avoid a bladder neck resection which may have disastrous results (e.g. the central uninhibited bladder of the elderly male mimicking bladder neck obstruction). One must be particularly careful in situations of unusual retention or of marked urgency incontinence.

Drugs are a particularly important cause of a neurogenic bladder. Any drug with an anticholinergic or α-sympathomimetic action can be responsible for bladder dysfunction.

Table III lists some of the causes of bladder dysfunction due to unrecognised neurological disease and table IV some of the common drugs disturbing bladder function.

Clinical Examination

A careful neurological examination is essential in all patients. The following features should be particularly assessed in patients with known neurological disease:

1) *In the hyper-reflexic bladder* the anal sphincter may be spastic on digital examination. The bulbocavernosus reflex (squeezing the glans penis produces contraction of the anal sphincter) is present and active as is the anal reflex (contraction of the anal sphincter on stimulating the perianal skin or hair).
2) *In the areflexic bladder* the anal sphincter is lax, with little or no tone, and bulbocavernosus and anal reflexes are weak or absent. Perianal and penile sensation is absent or impaired. An areflexic bladder is more commonly associated with impotence, whilst in the hyper-reflexic state reflex erectile activity is often retained.

Table III. Unrecognised neurological disease which may be present in patients with bladder symptoms

1. Retention of urine following specific surgery
   a) rectal excision
   b) radical hysterectomy
   c) retrovesical surgery
      These operations may affect the parasympathetic pelvic nerves; a significant degree of recovery is possible if overdistension is prevented
   d) aortic resection
      This may lead to ischaemia of conus medullaris

2. Multiple sclerosis
   Some 5-10% of multiple sclerosis patients present initally with bladder symptoms

3. Central prolapsed intervertebral disc
   The cauda equina, rather than the emerging lumbar nerve roots, is compressed producing sacral cord disturbance. This is one cause of neurogenic bladder which may be totally correctable. Back pain is a clue but not necessarily present

4. Uninhibited bladder from cerebral causes
   Dementia or cerebral dysfunction may not be obvious

5. Spinal cord tumour

6. Diabetes mellitus
   An autonomic neuropathy may occur as well as the more usually recognised peripheral neuropathy

7. Spina bifida occulta
   A common radiological finding but occasionally associated with a neurogenic bladder

8. Sacral agenesis
   A rare congenital absence of part of the sacrum and associated nerves

9. Tabes dorsalis

Table IV. Drugs that may produce neurogenic bladder dysfunction

Drugs with Anticholinergic Effects
1. Synthetic anticholinergic drugs (antispasmodics) which may be prescribed for peptic ulcer or irritable colon, e.g. propantheline, oxyphenonium bromide, penthienate bromide

2. Tricyclic antidepressants, e.g. imipramine, amitryptyline

3. Some other antidepressants and psychiatric drugs, e.g. phenothiazines such as perphenazine

4. Antihistamines, e.g. cypropheptadine

5. Drugs used to treat Parkinson's disease, e.g. amantidine, benzhexol

6. Some antihypertensives, particularly the ganglion-blocking drugs

7. Some antiarrhythmic drugs, e.g. disopyramide

Drugs with α-Sympathomimetic Effects
1. α-Sympathomimetic drugs used for bronchospasm, decongestion (vasoconstriction), e.g. ephedrine, phenylephrine

2. Appetite suppressants, e.g. mazindol, amphetamine-related drugs such as diethylpropion

**Special
Investigations**
*Radiological
Investigations*

The neurogenic bladder may be associated with many radiological changes but only two are specific to it:

1) *'Fir tree' bladder:* As seen in figure 191, there is gross trabeculation and sacculation of the bladder.
2) *A grossly dilated prostatic urethra,* due to a spastic external sphincter, which is easily displayed in a micturating cysto-urethrogram (fig. 192).

Urodynamic Studies

The cystometrogram, voiding flow rate, intravesical pressure measurements, sphincter electromyography and urethral pressure profiles (chapter IV) are essential investigations, particularly in diagnosing the pure uninhibited bladder, the atonic bladder and the areflexic bladder, and in assessing the effects of drug therapy on these states.

**Management of the
Neurogenic Bladder**

Management is based on the presenting symptoms and the urodynamic situation. Symptoms must be relieved and the urodynamic situation improved.

General Principles

The bladder which cannot empty, or empties poorly, must be investigated to determine why it has failed. In the rare absence of correctable factors the following methods are used to improve emptying:

1) Bladder training: This involves regular enhancement of reflux activity by tapping, straining and Crede manoeuvre (self-maintained suprapubic manual pressure) and, in some, external sphincter relaxation by anal sphincter stretching
2) Endoscopic surgery: External sphincterotomy and bladder neck resection
3) Drug therapy.

Where inadequate emptying persists or emptying without adequate continence occurs the following measures are necessary:

1) External collecting devices such as condom drainage
2) Intermittent clean self-catheterisation
3) Suprapubic catheter
4) Indwelling urethral catheter
5) Supravesical diversion (p. 194).

Where emptying is adequate but bladder function is impaired by frequency and urgency incontinence, drug therapy with anticholinergic drugs such as propantheline or imipramine may have dramatic effects (p. 357).

Some of these general principles are illustrated in more detail when applied to the acute neurogenic bladder

*Management of the
Acute Neurogenic
Bladder*

The bladder must be prevented from overdistension damage until spinal shock has resolved and the patient has learned to understand and effectively empty his bladder. This requires catheterisation with the attendant risks of infection and may be carried out by:

1) Intermittent urethral catheterisation
2) Suprapubic stab cystotomy
3) Indwelling urethral catheter.

The incidence of urinary tract infection and urethral trauma are more common with the third method but it is the least demanding of trained personnel.

When spinal shock has resolved, as indicated by a recovery of reflex activity in the cystometrogram (for the more common hyper-reflexic bladder), bladder training can begin. For these hyper-reflexic bladders this involves learning to trigger and enhance the reflex contractions of the bladder by suprapubic tapping, or stimulating other appropriate trigger areas. This tapping may cause detrusor contraction but also often external sphincter contraction; thus it must be persisted with until the external sphincter has tired, when emptying against minimal resistance may occur.

Relaxation of the external sphincter may also be achieved by manual stretching of the anal sphincter.

Neurogenic bladder cystograms.

191 Cystogram of a hyper-reflexic neurogenic bladder. The heavily trabeculated and sacculated bladder develops a characteristic 'fir-tree' shape. The balloon of the filling catheter is lying in the greatly dilated prostatic urethra.

192 Voiding cysto-urethrogram of a hyper-reflexic neurogenic bladder. The bladder neck is wide open and the prostatic urethra dilated, but the external sphincter is spastic and does not relax during detrusor contraction. Right-sided vesico-ureteric reflux is also shown.

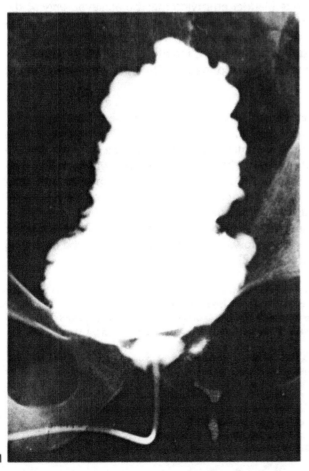

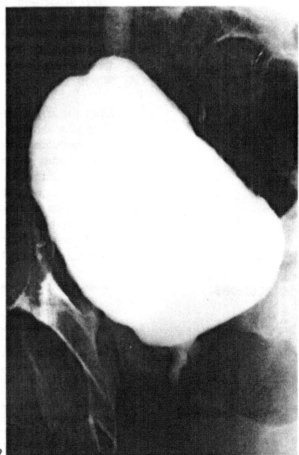

191   192

With areflexic bladders training involves increasing intravesical pressure by abdominal straining and associated Crede manoeuvre to initiate and maintain flow.

Satisfactory emptying, with continence, is achieved by some patients provided that a careful control of their fluid intake is observed. Unfortunately most patients continue to experience sudden reflex contractions and resultant incontinence. In the male an external incontinence device is worn (e.g. condom urinal and leg bag for men) for this reason. There is no satisfactory incontinence device for women (see chapter XV) so that continued use of a catheter is necessary. Intermittent, aseptic, self-catheterisation is undoubtedly the best technique for those with the manual dexterity and a permanent suprapubic catheter for those who cannot satisfactorily self-catheterise (p. 258). A permanent indwelling urethral catheter usually results in urethral dilatation and resultant bypass incontinence of urine.

Despite bladder training a significant number of neurogenic bladders will not empty effectively. In the hyper-reflexic situation this is due to dysneuria and in the areflexic situation to the inherent resistance of the sphincter mechanism (Rockswold and Bradley, 1977). Endoscopic surgery, in the form of external sphincterotomy and, less commonly, transurethral resection of the bladder neck and prostate, is often successful. The former operation involves incising deeply from the bladder neck to the urethral bulb in the anterior midline position.

All patients considered bladder-trained by these methods require diligent follow-up to detect deterioration in bladder function with time (Hackler, 1977). Apparently adequate bladder emptying may be achieved only at the cost of bladder hypertrophy and the development of excessive intravesical pressures, which leads to bladder diverticula, vesico-ureteric reflux, upper tract dilatation and recurrent or persistent infection. Delayed or repeat external sphincterotomy may be required to deal with these problems (Yalla et al., 1977).

Drug therapy in association with the above training may also be useful. Diazepam reduces somatic spasticity to some extent. Dantrolene sodium and baclofen also reduce somatic spasticity but side effects can be troublesome. α-Sympathomimetic blockers (e.g. phenoxybenzamine) may reduce the tone in the smooth muscle of the internal sphincter and anticholinergics (e.g. propantheline) may reduce reflex activity of the bladder in patients on intermittent self-catheterisation. Cholinergics (e.g. urecholine) have no place in an endeavour to empty a mechanically obstructive neurogenic bladder. They may however be of value in aiding the emptying of a purely atonic bladder (p. 258)

References

Hackler, R.H.: 25 year prospective mortality study in spinal cord injured patient: comparison with long-term living paraplegic. Journal of Urology 1117: 486 (1977).

Smith, J.C.: The function of the bladder; in Blandy (ed) Urology, p.672 (Blackwell, Oxford 1976).

Summers, J.L.: Neurogenic bladder in women with multiple sclerosis. Journal of Urology 120: 555 (1978).

Yalla, S.V.; Fam, B.A.; Gabilondo, F.B.; Jacobs, S.; Di Benedetto, M.; Rossier, A.B. and Gittes, R.F.: Anteromedian external urethral sphincterotomy technique, rationale and complications. Journal of Urology 117: 489 (1977).

Further Reading

Rockswold, G.L. and Bradley, W.E.: Use of sacral nerve blocks in evaluation and treatment of neurological bladder disease. Journal of Urology 118: 415 (1977).

Hinman, F. Jr.: Hydrodynamics of Micturition (Thomas, Springfield 1971).

Oyarsky, S.: The Neurogenic Bladder (Williams and Wilkins, Baltimore 1967).

Chapter XII

Upper Urinary Tract Obstruction

In 1897 Rose Bradford ligated dogs' ureters and studied the resultant changes. Hinman (1926) further studied the problem in dogs by performing 4 experiments. First, he unilaterally ligated a normal ureter for 2 weeks and then released the ligature and performed a contralateral nephrectomy. The ligated system, by hypertrophy compensation, recovered normal bodily function within 1 month. Secondly, he repeated the experiment but did not remove the ligature for 3 weeks. The ligated system was now able to recover only 50% of its normal function. Thirdly, he repeated the experiment but did not remove the ligature for 4 weeks. The ligated system was now unable to recover from this period of obstruction and the dogs died. Finally, he repeated the first experiment but delayed the contralateral nephrectomy for 3 months. While the contralateral kidney was *in situ* the now unobstructed system failed to undergo compensatory hypertrophy but when the contralateral kidney was removed such hypertrophy resulted in a size increase similar to that observed in the first group.

These findings indicate that compensatory renal hypertrophy will occur, dependent upon the quality of the remaining nephrons and the workload they are submitted to. In 1969 Hodson performed similar experiments using pigs which, like man, have a multi-pyramidal kidney. These experiments, and many clinical observations since, indicate that acute and chronic ureteric and renal obstruction results in:

1) Raised intra-tubular pressure with urine entering the renal lymphatic system at the calyceal fornices
2) Impaired glomerular filtration due to the raised intra-tubular pressure and associated ischaemia, resulting from compression of the renal vessels as they enter the hilum
3) Inflammation-infection at and proximal to the infected site
4) Calculus formation
5) Over-distension and damage to the pelvic and calyceal musculature
6) Rarely, squamous cell carcinoma of the pelvis

Pre-renal (Block, et al., 1953), renal and/or post-renal causes of nephron damage (see chapter XVI) result in varying degrees of temporarily or permanently impaired renal function. The early diagnosis and relief of any post-renal obstructive element greatly assists renal recovery. The attempted relief of bilateral upper urinary tract obstruction is aimed at encouraging the maximum hypertrophic potential of the remaining nephrons. This is the principal reason for initially correcting the worst of two chronically obstructed systems. Successful correction will enable optimal hypertrophy to occur on this side due to the lesser, but continuing, contralateral obstruction. Specific measurement of this hypertrophy over a period of several months will indicate the most suitable time for the contralateral operation.

Upper urinary tract obstruction of urine may be defined as mechanical and/or functional ureteric and/or renal obstruction which leads to progressive renal damage. *Hydronephrosis* traditionally implies obstruction of the system above the pelvi-ureteric junction whilst *hydro-ureter* implies obstruction of the ureter proximal to the obstructing cause. Hydronephrosis results in varying degrees of renal parenchymal obstruction and ischaemia (Anderson, 1963), with or without infection, calculus formation or haemorrhage.

Dilatation of the system (fig. 193) however does not necessarily mean obstruction (Whitaker, 1979) as there may be no significant delay in emptying and the dilatation may represent only a congenital anatomical or physiological abnormality and not obstruction. Such ureteric dilatation commonly occurs in women (Spiro and Fry, 1970) and in congenital disorders such as mega-calycosis (Gittes and Talner, 1972) and some megaureters (Murnaghan, 1979).

As indicated in figure 193 upper urinary tract obstruction may result from:

1) Obstruction within the lumen of the system
2) Pathological narrowing within the walls of the system or inefficiency in the calyceal-pelvi-ureteric conducting mechanism
3) Extrinsic lateral or inferior pressure on the system.

Acute unilateral or bilateral hydronephrosis and hydro-ureter are usually painful, but chronic obstructions, may be silent. An acute obstruction of all the renal parenchyma rapidly produces a uraemic anuria while chronic progressive obstruction eventually produces uraemia prior to oliguria or anuria (see chapter XVI). Pyonephrosis may complicate the obstruction and result in a serious illness.

Diagnosis

If the renal function is adequate the history and physical examination findings, together with an intravenous pyelogram, renography (O'Reilly et al., 1978) or gamma camera renography (Whitfield et al., 1978; Whitaker, 1979), may provide the diagnosis; if not, cysto-urethroscopy with a Braasch bulb retrograde pyelo-ureterogram is required. Occasionally open surgical exploration provides the only means of diagnosis.

193 The causes of upper urinary tract obstruction of urine. I within the lumen of the system; II within the walls of the system; III from extrinsic pressures.
Note — ureteric obstruction may be mechanical and/or functional, unilateral or bilateral and due to upper and/or lower tract causes.

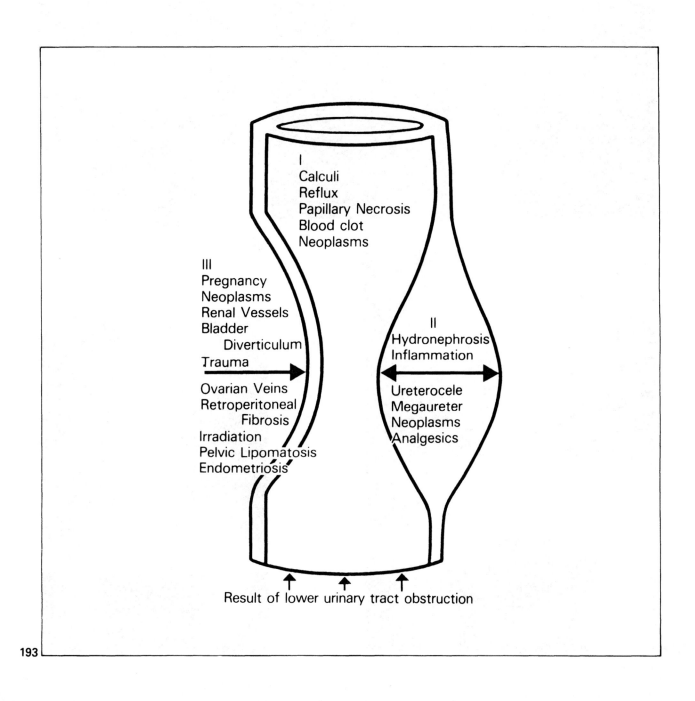

The specific treatment depends upon the particular cause. Figures 194-196 illustrate the difference between upper urinary tract dilatation and obstruction.

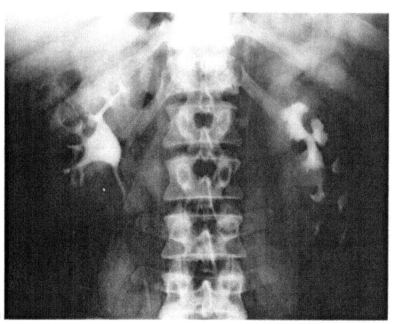

194a

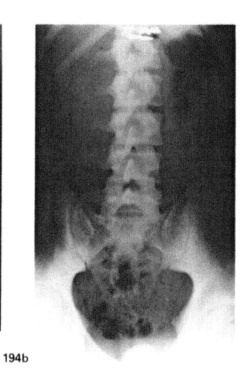

194b

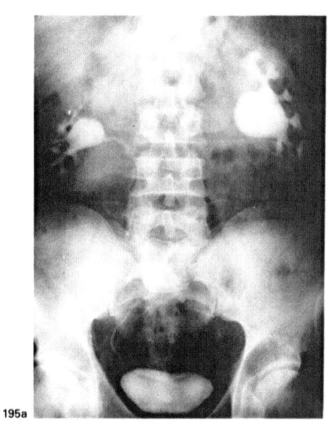

195a

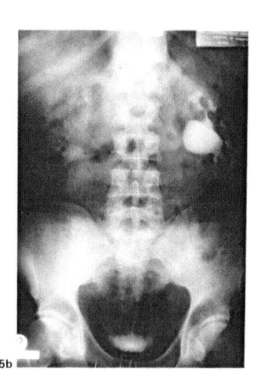

195b

Dilatation does not necessarily mean obstruction

194 This 45-year-old male presented with aching left lumbar pain. At 40 minutes an intravenous pyelogram (a) revealed left-sided uniformly dilated calyces but both systems drained equally within 75 minutes of injection of the dye (b) confirming the diagnosis of congenital left megacalycosis and proving that no significant obstruction was present.

195 This 45-year-old male also presented with aching left lumbar pain. The 40 minute intravenous pyelogram (a) again revealed a uniformly dilated left calyceal system, together with a dilated left renal pelvis. The 75 minute film (b), however, confirmed that the left side was both dilated and obstructed. A left pyeloplasty operation corrected the obstruction.

196 The ureter is commonly narrowed, but not obstructed, at the pelvi-ureteric junction, crossing the common iliac vessels and at the uretero-vesical junction. Some physiological dilatation is common proximal to these sites, particularly in females(a). The post-micturition film (b) indicates that there is a right-sided pelvi-ureteric obstruction in this patient but no other abnormality.

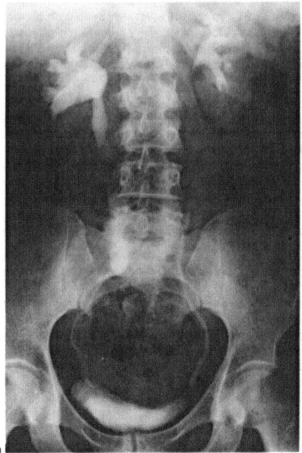

196a

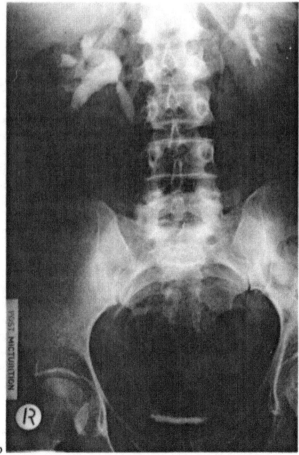

196b

Obstruction Above the Ureteric Orifices

Obstruction Within the Lumen of the System

Calculi: This is the most common cause of obstruction to the upper urinary system (fig. 197) but, even with large calculi, it is rare for a calculus to completely obstruct the ureter. See chapter IX.

Vesico-ureteric Reflux: The effects of vesico-ureteric reflux are identical to obstruction as the upper system never empties and, in severe reflux, is subjected to an intermittent high intra-tubular pressure. The reflux may be either vesico-ureteric or uretero-ureteric, which may occur in certain bifid systems joining before they enter the bladder (see chapter I fig. 9).

Renal Papillary Necrosis: The ingestion of large amounts of analgesics in susceptible patients, infection, arterial disease and diabetes may result in necrosis of the renal papillae and, if severe, sloughing of the necrosed tissue leading to:

1) Interference with the vital hyperconcentration functions of the papillae
2) Occasional impaction of the sloughed papillae in the ureter which may require basket (chapter IX fig. 168) or, rarely, open surgical extraction
3) Fibrosis which assists the subsequent radiological appearance of dilated blunt calyces (fig. 198)
4) Blood clot
5) Calyceal, pelvic and ureteric neoplasm.

Obstruction Within the Walls of the System

Obstruction may arise as a result of pathological narrowing within the walls of the system and/or inefficiency of the calyceal-pelvi-ureteric conducting mechanism. The ureter is normally narrowed at the pelvi-ureteric junction, as it crosses the common iliac vessels, and in its distal portion (fig. 196a).

Pelvi-ureteric Hydronephrosis: A congenital, mechanical (70% of cases) excess of fibrous tissue, or a 'functional' (of unknown aetiology) abnormality of the pelvi-ureteric junction (30% of cases), prevents the calyceal-pelvic system from emptying within a normal time period, leading to a hydronephrosis with vascular and back pressure obstructive damage to the renal parenchyma (p. 36).

An extra-renal pelvis may enlarge considerably and protrude between the main renal artery and the artery (division of main renal artery or separate branch to kidney) running to the lower pole (fig. 199), giving a false impression that the artery to the lower pole is the complete cause of the obstruction (Murnaghan, 1958). A so-termed 'high take-off ureter' represents the new site of the ureter after the pelvis has enlarged. In its altered and deformed position it may contribute secondarily to the obstruction.

Presentation: The inability to empty the calyceal-pelvic system efficiently may result in several types of clinical presentation:

1) Episodes of loin and/or abdominal pain, particularly related to excessive fluid intake (Bourne, 1966).
2) Dyspepsia and an uncomfortable epigastric sensation. These symptoms may result from the interrelated nerve supply of the kidney and the upper gut and/or from the close relationship of the duodenum and colon.
3) Silent atrophy which, if bilateral, may result in uraemia.
4) An asymptomatic or tender retroperitoneal mass (p. 340 for the differential diagnosis of retroperitoneal masses).
5) Rarely, painless haematuria may result from the obstructed renal venous system.
6) Abnormal kidneys rupture more readily than normal kidneys and the diagnosis is often made for the first time after such an accident.

197 Ureteric calculus obstruction. A ureteric calculus obstructing the right upper ureter and kidney. This is the most common cause of upper urinary tract obstruction but does not always require surgical correction.

198 Renal papillary necrosis. This may result from several causes. Note the almost total absence of papillae in both kidneys.

199 Primary functional pelvi-ureteric hydronephrosis. Note the absence of a mechanical stricture, which is usually present, and the mechanical, and possibly functional, secondary obstruction of the lower pole vessels.

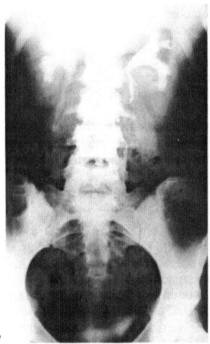

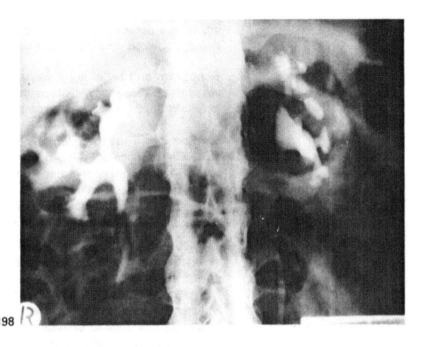

197

198

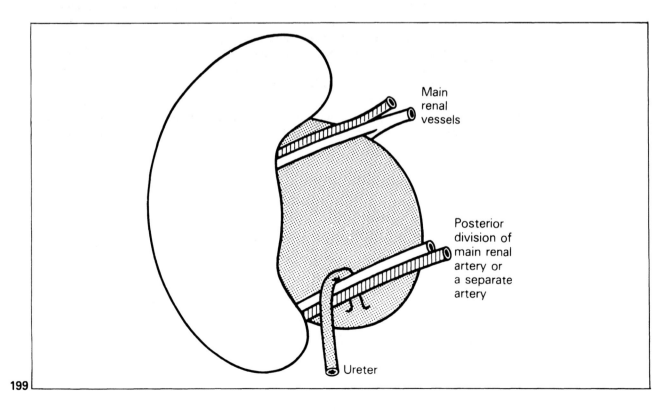

199

Diagnosis

Intravenous pyelogram. The inability to empty the calyceal-pelvic system, within a normal period of time, may be obvious or there may be sufficient suspicion to justify an intravenous pyelogram performed with an excessive fluid load thus magnifying the effects of the situation (fig. 200). Compensatory contralateral hypertrophy is not a contraindication to conservative surgery (Milewski, 1978).

Renal angiogram. This investigation is of value in deciding whether a poorly or non-functioning hydronephrotic kidney should undergo an attempted pyeloplasty operation or be removed. A 50% obstructive narrowing of the main renal artery and its branches indicates irreversible renal damage (Olssen, 1961) and justifies nephrectomy.

Renogram and renal scan. In patients who are allergic to iodine or who are uraemic these radio-isotope methods of diagnosis, with or without an excessive fluid load, are an alternative to intravenous pyelography.

Voiding cysto-urethrogram. This is often necessary in children, to exclude the presence of vesico-ureteric reflux which may have produced a secondary pelvi-ureteric hydronephrosis due to overloading of the system.

Treatment

Correction of the obstruction may be achieved by a pyeloplasty or an anti-reflux operation. There are several essential operative principles:

1) The decision to operate should be made in the light of the above investigations and not on the appearance of the pelvi-ureteric junction at operation. Woe betide the urologist who operates on an anatomically hypoplastic but not significantly functionally abnormal upper system.
2) After the anaesthetic has been administered a Braasch bulb retrograde ureterogram is done to exclude any associated ureteric pathology (p. 114).
3) An extra-peritoneal anterior loin incision is made and every care is taken to preserve all of the terminal renal arteries.
4) A complete pelvi-ureterolysis is made to display the particular (short or long mechanical stricture, no mechanical stricture, large flabby pelvis, multiple vessels etc.) anatomical situation (fig. 199).
5) A pyeloplasty operation which will correct all of these abnormalities and produce a dependent, wide pelvi-ureteric junction is then selected. The results of such surgery are very good.
6) Should an anti-reflux operation be necessary then this is performed and the resultant effect on the pelvi-ureteric junction observed radiologically before determining whether or not a pyeloplasty operation will be necessary.

Magnification diagnosis of pelvi-ureteric hydronephrosis
200a A possibly obstructed right pelvi-ureteric junction is indicated

200b A high fluid load confirms the diagnosis by exaggerating the inability of the right kidney to empty itself within a normal time period.

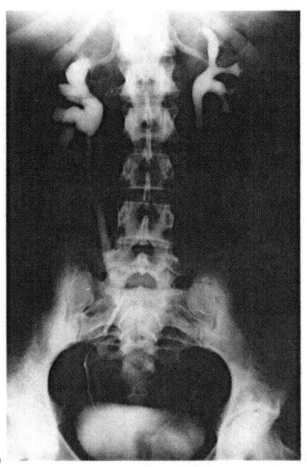

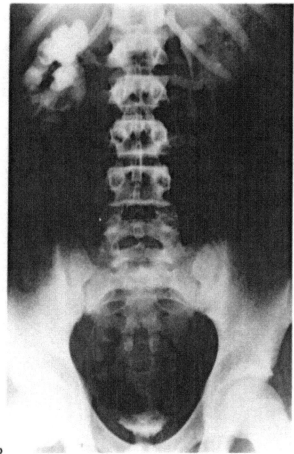

200a   200b

Surgical and Non-Surgical Trauma: Figure 201 indicates the result of inadvertent ligation of the ureter during a difficult hemi-colectomy operation. See chapter XIII.

Inflammation: Inflammatory causes include:

1) Tuberculous strictures at the distal or mid-ureter and the pelvi-ureteric junction
2) Physical inflammation after deep x-ray therapy which may fibrose the ureteric wall and the surrounding tissues
3) A ureteric calculus which has remained in the one position for many years may cause a stricture but this is always difficult to prove
4) Bilharziasis strictures may occur in the distal ureter.

Calyceal-pelvi-ureteric Neoplasm: The upper tract obstruction in figure 202 is due to a ureteric neoplasm situated in the upper ureter.

Ureterocele and Mega-ureter: A dilated mega-ureter (figs. 203-204) may not necessarily be obstructed although this may be difficult to confirm. Whitaker's test (p. 121) is designed to make this distinction and enables selection of those patients who would benefit from an attempted surgical correction.

Analgesic Abuse: In addition to causing papillary necrosis analgesic abuse may also result in a ureteric stricture (McGregor et al., 1979).

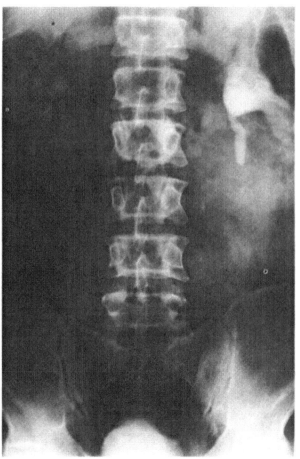

201

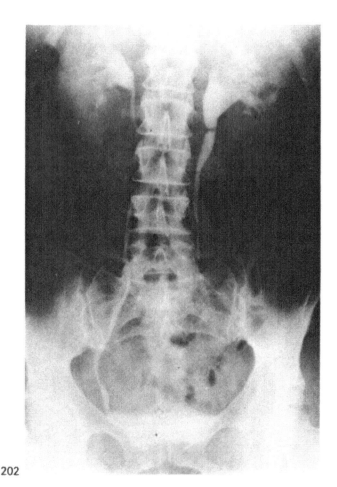

202

201 Traumatic obstruction. Inadvertent ligation of the left ureter during a difficult left hemi-colectomy operation. Fortunately the trauma was diagnosed in the early postoperative period and successful removal of the ligature and reconstruction of the damaged ureter undertaken.

202 Neoplastic obstruction. An upper ureteric neoplasm in a 50-year-old woman who presented with painless haematuria.

Mega-ureter

203 A supra-vesical dilated but non-obstructed primary mega-ureter usually requires no operative intervention.

204 A vesical obstructed primary mega-ureter (b) often requires surgical correction.

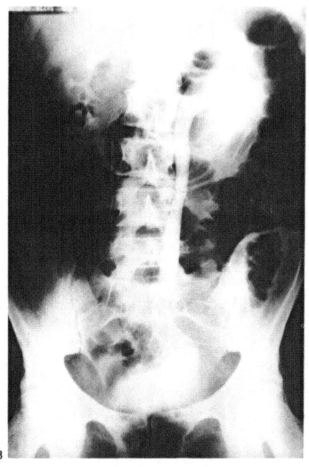

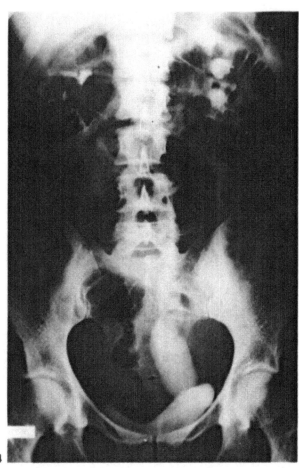

203   204

Extrinsic Pressure on the System

Pregnancy: The developing fetus progressively obstructs both ureters.

Pelvic or Retroperitoneal Neoplasm: Neoplasms in this area may infiltrate (fig. 205) and obstruct the ureter producing uraemia, which is a common form of death in advanced cancer. Large benign tumours, such as pelvic lipomatosis (Crane and Smith, 1977) or an aneurysm (Peters and Cowie, 1978) may also cause obstruction.

Bladder Diverticula: If large these may obstruct the terminal ureter (fig. 206).

Retrocaval Ureter: This is a rare condition in which the ureter passes behind the inferior vena cava (see chapter I fig. 23) and if severe obstruction is produced it may require surgical correction.

Ovarian Vein Syndrome: It has been postulated that a gross dilatation of the right ovarian vein can result in ureteric dilatation which may require surgical correction (Derrick et al., 1973).

Upper Ureteric Vascular Compression and Pulsation: Renal vessels may compress the pelvi-ureteric junction or the upper ureter. They may occasionally cause mechanical obstruction or their pulsation may cause functional obstruction by interfering with ureteric peristalsis. Such vessels are moved or sutured away from the new pelvi-ureteric junction following pyeloplasty operations.

Some extrinsic causes of upper urinary tract obstruction
205 Infiltration of the right ureter by a rectal carcinoma

206 Obstruction due to a large bladder diverticulum

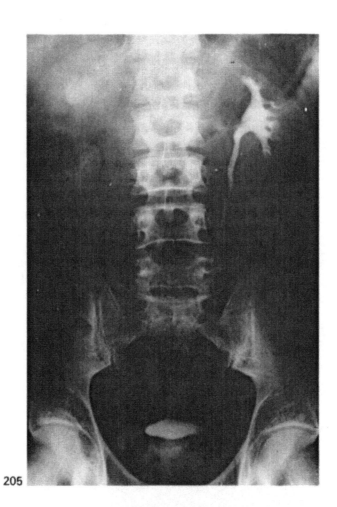

205

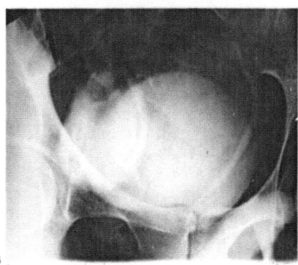

206

Idiopathic Retroperitoneal Fibrosis: This rare condition (fig. 207) presents between the age of 40 and 50 years with malaise, abdominal pains, backache and, later, uraemia and/or anuria (Ormond, 1948). Many cases of presumed idiopathic benign retroperitoneal fibrosis are eventually found, by local tissue biopsy or future clinical progress, to have neoplastic infiltration of the area. The condition results from fibrosis of the retroperitoneal tissue sufficient to obstruct the ureter. Similar fibrotic changes may occur in the ears, mediastinum and palms (Dupuytren's contracture). The aetiology is unknown but may be related to analgesic abuse or the antiserotonin drug methysergide which is used to treat migraine.

Diagnosis

Intravenous Pyelogram. Provided that the kidney is functioning sufficiently well, a medial deviation of the middle third of the ureter resulting from the fibrotic pull, is displayed, together with varying degrees of proximal hydro-ureter and/or hydronephrosis.

Treatment

Retrograde catheters often pass the obstructed level without difficulty (fig. 207) and temporary urinary diversion may be achieved by this procedure until such time as open surgical liberation of the ureters, with associated suture positioning well away from the scar tissue, is possible. Renal dialysis may be necessary if retrograde catheterisation diversion is not possible or if the patient is grossly uraemic upon initial presentation.

Deep X-ray Therapy: Attempted therapeutic irradiation of pelvic malignancies may result in severe pelvic and lower abdominal retroperitoneal fibrosis (Dean and Lytton, 1978) sufficient to cause upper urinary tract obstruction (p. 312).

207 Idiopathic retroperitoneal fibrosis. A 45-year-old male was admitted with gross uraemia and oliguria. The lack of renal concentrating ability prevented intravenous pyelography assessment. Panendoscopy revealed no lower urinary tract abnormality. Bilateral ureteric catheters passed easily to both renal pelves (a) and a rapid flow of urine occurred. These findings, together with the medial deviation of the ureters (b), was highly suggestive of retroperitoneal fibrosis, which was confirmed by open exploration and treated by bilateral ureterolysis with lateral ureteric fixation.

Note — that in this patient it was necessary to pass the catheters to the renal pelvis in order to obtain temporary urinary diversion drainage as well as carry out the calyceal-pelvi-ureterogram studies.

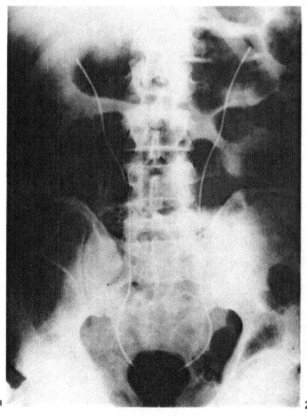

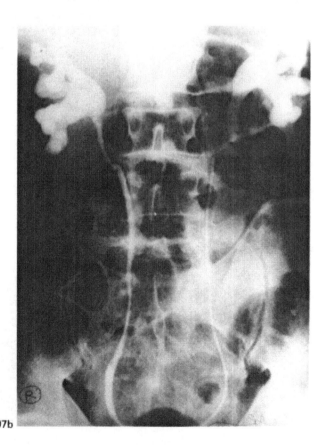

207a

207b

**Obstruction Below
the Ureteric Orifices**

All of the causes of lower urinary tract obstruction may, if allowed to progress, produce upper urinary tract obstruction (fig. 208).

Chyluria

This is a rare form of upper urinary tract obstruction characterised by the passage of milky white urine which often clots after voiding; microscopically it is shown to contain numerous fat globules. Chyluria may be associated with general symptoms of weight loss and anaemia.

208 Upper urinary tract obstruction commonly results from lower urinary tract obstruction. In this particular situation both systems are obstructed by a large benign prostate gland.

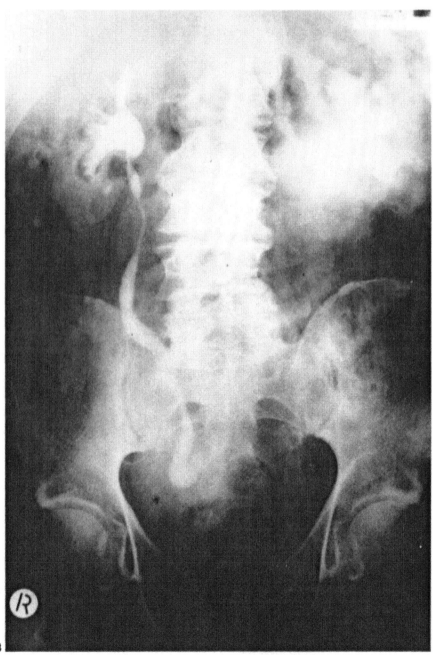

208

Aetiology

Obstruction to the abdominal lymph flow by filarial infection fibrosis (seen in South East Asia) or congenital lymphangiectasia (seen very rarely in Australia) may result in either raised urinary tract intraluminal lymphatic pressure, with chyle being forced into the urine, or abnormal lymph communications between the bowel and the urinary lymphatics, which may rupture into the urinary system.

Investigations

Intravenous pyelogram and/or retrograde pyelo-ureterogram may reveal a pyelolymphatic connection but lymphangiography is necessary to identify precisely the site and type of abnormality (Karanjavala, 1976).

Treatment

The lymphatic communication is usually renal and complete open surgical ligation of all lymph channels to the kidney, after they have been visualised by the pedal injection of blue violet dye, is usually successful.

Filarial infection is treated with diethylcarbamazine but such infestation is rarely detected at the fibrotic stage. The microcytic anaemia and/or other metabolic abnormalities resulting from the loss of lymph may also require correction.

References

Block, M.A.; Wakim, K.G. and Mann, F.C.: Appraisal of certain factors influencing compensatory renal hypertrophy. American Journal of Physiology 172: 60 (1953).

Bourne, R.B.: Intermittent hydronephrosis as a cause of abdominal pain. Journal of the American Medical Association 198: 1218 (1966).

Bradford, J.: Observations made upon dogs to determine whether obstruction of the ureter would cause atrophy of the kidney. British Medical Journal 2: 1720 (1897).

Crane, C.B. and Smith, M.J.V.: Pelvic lipomatosis: 5 year follow up. Journal of Urology 118: 547 (1977).

Dean, R.J. and Lytton, B.: Urological complications of pelvic irradiation. Journal of Urology 119: 64 (1978).

Derrick, F.C.; Rosenblum, R. and Brensilli, F.J.: Right ovarian vein syndrome: six year critique. Urology 1: 383 (1973).

Gittes, R.F. and Talner, L.B.: Congenital megacalices versus obstructive hydronephrosis. Journal of Urology 108: 833 (1972).

Hodson, C.J.; Craven, J.D.; Lewis, D.G.; Metz, A.R.; Clarke, R.J. and Ross, E.J.: Experimental obstructive nephropathy in the pig. British Journal of Urology 41: 1 (1969).

Karanjavala, D.K.: Lymphography in the management of filarial chyluria. Annals of the Royal College of Surgeons, England 46: 267 (1970).

McGregor, B.; Saker, B.M. and England, E.J.: Ureteric stricture associated with analgesic nephropathy. Medical Journal of Australia 1: 287 (1979).

Milewski, P.J.: Radiograph measurements and contralateral renal size in primary pelvic hydronephrosis. British Journal of Urology 50: 289 (1978).

Murnaghan, G.F.: Mechanisms of congenital hydronephrosis with reference to factors influencing surgical treatment. Annals of the Royal College of Surgeons, England 23: 25 (1958).

Murnaghan, G.F.: Experimental studies of the hydrodynamics of the dilated ureter with reference to surgical treatment. Report of the Societe Internationale d'Urologie, p. 251 (1979).

O'Reilly, P.H.; Testa, J.H.; Lawson, R.S.; Farrar, D.J. and Edwards, C.E.: Diuresis renography in equivocal urinary tract obstruction. British Journal of Urology 50: 76 (1978).

Peters, J.L. and Cowie, A.G.A.: Ureteric involvement with abdominal aortic aneurism. British Journal of Urology 50: 313 (1978).

Spiro, F.I. and Fry, J.K.: Ureteric dilatation in non-pregnant women. Proceedings of the Royal Society of Medicine 63: 462 (1970).

Whitaker, R.H.: The Whitaker test. The Urologic Clinics of North America 6: 529 (1979).

Whitfield, H.N.; Britton, K.E.; Hendry, W.F.; Nimmunm, C.C. and Wickham, J.E.A.: The distinction between obstructive uropathy and nephropathy by radioisotope transit times. British Journal of Urology 50: 433 (1978).

Further Reading

Anderson, J.C.: Hydronephrosis (Heinemann, London 1963).

Hinman, F.: Renal counterbalance. AMA Archives of Surgery 12: 1105 (1926).

Hultengren, N.: Renal papillary necrosis. A clinical study of 103 cases. Acta Chirurgica Scandinavica (Suppl.): 277 (1961).

Notley, R.G.: Ureteric obstruction; in Blandy (Ed) Urology, p. 568 (Blackwell, Oxford 1976).

Olsson, O.: Renal angiography; in Abrhams (Ed) Angiography vol. 2, p. 539 (Little, Brown, Boston 1961).

Smart, W.R.: Hydronephrosis; in Campbell (Ed) Urology, Vol. 3, p.2372 (Saunders, Philadelphia 1963).

Chapter XIII

Genitourinary Trauma

Non-penetrating road, industrial or sporting trauma accounts for most renal, bladder and urethral injuries but most ureteric injuries and some bladder and urethral injuries are caused by medical practitioners. Improvements in both equipment and techniques have meant that significant irradiation trauma is now uncommon.

Most genitourinary injuries do not require immediate surgery and, in civilian practice, time is usually available to transfer such patients to a major centre unless, uncommonly, life-saving nephrectomy or severe penetrating wound exploration is necessary. High speed missile or blast trauma may cause shock wave injuries far distant from the entry or exit wounds.

Renal Trauma

Trauma of the kidney may be classified as:

1) Blunt non-penetrating
2) Penetrating
3) Iatrogenic.

Most renal trauma is of the blunt non-penetrating type and results from motor vehicle, sporting or industrial accidents.

Excessive force is usually necessary to damage normal kidneys as they are well protected by the rib cage, vertebrae and related muscles, in addition to possessing a high degree of mobility, an envelope of shock absorbing perirenal fat and strong Gerota's fascia (fig. 209). A pathological kidney, because of its abnormal architecture, is more easily damaged and 12% of all traumatised kidneys are retrospectively found to be pathological, with pelvi-ureteric hydronephrosis being the most commonly found abnormality.

Associated non-genitourinary injuries occur in 30% of cases.

Penetrating renal injuries are uncommon but serious renal injuries may result from small penetrating stab wounds. Iatrogenic injuries usually result from renal biopsies and, rarely, from retrograde pyelography.

Pathology

Figure 209 shows the various types of renal trauma and table I lists the incidence of the early consequences. Varying degrees of bleeding and urinary extravasation may be present in addition to renal parenchymal damage. A life-saving emergency nephrectomy is necessary in 4% of patients in order to control massive early bleeding. Less severe bleeding and urinary extravasation is usually controlled by the tamponading effect of Gerota's fascia. This means that the vast majority of cases of renal trauma can be managed successfully by bed rest and constant observation (Badenoch, 1950a).

209 Types of renal trauma including incomplete and complete fissure and the rare ureteric and renal pedicle fissure. Note the importance of Gerota's fascia.

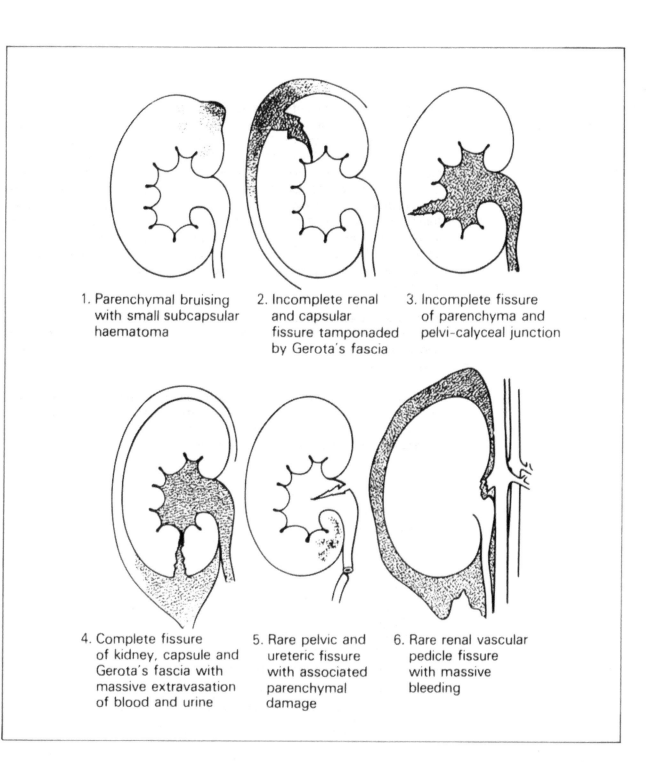

1. Parenchymal bruising with small subcapsular haematoma

2. Incomplete renal and capsular fissure tamponaded by Gerota's fascia

3. Incomplete fissure of parenchyma and pelvi-calyceal junction

4. Complete fissure of kidney, capsule and Gerota's fascia with massive extravasation of blood and urine

5. Rare pelvic and ureteric fissure with associated parenchymal damage

6. Rare renal vascular pedicle fissure with massive bleeding

Table I. The early complications of renal trauma

Complication	Incidence (%)
Parenchymal bruising	100
Subcapsular haematoma (mostly small)	60
Partial fissure (peri-renal and/or pelvic)	30
Complete fissure — polar avulsion	15
Pulped kidney	2
Major arterial and/or venous damage	1
Pelvic or ureteric split or division	1
Acute tubular necrosis	

The later complications of renal trauma are listed in table II. Most of the late complications are due to traumatic or secondary infective fibrotic changes which may be diagnosed radiologically. Tissue calcification may result. A peri-renal pseudocyst represents a persistent extravasated collection of blood and urine with a pseudo-capsule of fibrous tissue (p. 35). A relatively large subcapsular haematoma may be difficult to diagnose until it presents dramatically as a delayed rupture or as the cause of hypertension. Renal trauma resulting from sporting injuries is often not diagnosed at the time of injury unless haematuria occurs. It is not possible, or necessary, to prevent all of these late complications by surgical intervention and any such attempt may be associated with a further loss of renal tissue (Thompson et al., 1977).

Diagnosis

History and Examination: Patients present with haematuria, loin pain and tenderness and a degree of shock relative to the trauma sustained. The degree of haematuria is not always related to the severity of the injury and may be delayed for hours or, uncommonly, days.

Physical Examination: This may reveal pain and tenderness to palpation in the traumatised loin together with the later development of a loin mass and visible bruising. A relatively normal physical examination does not necessarily exclude severe renal or ureteric injury.

Table II. The later complications of renal trauma

1. Delayed haemorrhage

2. Fibrosed subcapsular haematoma

3. Renal and ureteric fibrosis
    Parenchymal
    Calcyceal
    Pelvi-ureteric (pseudo-hydronephrosis)
    Ureteric

4. Arterial and/or venous fibrosis and narrowing

5. Encysted urinary extravasation (para-renal pseudocyst)

6. Renal hypertension (due to renal parenchymal or subcapsular fibrosis and/or to delayed renal artery stenosis)

All patients presenting with such a history and/or physical signs should be suspected of having renal injury, particularly if there is any evidence of a fractured lower rib, and should have an intravenous pyelogram as soon as their systolic blood pressure is sufficient to enable adequate contrast medium concentration to occur. The major, but uncommon, risk to the patient at this early stage is death resulting from uncontrollable bleeding and it is therefore essential to determine, as early as is possible, whether or not the opposite kidney is normal in case an emergency nephrectomy is required. (Blood should be typed and two units cross-matched although most patients will not require a blood transfusion.)

Special Investigations. *Abdominal and Pelvic X-ray:* Straight abdominal and pelvic x-ray (fig. 210) may show a loss of the psoas shadow, due to blood or urinary extravasation, in addition to lumbar scoliosis, due to contraction of the lumbar muscles on the traumatised side. It may also show small, normal or enlarged (e.g. polar avulsion, subcapsular haematoma) renal outlines as well as calcifications, foreign bodies and evidence of skeletal or intra-peritoneal trauma.

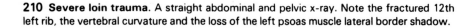

210 Severe loin trauma. A straight abdominal and pelvic x-ray. Note the fractured 12th left rib, the vertebral curvature and the loss of the left psoas muscle lateral border shadow.

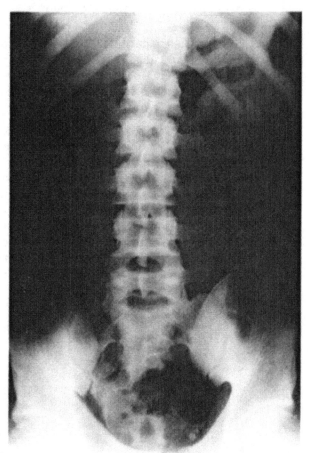

210

Injection phase of the pyelogram: Pyelography is performed principally to determine whether or not there is a normally functioning kidney on the non-traumatised side (fig. 211). Because of the impairment of function on the injured side, and occasional extravasation of the contrast medium, it is not usually possible, or necessary, to obtain precise anatomical details of the trauma at this stage. High dose medium injection may be necessary if there has been severe blood loss.

Management

Once the clinical state and the intravenous pyelogram has been assessed the patient is admitted to hospital with a diagnosis of:

1) Minor or moderate renal trauma ± associated injuries
2) Major renal trauma ± associated injuries.

Most cases of renal trauma fall into the first category and these patients are treated with bed rest, suitable analgesic and sedative therapy and continued observation of all vital signs, together with macroscopic examinations of all urine specimens passed. The patient is allowed up and discharged after resolution of the macroscopic haematuria with a review intravenous pyelogram appointment in approximately 1 month's time. Further follow-up is continued for a *minimum of 10 years.*

A small percentage of cases (4%) require an emergency nephrectomy because of uncontrollable bleeding. Should this be necessary it is performed through a transperitoneal abdominal incision, as this will enable control of the renal pedicle before Gerota's fascia is opened and will also enable a detailed laparotomy. All penetrating injuries should be surgically explored after the appropriate special investigations (see later) have been performed (Glenn and Harvard, 1960).

A further group of patients (35%), who initially are not bleeding sufficiently to justify an emergency nephrectomy, nevertheless do not make continued improvement despite adequate bed rest and sedation. Under these circumstances further specialised investigations are necessary (Hai et al., 1977). The causes of this failure to improve include:

1) Continued excessive bleeding, which is usually extra-renal, but may be intra-renal (e.g. arterio-venous fistula). Occasionally the continued bleeding results in a large subcapsular haematoma which may present as a renal mass, hypertension, or as a delayed, dramatic rupture.
2) Extensive urinary extravasation which, often combined with bleeding, presents as a progressively increasing loin mass.
3) Persistent complete or partial non-function or persistent poor function, which may result from either a severely damaged kidney, a severed or traumatised vascular pedicle, or a pre-existing abnormal lesion.
4) The rare development of renal hypertension (see chapter XVII).

211 Severe right renal trauma. An intravenous pyelogram. Note the large urinary extravasation which was drained 5 days after the injury.

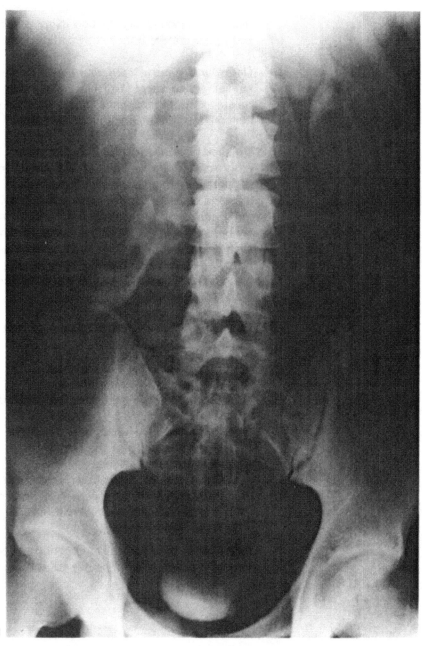

211

Further Special Investigations: Further special investigations are necessary in those patients who do not improve clinically.

Selective renal angiography: This investigation provides the only means of accurately diagnosing vascular injuries such as renal pedicle trauma, arteriovenous fistula formation (fig. 212), renal infarction, ischaemia and aneurysm. Early and delayed renal parenchymal damage is displayed in more detail than in the intravenous pyelogram. This particularly applies to avulsion of one or both renal poles. Major renal pedicle trauma usually means death of the kidney unless it is corrected within at least 6 hours of onset.

Retrograde pyelo-ureterogram: The possible risk of introducing infection and creating further renal damage, together with the inadequacy of the information gained (compared with angiography) means that there is little place for this investigation in the diagnosis and management of renal trauma. However, it is occasionally of value in excluding or diagnosing the rare upper ureteric penetration injury (see later), when poor renal function and upper urinary tract extravasation may obscure the correct diagnosis.

Ultrasound, gamma camera studies: As discussed in the chapter III these studies are of value in displaying the normality or otherwise of the contralateral kidney and occasionally in providing specific, progressive diagnostic information concerning the traumatised kidney.

Delayed Renal Surgical Exploration: Depending upon their clinical progress and the results of the above specialised investigations some patients may require a delayed exploration of the kidney. This may involve drainage of large extravasated collections, a partial or complete nephrectomy, the repair of major vessels, ureteric reconstruction, or specific surgery related to any pre-existing abnormal renal pathology. The timing of any such delayed surgery is dictated by the clinical situation but it is best performed 5 to 7 days after the injury as much of the smaller vessel primary bleeding has ceased by this time and the tissue planes have not yet become fibrosed.

Indications: Delayed renal surgical exploration is indicated under the following circumstances:

1) Continued excessive bleeding
2) A large urinary extravasation
3) A progressively increasing loin mass due to blood and/or urinary extravasation
4) Persistent non-function or persistent poor function of part, usually a renal pole, or all of the kidney
5) All penetrating injuries
6) Detection of potentially correctable pre-existing abnormal renal pathology such as a pelvi-ureteric hydronephrosis
7) A large subcapsular haematoma
8) Renal hypertension.

As indicated previously all emergency and early renal trauma surgery is performed through a trans-peritoneal abdominal incision.

212 Stab wound to left loin. Continuing profuse haematuria, following a small penetrating stab wound, necessitated a left selective renal angiogram, which displays a large left arteriovenous fistula subsequently treated by nephrectomy.

Penetrating stab wounds must always be surgically explored after appropriate special investigations have provided as much pre-operative information as is necessary.

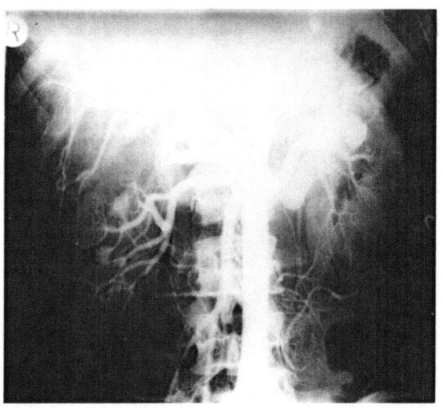

212

Delayed surgical findings of retroperitoneal haematoma: Occasionally a large, previously unsuspected retroperitoneal haematoma is found during an emergency post-traumatic laparotomy. The haematoma should not be 'explored' unless it is felt to be the reason for an, as yet unexplained hypotension, as the incising of Gerota's fascia releases its tamponading action and usually results in a nephrectomy. If possible an intravenous pyelogram should be obtained on the operating table prior to or during such an exploration, to assess the appearance and function of the kidneys more accurately.

Follow-up

It is essential that all patients be regularly reviewed for at least 10 years following renal trauma so that uncommon delayed complications, such as hypertension, can be detected and treated.

Ureteric Trauma

Because of its size, position, mobility and relatively thick wall the ureter is rarely damaged. The vast majority of such injuries result from surgical accidents. The presence of local peri-ureteric pathology, such as inflammation, obstruction, degeneration, irradiation changes, neoplasia or other masses, increases the chances of such trauma.

Surgical accident to the ureter may result in its being partially or completely divided, ligated, crushed, diathermised or devascularised. The injury may be single or multiple and may involve one or both sides.

Clinical Presentation

There is usually a history of a recent operation or, uncommonly, a history of blunt or penetrating external trauma (Carlton et al., 1971) or irradiation (p. 340).

Physical examination indicates that in the early post-traumatic period the patient is more restless and febrile than could be explained by the particular operation, with unexplained or unusually severe loin or wound pain and tenderness, or a presenting fistula.

As urinary extravasation increases abdominal distention, ileus, oliguria, anuria or septicaemia may occur. In the author's series of 71 referred cases the majority (89%) were diagnosed at least 4 days after the initial trauma (Brown, 1977). This delay is due to confusion of the early symptoms and signs with those of the particular operation performed or because concurrent external trauma soft tissue damage confuses the picture.

Diagnosis

A diagnostic intravenous pyelogram, with associated pyelo-ureterogram studies, are essential investigations in the clinical situations described above. Many medico-legal actions would not have taken place if the patient's postoperative complaints of excessive wound or related loin pain had been investigated at the time (fig. 213):

What therefore god has joined together let no man put asunder   *Matthew, 19.6*

213 Surgical trauma. A 50-year-old man complained of severe loin pain 48 hours after a left lumbar sympathectomy operation. The intravenous pyelogram revealed an obstructed left kidney, with gross extravasation of urine into the retro-peritoneal space. Reconstruction of the ureter was possible because of the early diagnosis.

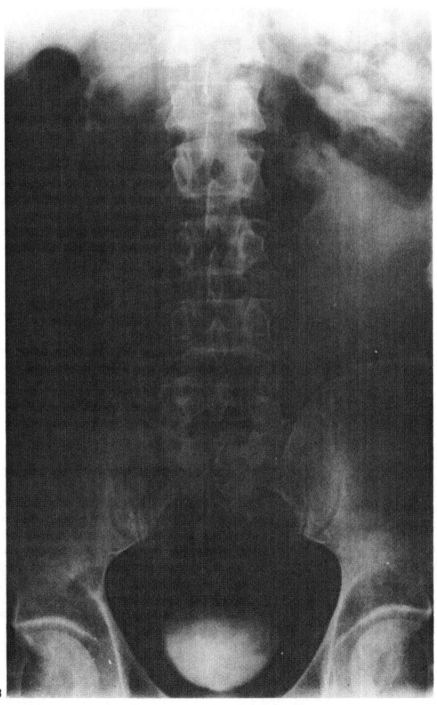

213

Table III. Cause of ureteric trauuma in the author's series of 84 patients

Cause	No. of patients
Surgery	
Gynaecology	18
Renal homo-transplantation	16
Open urological	10
Large bowel	9
Ureteric ligation	7
Endoscopic urological	7
Vascular	2
Orthopaedic	1
Appendicectomy	1
External penetration or blunt injury	3
Deep x-ray therapy	
Acute	4
Chronic	6

Aetiology

The causes of ureteric trauma in a series of the author's patients is shown in table III.

Treatment

The risk of iatrogenic damage to the ureter is lessened if the correct choice of operation is made, faults in technique avoided and, in situations involving large related masses or difficult operations such as secondary or tertiary procedures, preoperative intravenous pyelography and/or ureteric catheterisation performed. When damage has occurred the appropriate treatment will depend upon the following factors:

a) Type of injury
b) Delay in diagnosis
c) Total renal function and pathology
d) The patient's general condition
e) The site of injury
f) Life expectancy (e.g. incurable pelvic malignancy)
g) The surgeon's skill and experience.

Early diagnosis is essential as delayed recognition (longer than 2 weeks) of upper ureteric injuries usually results in a nephrectomy. Delayed finding of lower ureteric injuries however may not be so serious as these can often be by-passed.

The principle considerations in ureteric repair surgery are outlined below.

Management After Early Diagnosis

1) Because of the resultant inflammatory-infective tissue reactions any repair should be attempted either within the first 2 weeks of injury or, depending upon the particular circumstances, 2 months later.
2) Within the first week of a ligation injury it may only be necessary to remove the suture and insert a prophylactic drain tube, but this depends upon the precise circumstances (Raney, 1978).
3) Minimal partial ureteric injuries can occasionally be treated by the early endoscopic passage of a splinting and draining ureteric catheter, which is then left in situ for 10 to 14 days (Brown, 1977).

4) Penetrating injuries, which are rare, must be explored as soon as adequate (intravenous pyelogram with or without retrograde ureterogram) investigations have been performed. Extensive debridement is often necessary because of devitalisation of the ureter (Liroff et al., 1977). It is usually possible to excise up to 2.5cm of a ureter and still achieve a tension-free anastomosis.

5) Surgical injury usually does not require extensive debridement. The anastomosis should be performed obliquely end-to-end, in an endeavour to minimise stricturing, using fine 4/0 chromic cat gut interrupted sutures, over a splinting silastic 5F 'tissue inert' ureteric catheter, which should extend from the renal pelvis to the bladder and remain *in situ* for 10 days, if possible, thereby overcoming the problem of a possible undiagnosed second distal and/or proximal injury (Sieben et al., 1978).

If suture of the defect is not possible then the ureter is allowed to heal around the splint provided that it is left *in situ* for at least 8 weeks (Davis et al., 1948). The ureter should never be ligated in the hope that silent atrophy of the kidney will follow. Ligation may result in a septicaemic pyonephrosis or latent bursting of the suture, resulting in a difficult secondary nephrectomy.

6) Low ureteric injuries may be better treated by directly re-implanting the ureter, in an anti-reflux tunnel, into the bladder. This may require bladder mobilisation (Turner-Warwick, 1965) or even a bladder tube flap (Gow, 1968) to achieve continuity. A transuretero-ureterostomy operation (Hodges et al., 1963) overcomes the occasional difficulty of inadequate healthy distal ureteric length as does the rare operation of distal renal autotransplantation.

7) Adequate dependent drainage must be provided at the site of repair.

8) Proximal urinary diversion is often necessary, either as a primary independent procedure or as part of the repair, and may be achieved by performing a separate or combined splinting nephrostomy or proximal ureterostomy (see chapter VIII).

Management After Delayed Diagnosis

If the extravasated urine is infected then urgent adequate drainage of this area, combined with a proximally diverting nephrostomy, is performed until such time as a repair operation or a nephrectomy is undertaken. If the trauma is so severe that either delayed ureter-to-bladder or transuretero-ureterostomy by-pass operations are not possible, then the upper ureter or pelvis can be joined to the bladder by using a small bowel conduit (Boxer et al., 1979). An initial diverting nephrostomy operation is usually necessary in these situations and only removed after successful kidney-bowel-bladder continuity has been proved radiologically.

Lower Genitourinary Tract Trauma

Non-penetrating, high-speed motor vehicle trauma, industrial accidents and, rarely, surgical misfortune, account for most cases of lower genitourinary tract trauma. Modern pelvic war injuries are usually penetrating, multi-visceral, associated with severe soft tissue trauma and, usually, heavy contamination (Brown et al., 1980).

Depending upon the severity of the injury and factors such as infection, blood loss and associated trauma the damaged bladder or urethra heals by primary intention or by delayed secondary intention. The resulting fibrosis is rarely of concern in the bladder, because of its large capacity, but in the smaller lumen urethra the occurrence of fibrosis dominates the management.

Classification

Lower genitourinary tract trauma may be classified as:

1) Anterior urethral surgical and non-surgical trauma
2) Severe pelvic and lower abdominal trauma
3) Open or closed surgical or obstetric intra-peritoneal and/or extra-peritoneal bladder trauma
4) Genital trauma

Aetiology and Management

Anterior Urethral Surgical and Non-surgical Trauma. *Penetrating internal surgical trauma:* Surgical trauma accounts for the majority of urethral injuries (figs. 214-215). A life-long urethral stricture or death from septicaemia may result from the incompetent or rough passage of endoscopic equipment. Sharp, small calibre instruments should rarely be used and inability to pass the instrument selected should indicate the need to seek more experienced help (p. 240). Urethro-vaginal fistulae are rare but may result from forceful patient or medical instrumentation penetration.

Non-penetrating external (straddle) trauma: External urethral trauma (figs. 216-217) occurs following straddle injuries, motor car accidents, fighting or sporting accidents (surfboards, skis). The urethra may be divided partially or completely, with resultant corpora bleeding and urinary extravasation if the injury is severe and the patient has voided following the accident.

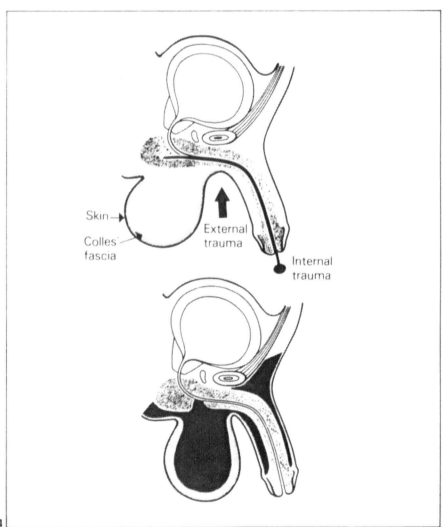

214

Urethral trauma

214 Extravasation following severe anterior external or internal urethral trauma.

215 Surgical trauma accounts for the majority of urethral injuries. Be careful and gentle and never use small, rigid, sharp-headed instruments.

216 Straddle anterior urethral trauma resulting from a fall on a construction site. The patient was unable to void and required a diverting and splinting silastic urethral catheter.

217 A severe straddle injury of the anterior urethra. Note the areas of extravasation and the suprapubic drainage. This injury required open surgical reconstruction.

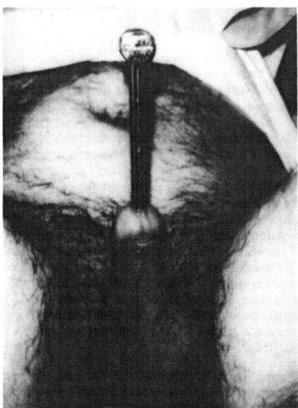

215

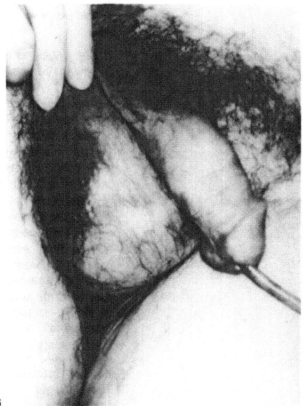

216

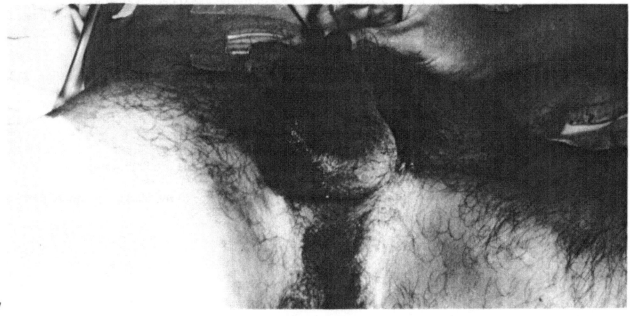

217

Self-induced Trauma: Patients occasionally attempt to insert foreign bodies or chemically irrigate their urethras, often with disastrous results.

Treatment: The aims of treatment are:

1) To prevent extravasation of urine
2) To drain extravasated urine and large haematomas
3) To control infection
4) To achieve urethral continuity without stricturing.

Many injuries require a diagnostic urethrogram and, depending upon the clinical progress and the result of this investigation, the following steps are taken:

1) The patient is allowed to void spontaneously under supervision.
2) Any instrument or foreign body is removed if this can be accomplished gently and without further complications. In many cases the foreign body is impacted and a general anaesthetic with either endoscopic or open surgical extraction is required.
3) The patient is given suitable analgesic and broad spectrum chemotherapy to combat any possible bacteraemia and local infection.
4) Should the patient not be able to void, a urethral silastic catheter is inserted to act as a healing splint and to relieve urinary retention (fig. 216).
5) If the injury is so severe that urethral catheterisation cannot be achieved then a suprapubic cystostomy is performed, prior to evacuation of the usually large perineal haematoma, and open repair of the partial or complete urethral separation carried out through a vertical perineal incision, using 2/0 chromic cat gut interrupted sutures. A splinting and draining silastic urethral catheter is left *in situ* for 3 weeks. If satisfactory voiding occurs with the suprapubic catheter clamped then it also is removed.
6) Follow-up urethral bouginage is performed at progressively increasing intervals of time and resultant severe urethral stricture treated by a urethroplasty operation (p. 256).

Severe External Penetrating Anterior Urethral and Perineal Injuries:
These injuries usually result from bomb blasts and require both suprapubic cystostomy drainage and extensive wound debridement. Primary repair of the injury is not usually possible because of the extent of urethral loss. A mucosa-to-skin anastomosis of the debrided healthy margins of the defect is made and the resultant hypospadias corrected when the area has healed. Associated perineal and rectal trauma is common and a proximal diverting colostomy is usually also necessary.

Severe Pelvic and Lower Abdominal Trauma: These injuries (figs. 218, 219-225) may be classified as:

a) Penetrating
b) Non-penetrating extra-peritoneal bladder rupture
c) Non-penetrating intra-peritoneal bladder rupture
d) Non-penetrating prostato-membranous urethral rupture
e) Combinations of the above
f) Non-penetrating, non-rupture injuries of the bladder, posterior urethra and related viscera.

218 Severe, external non-penetrating pelvic injury. Differential diagnosis and management.

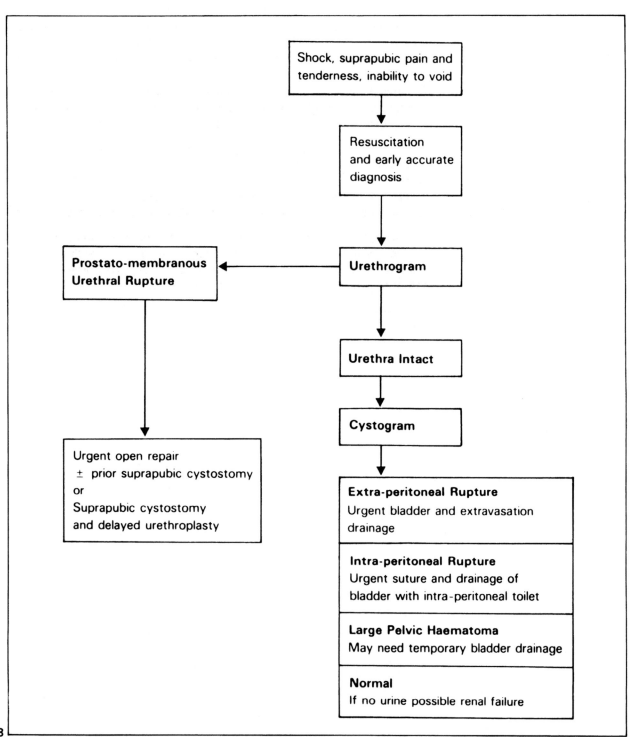

218

Penetrating Injuries: These injuries are rare in civilian life but are not uncommon in war time. They require immediate blood replacement and associated resuscitation, followed by urgent open exploration of the area. Proximal diversion of both the urinary stream (suprapubic cystostomy, ureterostomy or nephrostomy) and the bowel (colostomy or, less commonly, ileostomy), together with adequate debridement, drainage and removal of any foreign bodies are usually necessary. Associated reduction and stabilisation of any pelvic bone fracture may also be called for.

All severe penetrating injuries in this area require the passage of a urethral catheter (22F Foley), both to ensure the integrity of the urethra and bladder and, depending on the method of proximal urinary diversion, to measure the urinary output. Should there be any doubt about the integrity of the bladder a distension dye (radiological or visual) cystogram should be done.

Differential Diagnosis: Although an adequate history, a thorough physical examination and straight abdominal and pelvic x-rays may enable an accurate diagnosis it is often not possible to distinguish clinically between:

1) Moderate or major low abdominal and/or pelvic trauma, without bladder or posterior urethral injury
2) Extra-peritoneal bladder rupture and/or a prostato-membranous urethral separation, with or without associated trauma
3) Intra-peritoneal bladder rupture, with or without associated trauma.

Bleeding appearing at the external urinary meatus indicates lower genitourinary tract trauma whilst low abdominal *pain* and tenderness indicates that bone and soft tissue damage must be excluded, irrespective of whether or not the patient has voided clear urine.

External pelvic trauma (219 to 225)
219 Types of severe external pelvic trauma. Intra-peritoneal rupture of the bladder is a rare injury. All three types usually result from high-speed motor vehicle accidents.

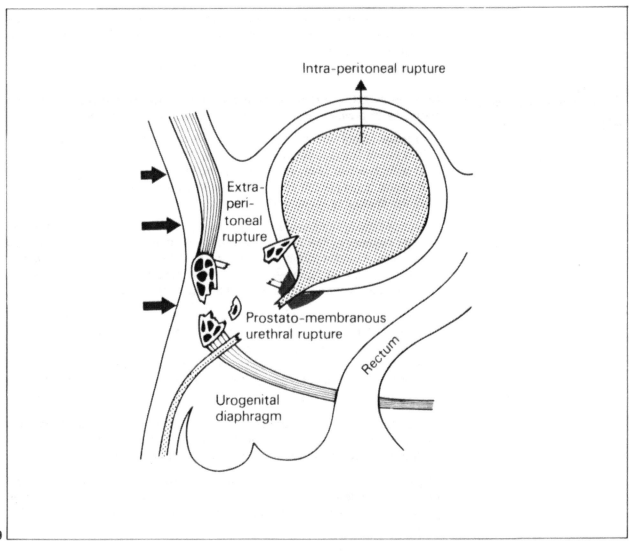

Major injuries result from severe pelvic bone or foreign body penetration of the pelvic tissues and bladder and/or separation of the prostato-membranous urethra, as the bladder and prostatic urethra is forced backwards by the pelvic fracture-dislocation. Such serious injuries occur in 10% of all non-penetrating pelvic fracture-dislocations (Coffield and Weems, 1977). This figure is high enough to justify all patients presenting with a fractured pelvis being suspected of having sustained bladder and/or urethral trauma until proven otherwise.

The severity of these injuries is illustrated by the fact that 80% sustain other severe injuries, including head and chest trauma, ruptured bowel, diaphragm and limb fractures. An early intravenous pyelogram assessment is essential as associated upper urinary tract injuries are common. Up to 20% of patients die as a result of these combined injuries (fig. 220).

An early, accurate diagnosis is essential and usually a diagnostic urethrogram and cystogram are necessary. Failure may result in death or severe long term complications. The differential diagnosis and management of severe, external non-penetrating pelvic injury is depicted schematically in figure 218.

Indications for urethrography: A urethrogram is indicated in the following circumstances:
1) Failure to void satisfactorily or improve clinically. If a prostato-membranous urethral rupture is excluded, a bladder catheter is passed and a distension cystogram obtained.
2) Moderate to severe anterior urethral injuries (p. 298).

Prostato-membranous Urethral Rupture

Non-penetrating Prostato-membranous Urethral Rupture: A clinical diagnosis of a *ruptured prostato-membranous urethra* is made if:

    a) lower abdominal pain and tenderness is present and progressive
    b) a pelvic fracture is present
    c) urine has not been voided since the injury
    d) blood is present at the external meatus (fig. 220)
    e) the bladder is distended.

This uncommon multi-system injury usually requires temporary suprapubic bladder catheterisation until such time as definitive surgical repair can be undertaken. A urethrogram will confirm the diagnosis although there is occasionally doubt as to whether the injury is at the bladder neck or the prostato-membranous urethral junction (fig. 220, 221).

Should the patient's general condition permit it an attempted open re-alignment of the ruptured urethra is performed immediately; however, in view of the high incidence of associated injuries and the inevitable time delays, it is usually necessary to perform suprapubic urinary diversion until the patient's general condition permits either early open re-alignment of the rupture or a delayed urethroplasty operation for the resultant stricture.

In the presence of an associated colo-rectal injury infection of the area is inevitable and usually severe. Such combined injuries require a proximal diverting colostomy in addition to a suprapubic cystostomy.

The traumatised area rapidly fibroses and attempted open or endoscopic reconstruction (Mitchell, 1968) must be performed within 2 weeks of injury, or the area left to heal for 3 months before a posterior urethroplasty is attempted.

External pelvic trauma (continued)
220 Severe pelvic and lower abdominal trauma is usually not an isolated injury and this accounts for the overall mortality rate of 20%. Note the suprapubic bladder drainage.

221 A prostato-membranous urethral rupture diagnosed by a urethrogram.

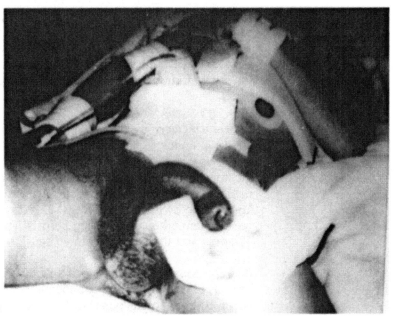

220

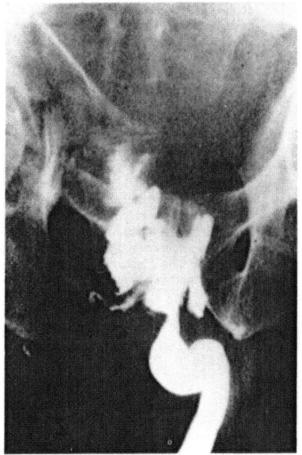

221

If the patient's general condition permits an attempted open surgical re-alignment of the ruptured urethra, the patient is anaesthetised and placed, if possible, in a slight Trendelenburg position. In view of the high incidence of associated injuries an initial laparotomy is performed before the bladder and associated retropubic haematoma is displayed. Large blood clots are removed and a 'tissue inert' fenestrated (Turner-Warwick, 1973) silastic Foley catheter (chapter X; fig. 170) is passed along the urethra into the retropubic space. The bladder is then opened and a Nelaton catheter passed through the bladder and into the retropubic space. The catheters are sutured together and the Nelaton catheter pulled backwards, so that the silastic catheter enters the bladder. The Nelaton catheter is removed, the cystostomy incision closed, and the retropubic space drained for 48 hours.

In severe injuries, in case the silastic catheter blocks, it is wise to use a second suprapubic Foley drainage catheter for the first 48 hours after operation. This operation has approximated the ruptured urethral margins but, in most injuries, the anastomosis is under excessive tension, because of the pelvic bone fracture-dislocation. An associated orthopaedic reduction-stabilisation of this fracture (figs. 222a,b) usually reduces this tension and the resultant amount of healing fibrosis. The retropubic space is drained for 48 hours and the catheter left *in situ* for 2 months.

It is not possible to visualise the ruptured urethral margins retropubically and this prevents accurate debridement and suture apposition of the edges; however, this is partly possible if a second perineal incision is made and the ventral and lateral urethral margins displayed. In the author's experience the patient's associated injuries and general condition usually prevent this second operation and the technical difficulty of maintaining the sutures in position, because of the inflammatory oedema present, have made it disappointing in those in whom it has been attempted.

Cysto-urethroscopy: Mitchell (1968) has stressed the importance of this procedure in partial prostato-membranous urethral injuries, as it may enable endoscopic splinting catheterisation of the bladder without opening the retropubic space. Cysto-urethroscopy should be attempted initially in those injuries where operative reconstruction has been delayed 4 to 14 days. This delay enables some resolution of the infalmmatory tissue oedema although fibrosis rapidly occurs and the area soon resembles a 'brick wall'. When the catheter is removed the urethra should be gently dilated, at least weekly for the next 2 months, once a fortnight for a further 2 months and then monthly for the next 6 months, under strictly aseptic conditions, in order to minimise severe stricturing of the traumatised site. Further dilatations are usually necessary at progressively increasing intervals of time for the rest of the patient's life (Myers and DeWeerd, 1972). Despite this treatment severe posterior urethral strictures often result from this injury.

External pelvic trauma (continued)

222a Prostato-membranous urethral separations result from severe pelvic bone trauma. This patient has sustained a wide separation-fracture of the pelvic girdle.

222b Orthopaedic reduction and stabilisation of the fracture enables a tension-free anastomosis of the ruptured urethral margins to be achieved, diminishing the severity of the secondary intention healing fibrosis.

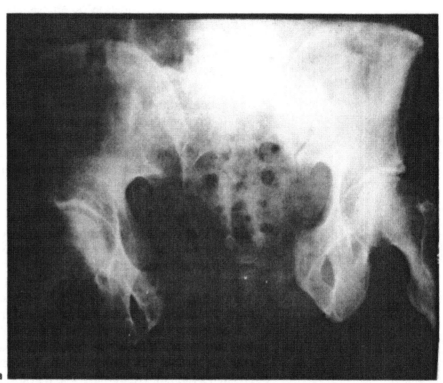

222a

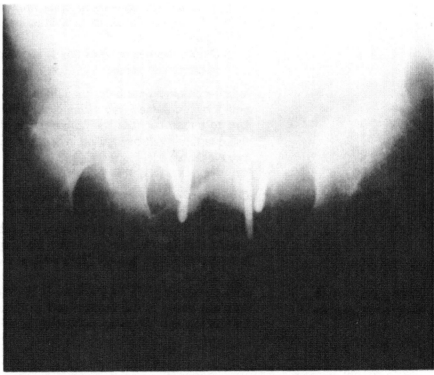

222b

Delayed Posterior Urethroplasty: If early open surgical repair of the injury is not possible then the suprapubic cystostomy catheter is left *in situ* for 3 months, until the area has healed, and then a posterior urethroplasty operation performed. In contrast to anterior urethroplasty operations posterior urethral stricture repair is difficult. Posterior urethroplasties may entail:

1) Removal of the anterior portion of the pubis, excision of the stricture and either end-to-end anastomosis of the non-narrowed urethral margins or a by-pass anastomosis (Moorehouse and McKinnon, 1969; Pierce, 1972; Coffield and Weems, 1977).
2) A ventral excision of the stricture and the utilisation of a scrotal skin flap to achieve continuity (Blandy et al., 1971); Turner-Warwick, 1977).
3) A pull-through operation (Badenoch, 1950b).

Impotence resulting from severe pelvic trauma: Although impotence usually results from vascular and nerve damage at the traumatised site it is often difficult to assess. Most people are impotent following prostato-membranous urethral separations but there are some who gradually recover at least partial erection. No prognosis should be given for at least 2 years following the accident (Gibson, 1970).

Indications for catheterisation and cystogram: Although a urethrogram may have excluded a urethral rupture the patient's symptoms, signs and clinical progress may indicate the need for diagnositc bladder catheterisation and cystogram evaluation.

The passage of the catheter (22F 2-way silastic Foley catheter for adults) along the urethra is performed gently and under strictly aseptic conditions. The sudden appearance of urine in a reasonable quantity usually indicates that the urethra is intact (as previously indicated by the urethrogram) and that the bladder has been reached. The catheter balloon is inflated and a preliminary straight abdominal and pelvic x-ray done. This preliminary x-ray may:

1) Indicate the presence of bone fractures
2) Indicate soft tissue abnormalities including associated intra-peritoneal injuries
3) Detect the presence of any foreign bodies or calcified material in the abdomen or pelvis.

Iodine-containing contrast medium is now slowly inserted into the bladder until a high volume x-ray series cystogram has been achieved. It is important to remember that the normal adult bladder holds at least 400ml and this quantity must be instilled in order to eliminate the possibility of a small extravasation.

Cystogram evaluation: If progressive clinical improvement occurs and/or the urethrogram and cystogram reveal no rupture, it can be assumed that no major bladder or urethral injury is present although compression and elevation of the bladder ('tear drop bladder') may result from a large pelvic haematoma which usually takes several months to resolve.

Extra-peritoneal Bladder Rupture

Non-penetrating Extra-peritoneal Bladder Rupture (figs. 223-224): Occurs low down in the bladder and is diagnosed by contrast medium extravasation into the extra-peritoneal tissues, with associated severe pain.

External pelvic trauma (continued)
223 An extra-peritoneal bladder rupture diagnosed by a distension cystogram.

224 An extra-peritoneal bladder rupture usually results from pelvic bone penetration. Orthopaedic reconstruction may be necessary.

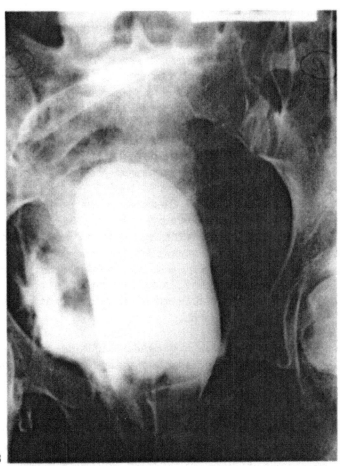

223

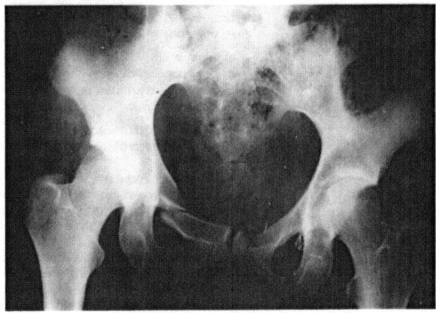

224

Management: The extravasated urine is stab drained for 48 hours and a Foley haematuria catheter left indwelling on continuous drainage for 10 days, dependent upon the patient's general condition. The catheter maintains apposition and healing of the separated bladder margins. Attempted suture apposition is not necessary and may cause further trauma to related structures.

Intra-peritoneal Bladder Rupture

Non-penetrating Intra-peritoneal Bladder Rupture (fig. 225): This rare injury occurs at the fundus of a previously distended bladder and the cystogram reveals a partly filled bladder with extravasation of the contrast medium within the intra-peritoneal pelvis, producing an hour-glass appearance. An immediate laparotomy is performed and the extravasated urine removed from the peritoneal cavity and the bladder rupture sutured with 2 layers of interrupted O chromic cat gut. A laparotomy is always performed at the same time to detect the presence of any associated injury. The urethral haematuria catheter is left indwelling on continuous drainage for 10 days and then removed, provided the patient's clinical state permits.

Surgical or Obstetric Intra-peritoneal Bladder or Posterior Urethral Trauma: Extensive, difficult pelvic surgery, or the unsuspected presence of a bladder protrusion into an inguinal hernia, may result in inadvertent trauma. Transurethral prostatic or bladder neoplasm resection (p. 176) may also, rarely, penetrate the full thickness of the prostatic capsule and/or the bladder wall. Treatment consists of primary suture of any bladder penetration and drainage of the area and/or continuous bladder catheter drainage for 10 days.

Vesico-vaginal fistula: Obstetric pressure necrosis, due to obstructed labour, causes most traumatic vesico-vaginal fistulae in less affluent countries; in other parts of the world it is a rare complication of abdominal or vaginal hysterectomy (Kelly, 1979).

Once a fistula has occurred it is preferable to attempt to repair it either within the first 2 weeks or to wait 3 months for the infection and inflammation to resolve. A combined trans-vesical and vaginal approach, with 2 surgeons assisting each other to obtain a no-tension, firm, mucosa-to-mucosa anastomosis of both the separated bladder and vaginal mucosal layers, using 2/0 chromic cat gut, is successful in 90% of patients. However, the repair of complicated fistulae, which may be characterised by

a) large defect
b) long-standing defect
c) previously attempted repair operation
d) irradiated tissue

results in diminishing success rates, even if pedicle fat grafts (Maritus, 1939) are interposed between the two mucosal layers.

Other Bladder Fistulae: Vesico-colic fistulae may result from either severe colonic peri-diverticulitis or from an invasive sigmoid carcinoma. Severe cystitis results, often with pneumaturia, and occasionally the passage of solid material per urethra. If possible the diseased bowel is resected, with or without a temporary or permanent colostomy, and the bladder fistula repaired. Vesico-caecal and vesico-ileal fistulae may result from Crohn's disease and are similarly treated after barium radiological identification and cystoscopic assessment (p. 160). Vesico-uterine fistulae are very rare and result from uterine neoplastic invasion of the bladder

225 An intra-peritoneal bladder rupture diagnosed by a distension cystogram.

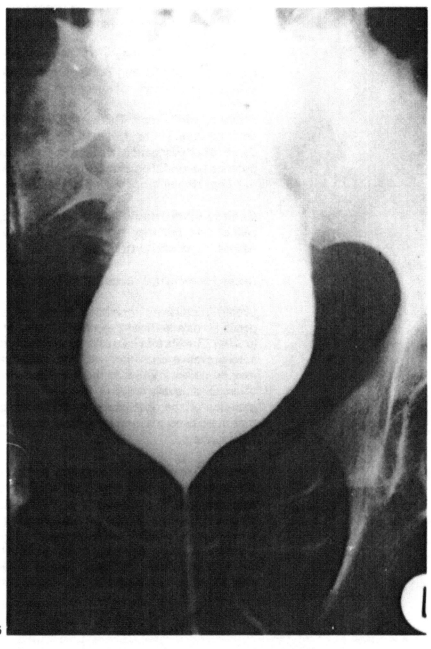

225

resulting again in a severe cystitis and, in younger patients, haematuria at the time of menstrual periods. It is most unusual for a bladder neoplasm to be the cause of any of the above fistulae.

Genital Trauma: Injuries to the penis, scrotum, testes and spermatic cord need control of haemorrhage, conservative debridement and early repair. Extensive penile denudation may need to be treated by suprapubic cystostomy drainage and implantation of the penis into a scrotal tunnel until a specialised plastic repair can be attempted.

Testicular injuries: The high mobility of the testis safeguards against injury but should the tunica albuginea be torn then a haematocele develops. This must be evacuated, and careful point diathermy of the bleeding vessels and repair of the divided tunica margins carried out.

Scrotal injuries: Should the scrotal skin be completely avulsed then the testis can be temporarily placed under the related abdominal or thigh skin. A testicle should never be removed unless it is dead.

Post-surgical haematocele: Open evacuation is usually necessary as the condition is painful and resolves spontaneously only at a very slow rate with a high incidence of secondary infection.

Fractured penile shaft: This rare injury (p. 68) occurs following trauma to an erect penis and is best treated by open surgical repair of the split corpora sheath after evacuation of the clot. The incidence of partial or complete impotence beyond the point of fracture is high and the patient should be told this prior to any proposed operation (Gross et al., 1977).

Genitourinary Irradiation Trauma: Therapeutic irradiation may destroy cancer cells but may also damage the genitourinary system and related tissues (Dean and Lytton, 1978).

Renal: Parenchymal fibrosis may occur but this is now very rare.

Ureter: Therapeutic irradiation of the pelvis for malignancy may result in pelvic fibrosis sufficient to obstruct one, or more commonly both, ureters (p. 294). The fibrosis is usually so extensive that it is not possible to perform a conservative operation and, with unilateral involvement, a nephrectomy may be necessary but, in the more common bilateral involvement, urinary diversion is usually required. Every effort should be made at the time of exploration of the obstruction to obtain adequate tissue biopsies to ensure that there is no malignancy present before attempting major urinary diversion surgery.

Bladder: Telangiectasis, ulceration or fibrosis of the bladder may occur. Telangiectasia or ulceration may result in severe bleeding, which usually responds well to Helmstein's (p. 178) balloon distension application, intravesical formalin instillation (Likourinas et al., 1979) or to diathermy. A small capacity bladder can be enlarged by performing an ileocystoplasty or a colocystoplasty operation or by suprapubic urinary diversion. The incidence of significant irradiation injuries has decreased markedly during the past 10 years with improved equipment and techniques.

References

Badenoch, A.W.: Injuries of the kidney. Medicine Illustrated 4: 53 (1950a).

Badenoch, A.W.: Pull-through operation for impassable traumatic stricture of the urethra. British Journal of Urology 22: 404 (150b).

Blandy, J.P.; Sing, M.; Notley, R.G. and Tressinder, G.C.: The results and complications of scrotal flap urethroplasty for strictures. British Journal of Urology 43: 52 (1971).

Boxer, R.J.; Fritzsche, P.; Skinner, D.G.; Kaufman, J.J.; Belt, E.E.; Smith, R.B. and Goodwin, W.E.: Replacement of ureter by small intestine: clinical application and results of ileal ureter in 89 patients. Journal of Urology 121: 728 (1979).

Brown, R.B.: Surgical and external ureteric trauma. Australian and New Zealand Journal of Surgery 47: 471 (1977).

Brown, R.B.; Cantamessa, S. and Nunn, I.: Genito-urinary War Injuries. Australian Army Handbook (in press).

Carlton, C.E. Jr.; Scott, R. Jr. and Buthrie, A.G.: The initial management of ureteral injuries: a report of 78 cases. Journal of Urology 105: 335 (1971).

Coffield, K.S. and Weems, W.L.: Experience with management of posterior urethral injury associated with pelvic fracture. Journal of Urology 117: 722 (1977).

Davis, D.M.; Strong, G.H. and Drake, W.M.: Intubated ureterotomy: experimental work and clinical results. Journal of Urology 59: 851 (1948).

Dean, R.J. and Lytton, B.: Urological complications of pelvic irradiation. Journal of Urology 119: 64 (1978).

Gibson, G.R.: Impotence following fractured pelvis and ruptured urethra. British Journal of Urology 42: 86 (1970).

Glenn, J.F. and Harvard, B.M.: The injured kidney. Journal of the American Medical Association 173: 1189 (1960).

Gow, J.G.: The results of reimplantation of the ureter by the Boari technique. Proceedings of the Royal Society of Medicine 61: 128 (1968).

Gross, M.; Arnold, T.L. and Peters, P.: Fracture of penis with associated laceration of urethra. Journal of Urology 117: 725 (1977).

Hai, M.A.; Pontes, J.E. and Pierce, M.J. Jr.: Surgical management of major renal trauma: review of 102 cases treated by conservative surgery. Journal of Urology 118: 7 (1977).

Hodges, C.V.; Moore, R.J.; Lehman, T.H. and Behman, A.M.: Clinical experience with transuretero-ureterostomy. Journal of Urology 90: 552 (1963).

Kelly, J.: Vesicovaginal fistulae. British Journal of Urology 51: 208 (1979).

Lang, E.K.; Trichel, B.E.; Turner, R.W.: Renal arteriography in the assessment of renal trauma. Radiology 98: 103 (1971).

Likourinas, M.; Cranides, A.; Jiannopoulos, B.; Kostakopoulos, P. and Dimopoulos, C.: Intravesical formalin for the control of intractable bladder haemorrhage secondary to radiation cystitis or bladder cancer. Urological Research 7: 125 (1979).

Maritus, H.: Gynaecological operations and their topographic-anatomic fundamentals. Canterbury Press Chicago: 271 (1939).

Mitchell, J.P.: Injuries to the urethra. British Journal of Urology 40: 649 (1968).

Moorehouse, D.P. and MacKinnon, K.G.: Urological injuries associated with pelvic fractures. Journal of Trauma 9: 479 (1969).

Myers, R.P. and DeWeerd, J.H.: Incidence of stricture following primary realignment of the disrupted proximal urethra. Journal of Urology 107: 265 (1971).

Pierce, J.M. Jr.: Management of dismemberment of prostatic membranous urethra and ensuing stricture disease. Journal of Urology 107: 259 (1972).

Raney, A.M.: Ureteral trauma: effects of ureteral ligation with and without deligation — experimental studies and case reports. Journal of Urology 119: 326 (1978).

Sieben, D.M.; Howerton, L.; Amin, J.; Holt, H. and Lich, R.J.: Role of ureteral stenting in management of surgical injury of ureter. Journal of Urology 119: 330 (1978).

Thompson, I.M.; LaTourette, H.; Montie, J.E. and Ross, G. Jr.: Results of non-operative management of blunt renal trauma. Journal of Urology 118: 522 (1977).

Turner-Warwick, R.: The Psoas Hitch Procedure. Institute of Urology Film, London (1965).

Turner-Warwick, R.: Observations on the treatment of traumatic urethral injuries and the value of the fenestrated urethral catheter. British Journal of Surgery 60: 775 (1973).

Turner-Warwick, R.: Complex traumatic posterior urethral strictures. Journal of Urology 118: 564 (1977).

Further Reading

Bonnin, N.J.; Brown, R.B.; Hall, R.J. and Jose, J.S.: Urological Injuries. The Management of Road Traffic Injuries. Royal Australasian College of Surgeons Handbook (McCarron-Bird, Melbourne 1969).

Liroff, S.A.; Pontes, J.E.S. and Pierce, J.M. Jnr.: Gunshot wounds of the ureter: 5 years experience. Journal of Urology 118: 551 (1977).

Chapter XIV

Paediatric Urology

In this short review of paediatric urology space permits only a summary of some distinctive differences from the concepts of adult disease and a brief synopsis of some of the more important lesions encountered in children. Reference should be made to the chapter on Embryology and Congenital Abnormalities (chapter I) and the suggested Further Reading as well as to the appropriate chapters on specific conditions.

Paediatric Compared to Adult Practice

Symptomatology

In adult urology urinary symptoms almost always indicate urological disease. In children urinary symptoms are often misleading; frequency, scalding and wetting, in the absence of toxaemia, more commonly indicate a functional or nervous state than they do infection. When such symptoms are accompanied by a positive urinary culture, on an inadequately collected specimen of urine, it is not surprising that the complex is misinterpreted as 'infection' and a train of unnecessary investigations set in motion. On the contrary, children with true urinary infection characteristically have a predominence of nonspecific symptoms — fever, lethargy, anorexia, vomiting, and abdominal pain. This is especially so of infants and toddlers, in whom failure to thrive, vomiting and diarrhoea may be the only manifestations; in the older the child, the more characteristic 'adult' urinary symptoms are added to the story.

The fact that the emotional response of a child to stress or personality disturbance is to produce urinary symptoms is doubly confusing. Such a child may, in addition, develop a fever or toxaemic symptoms and be found to have a genuine urinary infection; investigations may then reveal an organic urinary abnormality. An assurance is given that the 'cause' has been found, and disappointment and disillusion follow when, after treatment of the organic anomaly, the child continues to wet or complain of dysuria. This double pathology is a common occurrence in children.

Infection in the Absence of Recognisable Pathology

In female children, with unequivocally proven urinary infection, no identifiable organic lesion can be found in about 60% of patients. In the first year of life, in both sexes, only 50% have an identifiable anomaly. These infections are predominantly urethro-trigonitis, confined to the lower urinary tract, and pyelonephritis is rarely found. The background to these lower tract infections is very commonly poor perineal hygiene or the repeatedly wet state of a child who has not yet gained urinary control, the moist vulva and perineum offering a good culture medium for organisms. The functional wetting is itself a contributing cause of infection. The reluctance to accept these facts leads some urologists to find some supposed organic basis to the infection and the symptoms, such as bladder neck or urethral 'stenosis'.

Another example of misinterpretation is the finding of double ureters on intravenous pyelography in a child with urinary symptoms, or actual infection, when the former is assumed to be the cause of the latter. Under certain defined circumstances this may be so (see later), but many double systems are accidental discoveries of no significance, and the infection is a localised urethro-trigonitis, or the symptoms are functional and quite unrelated to the ureteric anatomy.

Functional Stasis Versus Obstruction

Although quite specific obstructive lesions occur in children (pelvi-ureteric obstruction, ureteric strictures, urethral valves, etc.), with the same dire consequences as in adult pathology, a large component of paediatric urology deals with disturbance to emptying, which depend on abnormalities of peristalsis, or on hypo-muscularity of the tissues. Further, these disturbances may change or evolve with time, so that an understanding of the natural history of disease in which the process either progresses or cures itself, is necessary. These concepts fundamentally affect treatment in which operative surgery is not always applicable. Many examples may be cited: vesico-ureteric reflux due to deficiency of terminal ureteric musculature, which may or may not spontaneously recover; megaureter with neither vesico-ureteric obstruction nor reflux but gross hypo-dysplasia; calyceal and renal anomalies due to developmental dysplasia and not secondary to distal obstruction or infection; disturbed flow in bifid systems; stasis in non-stenotic bladder or urethral diverticula; neuropathic bladders of a lower motor neurone type with flaccid sphincters; the triad syndrome ('prune belly') with gross hypo-dysplasia of several areas of the urinary tract in addition to absent abdominal and intra-abdominal muscles.

Congenital Versus Acquired Disease

Although in children we see a number of acquired lesions (tumour, calculi, infection, etc.) paediatric urology includes a high preponderance of congenital lesions. This involves several important considerations:

1) Is it an isolated congenital lesion? Is this part of a syndrome? Is there a genetic basis and will the parents need genetic counselling? Should the other siblings be investigated?
2) The lesions more commonly require reconstructive surgery rather than excisional ablation. The technique employed has to meet a functional result often years ahead, in tissues that change with growth. Examples include hypospadias, epispadias, ectopia vesicae, intersex states, cryptorchidism.
3) The functional result is dependent on the integrity of the given tissues and the prognosis is accordingly very variable (e.g. the available sphincters in ectopia vesicae or epispadias; the severity of intrauterine damage to the kidney in posterior urethral valves; or the degree of renal dysplasia associated with vesico-ureteric reflux, duplex systems or ureteroceles). The prognosis must be projected over several decades rather than years.

The Emphasis in Investigations

The particular nature of paediatric lesions dictates some variations in the investigational plans compared with adults. In the investigation of urinary infection, an intravenous pyelogram is necessary to study the upper tract and a micturating cysto-urethrogram is mandatory. This is because of the predominance of vesico-ureteric reflux in the organic causes of infection and the fact that this lesion is not always identifiable with intravenous pyelography. Moreover, a post-intravenous pyelogram voiding cystogram (in an attempt to avoid a micturating cysto-urethrogram) is a poor compromise, as the detail is inadequate to show other bladder and urethral lesions. High quality urethrograms are essential in the identification of subtleties of urethral shape, which are frequently misinterpreted at endoscopy.

In the investigation of haematuria the infrequency of paediatric bladder lesions makes cysto-urethroscopy of less importance than renal biopsy. In the presence of a normal intravenous pyelogram and micturating cysto-urethrogram, the common childhood lesion is a focal nephritis.

Table I. Methods of urine specimen collection in children

Age group	Method	Reliability
Under 4 years	Suprapubic needle aspiration	Most reliable, simplest
	Bladder catheter	Reasonably reliable with good technique and careful interpretation (30ml 0.2% neomycin must be instilled afterwards to avoid infection)
	Paediatric urine collector	Unreliable
Over 4 years	Midstream specimen	Acceptable if taken with special precautions. Advised as routine method
	Suprapubic needle aspiration	Most reliable
	Bladder catheter	Reasonably reliable

Symptom Complexes

Urinary Tract Infection

In children under the age of 4 years it is almost impossible to obtain reliable mid-stream urines and suprapubic aspiration of the bladder is preferred.

Symptoms: Reference has already been made to the nonspecific nature of symptoms in children. The proof of infection requires an adequate specimen of urine. 'Ordinary' or bag specimens are useless and misleading, unless negative. Inadequately labelled and unrefrigerated specimens, are uninterpretable (see tables I and II).

Investigation: Essential investigations in proven infection include a blood urea estimation, intravenous pyelography and a micturating cysto-urethrogram. These should be performed in:

a) all infants with one proven infection
b) all males with one proven infection
c) females with recurrent infection
d) proven infection with haematuria
e) severe toxaemia
f) non-responders to chemotherapy.

Management Plan: This is shown in figure 226. Investigations will define 3 groups, those with:

A) Ureteric reflux
B) Other urinary anomalies
C) No identifiable cause.

Groups A and B are discussed later, discussion here being confined to group C, who are mainly females.

In the absence of loin pain the majority of these patients can be initially assumed to have vulvo-urethro-trigonitis and not pyelonephritis. Although a perineal source is presumed to be the origin of such infection the precise cause is unknown. Pathogenic organisms can regularly be found in the female urethra, yet only a few girls succumb to infection — probably those in whom there is a breakdown in host mechanisms in the bladder mucosa (p. 142).

Table II. Care of urine specimens ('Send the child, not just the urine, to the laboratory')

1. Label with:
    time of collection
    time of examination
    type of collection

2. Storage:
    deliver to laboratory within 20 min, keep in refrigerator
    (> 30 min without refrigeration invalidates specimen)

Treatment of this group of children consists of:

1) Intermittent courses of antibiotic therapy (1 week) for each episode, or if attacks are frequent, a 6-month course of a single dose at night is usually effective.
2) Frequent (2-hourly) voiding during the day to limit the time available for bacterial reproduction in the bladder.
3) Measures to improve perineal hygiene, such as showers rather than baths with adequate vulval washing; correct anal toilet, elimination of worms (which contaminate the vulva) and an antiseptic vulval cream.
4) The elimination of functional wetting if present.
5) If infection still continues, cysto-urethroscopy and ureteric catheterisation, with collection of urine from each renal pelvis (after thorough irrigation of the bladder) to localise the infection.

226 Management plan for confirmed urinary tract infection.

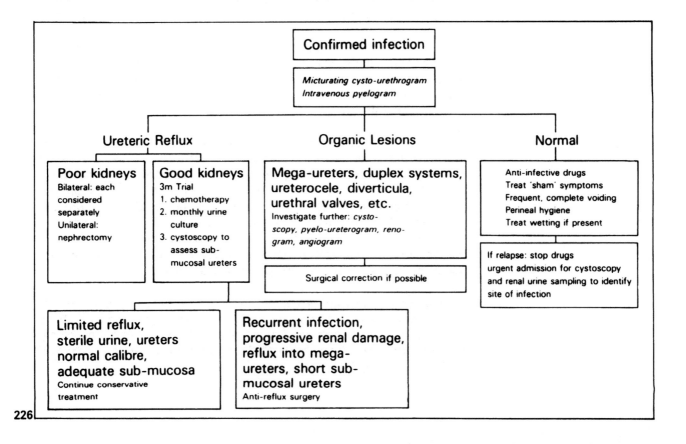

Despite these measures a number of girls will continue to have bacteriuria, with or without symptoms.

Haematuria

In contrast with adult practice, neoplasms make only a small contribution to the causes of haematuria in children. In most patients all investigations prove to be negative; the particular lesions found influence the investigational plan.

Clinical Findings: These, together with routine laboratory tests, may indicate a diagnosis of: a renal mass (Wilms' tumour, hydronephrosis); history of trauma; bleeding disorders; overt glomerulonephritis with albuminuria, oedema and hypertension; urinary infection or meatal ulcer.

Further Investigation: In the absence of clinical clues an intravenous pyelogram and micturating cysto-urethrogram are required. These may reveal calculi, hydronephrosis, polycystic kidney, mega-ureter with or without reflux, or diverticula.

Endoscopy is generally unrewarding, but is justified in children with persisting haematuria, as uncommonly a bladder tumour, haemangioma, or a small diverticulum is found.

In the majority of patients with negative investigation up to this point, the diagnosis is likely to be a focal type of glomerulonephritis, in which haematuria is precipitated by exercise or an intercurrent infection. Renal biopsy will confirm this diagnosis in half the patients, although that investigation carries some morbidity and is generally reserved for patients with repeated attacks.

Severe unexplained haematuria in older children may require selective renal angiography to diagnose a possible reno-vascular malformation (p. 96).

Urinary Incontinence

Wetting is an extremely common problem in paediatric practice and may be at night only, in the day only, or both. In those who only wet at night the cause is usually not organic and investigations are not required. The list of causes of wetting is formidable (table III) but by far the most common is the functional enuretic group.

In reaching a diagnosis some anomalies are obvious on inspection but in the remainder the clinical history is the most important clue to the cause. There are specific patterns of wetting and, when combined with clinical tests, a diagnosis can usually be reached, or at least a plan of investigation indicated. Some of these patterns are shown in figure 227. In *neurogenic* lesions the pattern is constant, day and night, and every day; indeed, when there is a history of intermittent dry days, a neurogenic cause is unlikely. The diagnosis is supported by the clinical signs of an expressible or palpable bladder, poor anal tone and perineal anaesthesia.

Wetting associated with *infection* is intermittent, coinciding with infection and improving with control of the infection; however, as described above, the prevalence of wetting as a functional symptom, and as a precursor to infection itself, sometimes leads to the persistence of wetting even after control of the infection.

Table III. Causes of urinary incontinence in children

1. Functional (enuresis)

2. Urinary infection (with all its underlying causes)

3. Structural anomalies
      Epispadias and ectopia vesicae
      Ectopic ureter
      Urethral valves
      Urethral diverticulum
      'Triad' or prune belly syndrome
      Phimosis

4. Neurogenic
      Myelomeningocele, spina bifida occulta and spina dysplasia
      Sacral agenesis
      Acquired spinal lesions (tumour, trauma, infection)

5. Traumatic injury to the bladder outlet sphincters (external violence or internal operative trauma)

Some of the *structural* lesions are obvious on inspection (epispadias, ectopia vesicae, and the post-voiding overflow from phimosis); the causes of others are hidden. An *ectopic ureter,* opening distal to the internal sphincter into the urethra, vestibule or vagina has a characteristic pattern — it only produces wetting in females with normal voiding, but there is a tiny dribble every few minutes, in a volume dependent upon the fluid load. It almost always occurs as the second ureter of a duplex system, draining the upper hemi-kidney, so an intravenous pyelogram will show a double set of calyces. Two difficulties may arise however; the finding of double ureters

227 The clinical patterns of wetting.

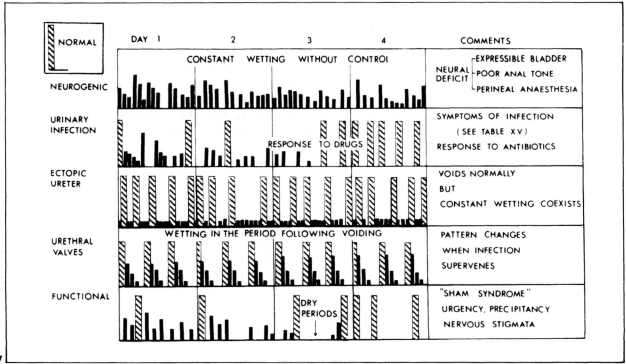

227

on an intravenous pyelogram in a child with wetting does not necessarily imply a relationship — the ectopic ureter will only be the cause if it can be shown to open below the internal sphincter. If the ureter opens into the bladder it is not the cause of the wetting, which is usually found to be an associated functional problem. The second difficulty is that, despite a classic history of an ectopic ureter, only one renal segment is seen in the intravenous pyelogram; the explanation may be that the function of the ectopic hemi-kidney is too poor to concentrate the dye (see chapter I figs. 6-7).

In the *urethral lesions* (valves, diverticula) the wetting tends to be in the period just after voiding and the stream may be thin and slow.

All the above organic causes account for only 5% of wetting children. The vast majority are *functional and nervous* in origin and no organic anomaly can be found. The clinical clue to this cause is the variability in the wetting pattern, from day to day, with some odd days of dryness, and fluctuations in volume and degree depending upon changes of environmental circumstance; there are occasionally other emotional stigmata and often some urinary frequency and urgency.

Where the clinical pattern strongly suggests a functional cause no investigations are required initially and treatment is begun along medical lines — reassurance, psychological advice, imipramine (at night) and hyoscine methobromide (by day), and/or sedation and tranquillisers and training to void 2-hourly 'by the clock'. Failure to respond, or doubt about the cause, calls for investigation by intravenous pyelography, micturating cysto-urethrography and, usually, cysto-urethroscopy.

Where the pattern suggests a structural or organic cause, or infection, obviously a full urological investigation is required.

Acute Retention of Urine

The lesions producing acute retention of urine in children are discussed in their appropriate chapters (X and XI).

Common Causes: *In either sex:*
1) Constipation is a common and often not thought of cause
2) Urethritis and/or cystitis, because of the constant pain
3) Oedema and pain after instrumentation or catheterisation
4) Intraluminal obstruction, by stone, clot, prolapsed ureterocele, foreign body, incomplete removal of the septum of a caeco-ureterocele (an ectopic ureterocele with urethral extension), neoplasm, neurogenic spasm

(especially with infection), Marion's disease (particularly if complicated by infection [p. 244]), and urethral stricture (inflammatory or traumatic)
5) Extrinsic pressure by a bladder base diverticulum (usually in males) or by a pelvic neoplasm.

Other causes in the male:
1) Balanitis, with or without phimosis or paraphimosis (common)
2) Meatal ulcer (common)
3) Urethral polyp (rare)
4) Urethral valves or membrane (rare)
5) Urethral diverticulum (rare).

Other causes in the female
1) Severe vulvitis (uncommon)
2) Urethral prolapse (rare).

The Urethral Obstruction Syndrome

This symptom-complex refers to the child presenting with wetting, frequency, burning, alterations to the stream, with or without infection, accompanied by the report of residual urine in the cystogram and by a collar at the bladder neck and some dilatation below. The latter is often interpreted as indicating distal obstruction.

Aetiological Concepts: Probably no area of paediatric urology has excited more controversy than the concept of outlet 'obstruction', in the absence of classically recognisable lesions such as urethral valves. The heat of the argument generated has usually been in inverse proportion to the scientific basis of the 'facts'. Until about 10 years ago the urological literature was full of such references and many thousands of children have had their bladder and urethra dilated or resected in a variety of ways. There remains a staunch band of urologists, usually those primarily adult orientated, who continue to stretch and cut; yet, by and large, paediatric urologists fail to find the lesions alleged to be responsible for the symptoms.

Anecdotally, surgeons insist the children are improved after dilatation; equally anecdotally the writer sees these same children, having been dilated repeatedly elsewhere, with no improvement whatever, and in whom one cannot see any evidence, endoscopically or radiologically, of any narrow zones; their symptoms are subsequently relieved by sedation. The protagonists of dilatation then argue that although one cannot 'see' a narrow zone, it is 'functionally abnormal', and dilatation produces a 'more linear axial flow'. It is perhaps significant that early reports referred mostly to alleged stenosis at the bladder neck. When this area seemed to lose its credibility the stenosis moved down to the distal urethra; it is hoped the next step will be to the knee joint, outside the range of the cystourethroscope.

To do justice to a critical review of the scientific evidence for and against the concept of stenosis would require a book in itself and only the conclusions are summarised here:

1) The radiographic appearances may only represent physiological variations in the response of the sphincters to the stress of the child at the time of the examination, or to the response to pain and discomfort on voiding in the presence of infection. Radiologists make much of 'residual urine' but many normal children find it difficult to empty the bladder in the strange conditions of an x-ray department. This is particularly so in an emotional child, whose sphincter behaviour can be quite extraordinary when observed on the television monitor during voiding. Figures 228 and 229 represent a few examples of the wide variation in urethral shapes in children presenting with wetting, or infection, but whose symptoms were relieved by either sedatives and/or chemotherapy. They are all variations of the normal. Many studies have now shown that vesico-ureteric reflux is rarely secondary to distal obstruction but is, almost always, due to a primary defect of the terminal ureter (p. 10). Many patients with posterior urethral valves do not have vesico-ureteric reflux.

2) The endoscopic appearances are often artifactual and represent degrees of bladder filling and water flow, both of which effect the shape of the bladder neck and posterior urethra. Trabeculation, so often interpreted as being solely due to obstruction, is frequently seen in children with infection alone, and in minor degrees of an occult neuropathic bladder (see chapters X and XI).

3) Studies on normal children (i.e. with conditions unrelated to the urinary tract) indicate a wide range of urethral calibrations, including sizes that protagonists would interpret as 'stenotic'.

4) The interpretation of bladder and urethral pressure-flow measurements has been subject to very extensive study; it is clear that a wide range of

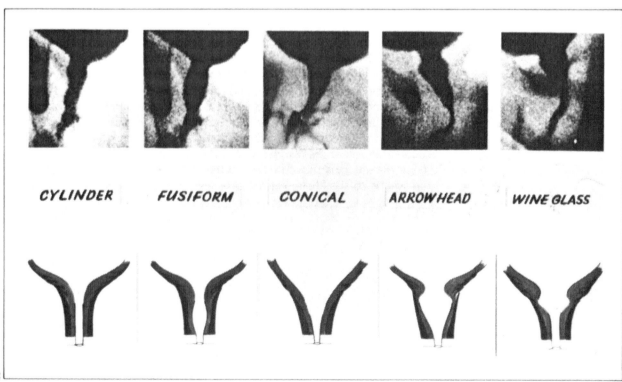

CYLINDER   FUSIFORM   CONICAL   ARROWHEAD   WINE GLASS

228

Variation in urethral shapes

228 Variation in girls. These are all normal and represent different degrees of contraction and relaxation of the urethral muscles during voiding (dark grey = striated muscle; light grey = smooth muscle). They should not be interpreted as 'urethral stenosis'.

229a to d Variations in boys. Although these are unusual shapes they are not abnormal and are caused by sphincter activity. None of these boys had 'obstruction' at the bladder neck or distally. Often a urethra will show alterations in shape in different phases of voiding.

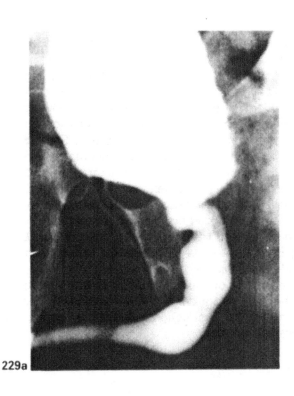

229a

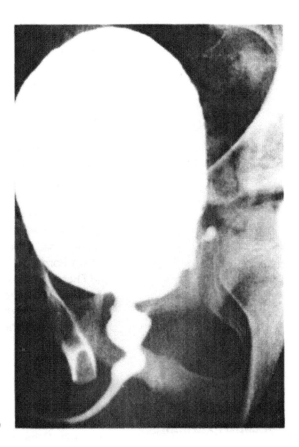

229b

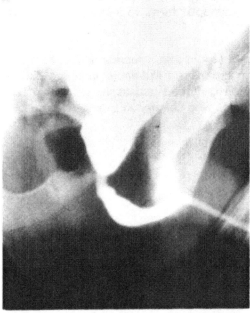

229c

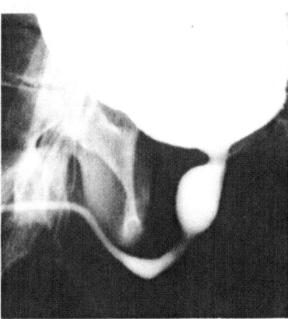

229d

pressures occur in normal children depending on many variables. The significant fact is that the sphincters themselves can alter every parameter of measurement, depending on their degree of contractility at the precise moment of measurement (p. 124).

Conclusions and Management

1) The explanation for the symptom complex of frequency-dysuria-wetting-infection (in the absence of recognisable urological disorders such as reflux, valves, etc.) *rarely* rests upon any concept of bladder neck or urethral stenosis. Most childrens symptoms can be explained on the basis of:

a) a functional disorder: most of these children are very active, busy children, 'highly strung', 'always on the go'; or, alternatively, timid and withdrawn. They fill our outpatient departments and our consulting offices, presenting their urological symptoms as a part only of a wider spectrum of recurrent short-lived abdominal pain, pallor, headaches, bedwetting, day pants wetting, etc. The wet female child more readily develops vulval excoriation, then sterile and later infected cysto-urethritis. Stephens et al. (1966) rightly call this the 'sham syndrome', as the symptoms mimic adult urological disease and can exhibit all the radiographic and cysto-urothroscopic appearances of so-called stenosis

b) urinary infection itself, with or without reflux and/or megacystitis.

c) uncommonly, varieties of an occult neuropathic bladder.

2) Patients who fail to respond to treatment on the basis of the above explanations, especially if infected, certainly require full urological investigation in order to exclude other causes.

3) There remains a small residue of patients who have a true stenotic lesion. Marion's disease in the male and a distal urethral stenosis in the female child, may produce mechanical obstruction sufficient to require surgical resection but these lesions are rare.

Synopsis of Paediatric Lesions

The number of congenital and acquired urological lesions in children is extensive; many conditions are rare and encountered only in specialised centres. Other paediatric texts (see suggested Further Reading) should be consulted for details. A few representative examples of the commoner lesions are given here, in synoptic form, to indicate the presentation and principles of management.

Lesions in the Upper Urinary Tract

Upper tract lesions present as loin pain, infection and/or haematuria. Some mechanically obstructing lesions are illustrated in figure 230 and lesions producing stasis based on disturbed peristalsis, without mechanical obstruction, in figure 231. (See also chapter XII).

Upper urinary tract lesions
230 Some obstructive lesions of the ureter, pelvi-ureteric junction, and calyces.

231 Stasis lesions of the upper urinary tract without significant obstruction.

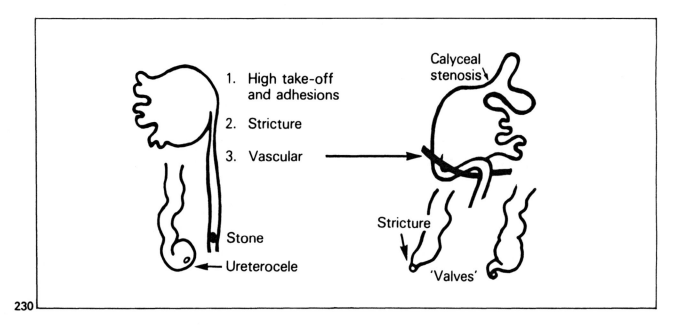

1. High take-off and adhesions
2. Stricture
3. Vascular

Stone
Ureterocele

Calyceal stenosis
Stricture
'Valves'

230

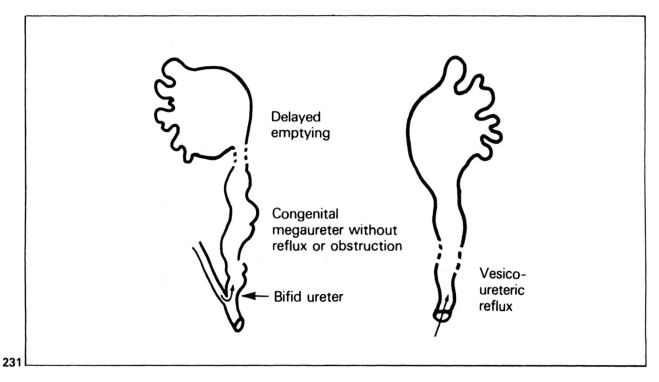

Delayed emptying

Congenital megaureter without reflux or obstruction

Bifid ureter

Vesico-ureteric reflux

231

Pelvi-ureteric Obstruction. *Aetiology:* Figures 232 and 233 illustrate some of the common causes of pelvi-ureteric obstruction. Mechanical or functional obstruction of the pelvi-ureteric junction produces dilatation of the renal pelvis, with further obstruction occasionally resulting from a related artery or a now abnormally high-insertion ureter.

Investigations and treatment: These are discussed in chapter XII page 276.

Calculi: These are discussed in chapter XI. In children:

1) Primary dietry deficient bladder calculi are common in certain endemic areas, such as the Middle East and Asia, but are otherwise rare
2) A demonstrable cause (foreign body, stasis, infection, metabolic) is found in less than 20% of cases
3) Stone basket ureteric removal is rarely necessary.

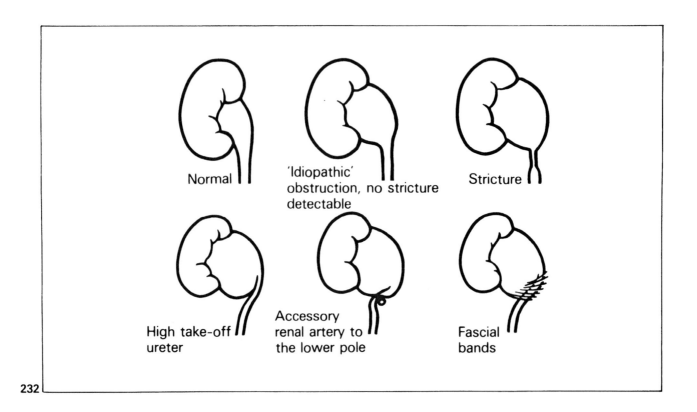

Normal

'Idiopathic' obstruction, no stricture detectable

Stricture

High take-off ureter

Accessory renal artery to the lower pole

Fascial bands

Pelvi-ureteric obstruction
232 Mechanisms of varying degrees of obstruction at the pelvi-ureteric junction.

233 Examples of obstruction causing hydronephrosis: (a) mechanical stricture; (b) non-contributing high 'take-off' ureter and (c) contributing vascular obstruction.

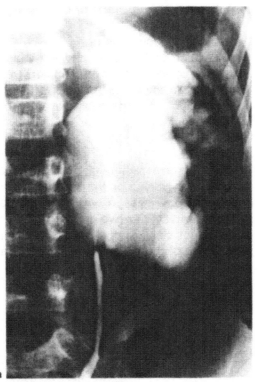

233a

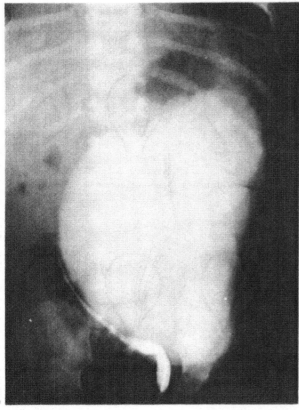

233b

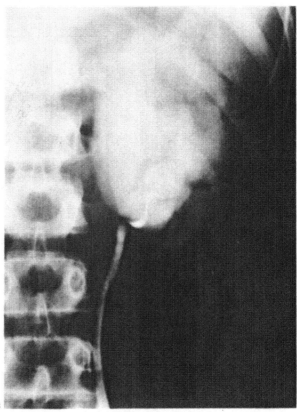

233c

Mega-ureters: This congenital abnormality is discussed in page 10. Mega-ureters may be present:

1) Without obstructional reflux
2) With a distal segment narrowing (fig. 234)
3) With reflux (see below)
4) Secondary to bladder or urethral obstruction.

Treatment: This consists of:
1) Correction of the cause and any infection, together with either re-implantation of the ureter into the bladder or a nephro-ureterphrectomy, depending upon the degree of renal damage.
2) Occasionally such children present with septicaemia, and may then require a temporary cutaneous ureterostomy urinary diversion (see chapter VIII).

Duplex Systems: Although double kidneys in the true sense do occur, i.e. two separate kidneys on the one side, the more common situation is that of a single kidney mass in which the calyces arrange themselves into two systems feeding into two ureters. The mere finding of a duplex system is, in iteslf, not significant, unless certain anatomical arrangements are present. Some of these significant situations are illustrated in figures 235-238.

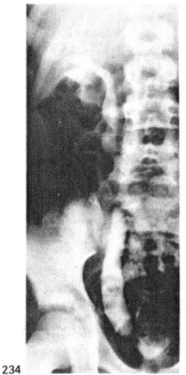

234

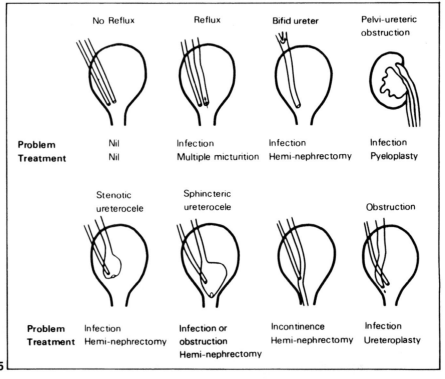

235

234 A mega-ureter with distal segment narrowing.

Duplex systems
235 Some variations in the arrangement of double ureters and their significance.

236 Bilateral duplex kidneys. On the right side the ureters are bifid, on the left both ureters enter into the bladder separately, without reflux. The renal segments are normal and the duplex systems are incidental findings of no significance.

237 Grade III reflux into double right ureters producing a urinary tract infection, and Grade I single ureter left reflux.

238 Bifid ureters with ureter-to-ureter reflux and infection. Filling the upper (ectopic) segment, via a ureteric catheter, immediately fills the lower (orthotopic) segment by reflux around the common junction.

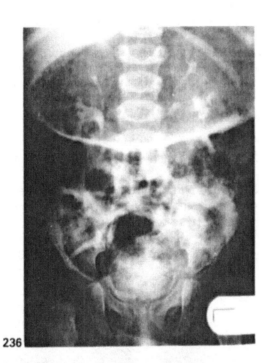

236

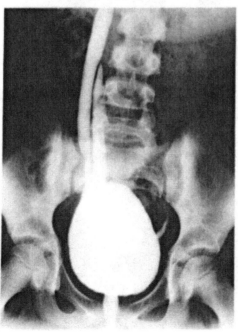

237

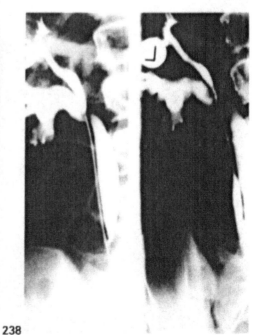

238

Bifid systems usually do not produce either symptoms or infection, but repeated infection by ureter-to-ureter reflux, with evidence of renal damage, may require conversion to a high uretero-pelvic anastomosis or a hemi-nephrectomy removal.

Duplex systems require thorough investigation with intravenous pyelography, micturating cysto-urethrogram and cysto-urethroscopy-retrograde pyelography, in order to assess the exact anatomy and significance. The anatomical arrangements are often complex.

Ureteroceles: A ureterocele (p. 12) is a cystic distension of the submucosal portion of a ureter. It may occur on a single ureter but in children 80% present in the ectopic ureter of a duplex system. The ectopic renal segment is frequently dysplastic or pyelonephritic or both.

Investigations: Intravenous pyelogram and micturating cysto-urethrogram to demonstrate a filling defect in the bladder or reflux. Figures 239-242 illustrate these features.. Cysto-urethroscopy is also indicated.

Treatment: This may consist of:

1) Open ureterocelectomy plus
2) Re-implantation of the ectopic ureter if there is adequate renal function or
3) Ectopic partial nephrectomy if there is poor renal function plus
4) Re-implantation of the orthotopic ureter, which usually refluxes after the ureterocele has been corrected.

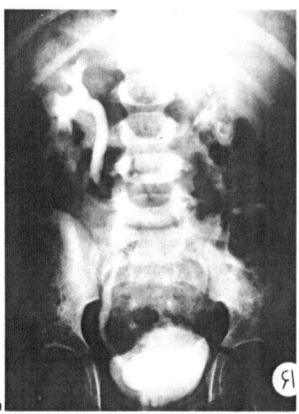

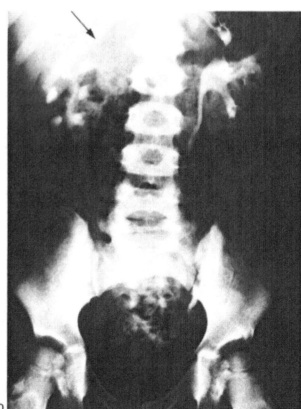

239   240

Ureteroceles

239 A ureterocele in the bladder with a stenotic orifice — the intravenous pyelogram dye becomes concentrated in the obstructed cystic cavity and the wall of the ureterocele shows as a black filling defect. In children, only 20% of ureteroceles occur in a single ureter-kidney system, as in this patient; the rest occur in duplex systems.

240 The more common situation in children of a ureterocele on the ectopic ureter of a duplex kidney, this renal segment usually being dysplastic. The upper or ectopic segment of the kidney (arrow) is poorly functioning on intravenous pyelography and its presence may be missed.

241 A sphincteric ureterocele (a) — one with a wide orifice in the sphincter zone of the bladder neck or urethra — showing as a filling defect on intravenous pyelography, because of the poor function in the subserving renal segment. Such a ureterocele usually refluxes (b), and the whole ectopic system is often grossly dysplastic.

242 A ureterocele may prolapse (arrow) through the bladder neck and cause urethral obstruction.

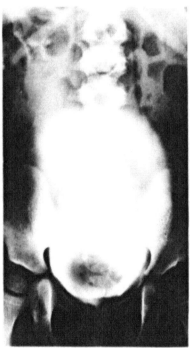

241a

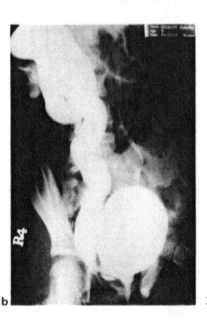

241b

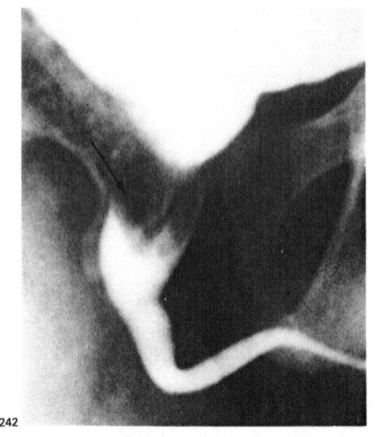

242

Lesions in the Lower Urinary Tract

Some of the internal mechanically obstructing lesions found in children are illustrated in figure 243, and other disturbances in figure 244.

Urachal Lesions: This abnormality (p. 16) may present as:

1) Discharge of urine at the umbilicus or
2) Sub-umbilical abscess.

The defect may be a:

a) patent urachus, not necessarily secondary to distal obstruction
b) urachal cyst or sinus
c) vesico-urachal diverticulum.

The treatment is excision.

Lower urinary tract lesions
243 Obstructive lesions of the lower urinary tract.

244 Stasis lesions in the lower urinary tract without significant obstruction. A neurogenic bladder is the most common. A recto-urethral fistula often occurs in patients with an imperforate rectum. (D = wide-necked stenotic diverticulum.)

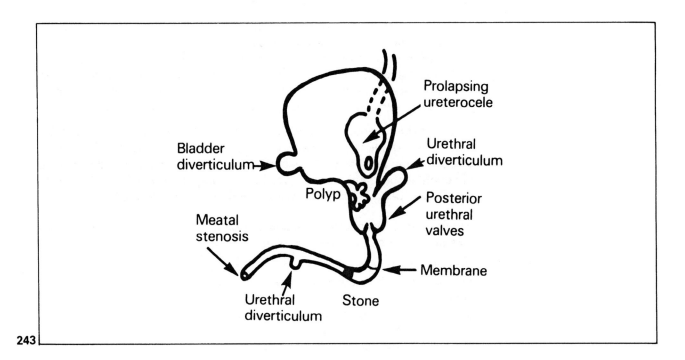

Prolapsing ureterocele
Bladder diverticulum
Urethral diverticulum
Polyp
Posterior urethral valves
Meatal stenosis
Membrane
Urethral diverticulum
Stone

243

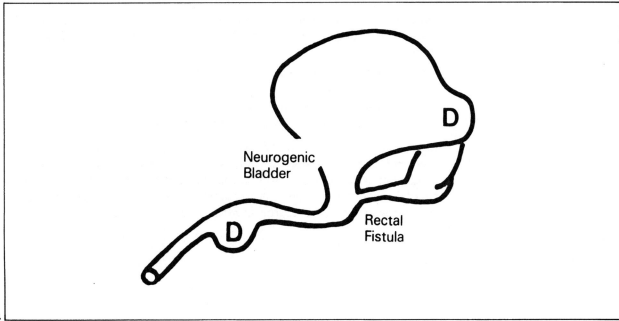

Neurogenic Bladder
D
Rectal Fistula
D

244

Vesico-ureteric Reflux: Reflux is usually due to a congenital shortness of the sub-mucosal ureter but may result from bladder inflammation, infection, trauma or outlet or uerthal obstruction (chapters I and V). It is the most common cause of paediatric pyelonephritis. Reflux may be graded as follows: (fig. 245-247)

Grade I	To lower ureter
Grade II	To the pelvis and calyces without permanent dilatation
Grade III	To the pelvis and calyces with moderate permanent ureteric and calyceal dilatation
Grade IV	To the pelvis and calyces with gross upper tract dilatation.

Diagnosis: This is based on the following:

1) A micurating cysto-urethrogram is essential as a post-intravenous pyelogram voiding film is inadequate
2) Serum urea and creatinine estimations
3) An intravenous pyelogram to assess total renal anatomy and function
4) Cysto-urethroscopy, to measure the length of the sub-mucosal ureter and to exclude uncommon primary obstructive pathology.

Natural history: Early, spontaneous, cessation of reflux is common (greater than 80% in grades I and II, 50% in grade III and 30% in grade IV in the first 5 years of life) but less so as puberty is approached. However, this chance of spontaneous 'cure' must be weighted against the risk of renal damage in the waiting period if silent or overt infection is allowed to continue.

Management: Management depends upon a balance of the following factors and no one criterion is absolute in itself.

a) grade of reflux
b) infection — frequency, severity
c) renal damage
d) cystoscopic assessment of the sub-mucosal ureter
e) age and sex
f) adequacy and feasibility of follow-up.

Conservative trial: Grades I and II reflux, in a child under 5 years of age who has normal kidneys, with easy control of infection and infrequent relapses, a long sub-mucosal ureter and adequate medical follow-up facilities requires:

1) Initial maintenance chemotherapy (3-6 months)
2) A trial without drugs
3) Regular 3-monthly urine cultures
4) Radiological reviews at 2 or 3-year intervals.

Grade III reflux, with minimal or no changes in the kidney, infrequent infection, and/or intermediate sub-mucosal ureteric length, also calls for nonsurgical management as described above, but anti-reflux surgery is indicated if the infection is difficult to control, renal damage occurs, or there is no improvement in the degree of reflux after the age of 5 years.

Grades of vesico-ureteric reflux. (Grade I is shown on the left side in figure 237)

245 Grade II. Reflux into normal ureters and pelvi-calyceal systems.

246 Grade III. Reflux into minimal or moderately dilated ureters; usually some associated renal changes.

247 Grade IV. Reflux into massive mega-ureters and hydronephrosis.

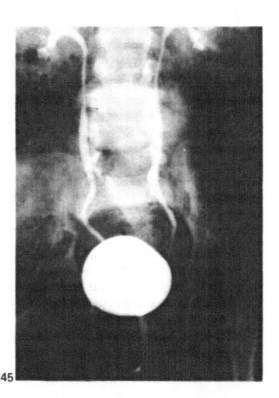

245

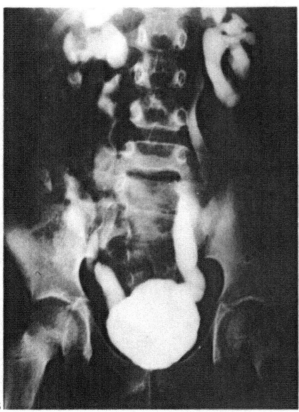

246

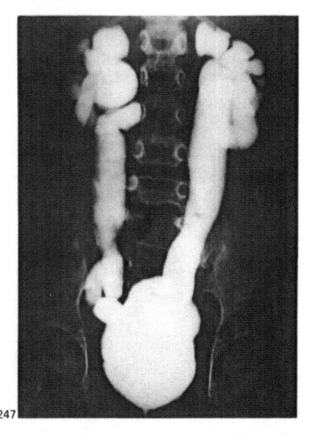

247

Immediate anti-reflux surgery: This is indicated in the following circumstances:

1) Grades III and IV reflux, with marked renal changes
2) Grade III reflux, with repeated infections
3) Grade II, III or IV reflux, with a very short sub-mucosal ureter
4) Any grade of reflux persisting near puberty
5) Any grade of reflux when medical follow-up is unavailable or inadequate
6) Any grade of reflux associated with a bladder diverticulum.

Nephro-ureterectomy: This is indicated in unilateral, grossly refluxing mega-ureter, with an absent or poorly functioning kidney.

Correction of cause: Surgical correction of any primary obstructive cause, such as posterior urethral valves, is necessary.

Bladder Diverticula: Bladder diverticula (p. 18) may have a narrow-necked stenotic orifice (fig. 248) or a wide necked orifice (fig. 249).

Secondary complications of diverticula may arise from:

1) Infection, which is more common in stenotic types
2) Ureteric reflux which may occur if the orifice of the ureter encroaches on to the wall of the diverticulum (fig. 250)
3) Ureteric obstruction which may occur if the ureter is kinked during filling of the diverticulum
4) Urethral obstruction from the pressure of a bladder base diverticulum (fig. 251).

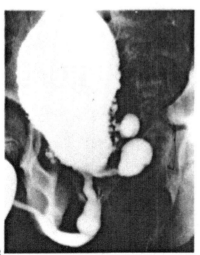

248

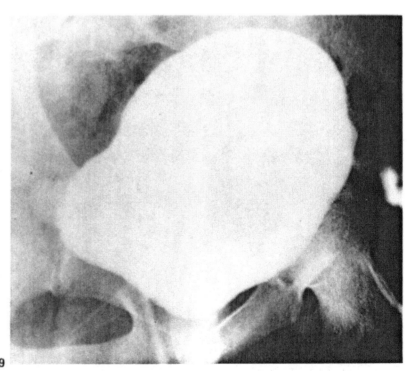

249

Diverticula

248 Narrow-necked stenotic bladder diverticula, producing infection. There is also a diverticulum in the posterior urethra.

249 A diffuse, wide-necked bladder diverticulum, often of no significance and not benefited by surgery.

250 A large stenotic diverticulum into which the ureter opens; such ureteric insertions always reflux (arrow) and show no tendency to improve spontaneously; surgery is always required.

251 A diverticulum near the bladder base may obstruct the urethra as it fills.

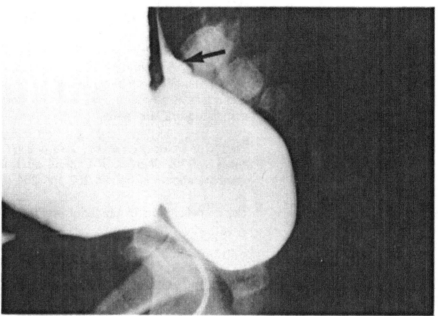

250

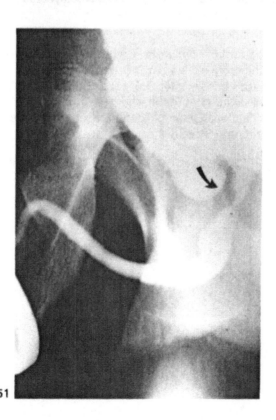

251

It should be stressed that diffuse lateral bladder bulges and multiple small saccules seemingly outside the bladder cavity (in a near empty bladder), are not true diverticula and are often found in normal children, or occur occasionally as a result of infection.

Investigations: These should include:

1) Micturating cysto-urethrography, to demonstrate the type of diverticulum, whether or not reflux is present, and the effects on the ureter.
2) Intravenous pyelography, to assess the effects on the upper urinary tract.
3) Cysto-urethroscopy, with or without retrograde pyelo-ureterograms, to asess the relationship of the diverticulum to the ureteric orifice and the presence of any distal obstructive lesions.

Treatment: Stenotic diverticula require excision but wide-necked diverticula, with no secondary effects need no treatment unless infection is present, when chemotherapy should be given. Excision is required if there is secondary obstruction and excision and anti-reflux surgery if there is associated ureteric reflux.

Posterior Urethral Valves: This is a lesion of male children which produces varying degrees of urethral obstruction (p. 22). Different types of valve are shown in figures 252 and 254.

The complications of posterior urethral valves are:

1) Bladder trabeculation and hypertrophy
2) Ureteric dilatation
   40% have reflux
   20% have vesuco-ureteric obstruction
   40% have dilatation secondary to the urethral obstruction
3) Hydronephrosis and hydrocalyectasis, which varies from minimal to gross renal damage.

Clinical Presentation: This is influenced by the degree of obstruction, with the more severe cases presenting at a younger age. Neonates present with gross urinary infection, septicaemia, uraemia, abdominal distension, palpable kidneys or ureters, while in infants there is failure to thrive, dribbling and infection. Older children present with wetting, haematuria and a poor strength stream.

Type I posterior urethral valves.
252a With the urethra opened, the valve fins (arrow) diverge from the verumontanum in the posterior urethra.

252b With the urethra reconstituted, the fins meet anteriorly and obstruct the urinary flow during voiding.

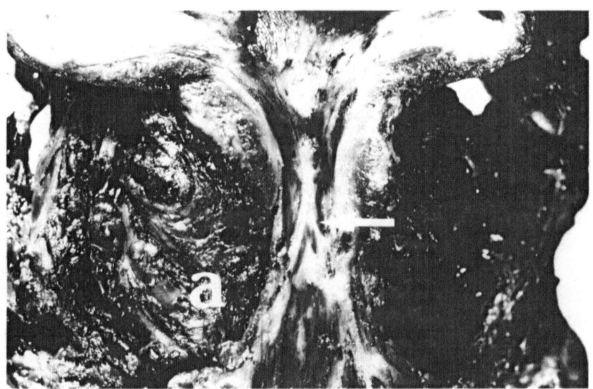

252a

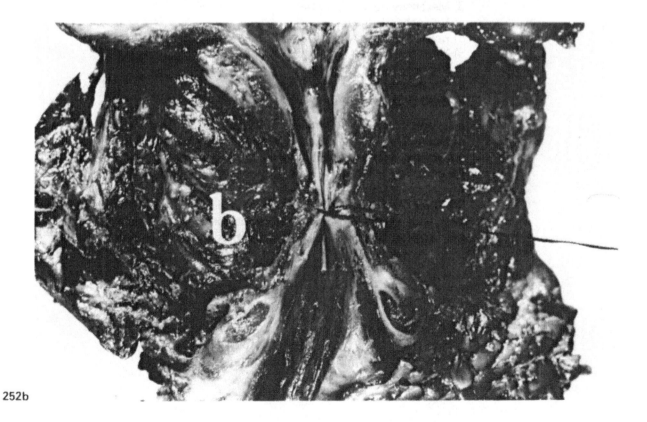

252b

Investigations and Diagnosis: The diagnosis is based on the results of:

1) Serum urea, creatinine and electrolyte estimations
2) Urine microscopy and culture
3) Micturating cysto-urethrogram (fig. 253-254)
4) Intravenous pyelogram
5) Cysto-urethroscopy, which is usually combined with valve resection.

Management: This consists of:

1) Correction of infection and electrolyte disturbances
2) Temporary urinary drainage:
   a) urethral catheter with regular neomycin irrigation
   b) occasionally cutaneous ureterostomy (see chapter VIII).
3) Definitive valve cysto-urethroscopic resection
4) Reconstructive surgery to upper tract:
   a) vesico-ureteroplasty for obstruction or reflux
   b) nephrectomy for gross renal damage.

Genitourinary Neoplasms

Nephroblastoma (Wilm's Tumour): This is the most common paediatric genitourinary neoplasm. See also chapter VII p. 166.

Over 60% of patients are aged between 1 and 4 years, with males predominating. The condition usually presents as a symptomless abdominal mass, in an otherwise healthy child, but abdominal pain and haematuria may occur. Hemi-hypertrophy of the limbs and aniridia are rare associated findings.

Diagnosis: The conditions which should be considered in the *differential* diagnosis of Wilm's tumour are:

1) Hydronephrosis
2) Multicystic kidney
3) Mesenchymal hamartoma
4) Horseshoe kidney
5) Renal vein thrombosis
6) Neuroblastoma
7) Retroperitoneal sarcoma
8) Phaemochromocytoma
9) Hepatoblastoma.

Macroscopically the tumour consists of a large, rounded, mainly homogeneous mass, which has partly replaced the compressed kidney substance. Microscopically, there are islands of packed epithelial cells, separated by loose connective tissue containing muscle, bone or cartilage.

The neoplasm may spread locally, to the para-aortic lymph glands and, even with small neoplasms, involve the renal vein. Pulmonary metastases are followed later by secondary growth in bones, brain and liver.

Posterior urethral valves on micturating cysto-urethrography.
253a Type I valves (arrow) showing dilatation of the posterior urethra, with a sudden calibre change to the membranous urethra, and associated vesico-ureteric reflux.

253b The valves shown in an antero-posterior view.

254 Type III valves. Gross urethral dilatation and obstruction in the membranous urethra. No fins demonstrable.

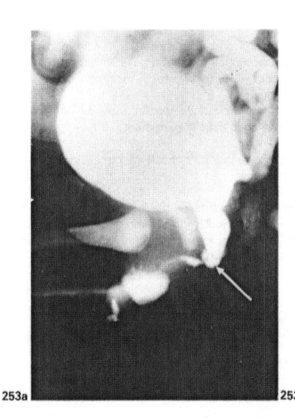

253a

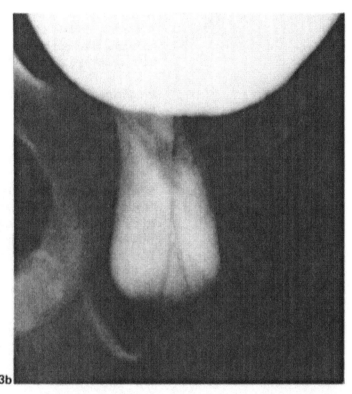

253b

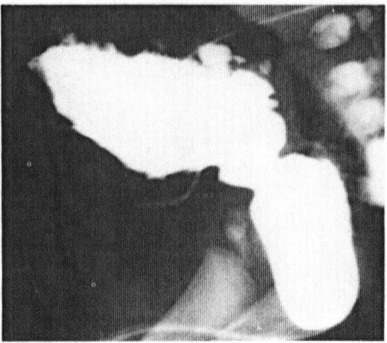

254

Investigations: These comprise those radiological studies, such as intravenous pyelogram, selective renal angiogram, inferior venacavagram, described in chapter III where the investigation of renal space occupying lesions is discussed (p. 94). A full blood examination is also undertaken, principally as a base line for cytotoxic therapy.

Treatment: This comprises radical nephrectomy, including renal lymph gland clearance and embolectomy of any neoplasm present in the inferior vena cava. Irradiation treatment is started 22 days after the nephrectomy.

A primary course of actinomycin D and vincristine, is given immediately following the nephrectomy and continued for 21 days. Repeated courses of both drugs are given at 10 weeks, 4, 6, 9, 12 and 15 months.

Prognosis: For stages I and II (tumour confined locally), there is an approximately 90% 2-year survival (which is usually permanent).

For stages III and IV (incomplete removal or distal metastases), at least 50% of children survive for 2 years.

Rhabdomyosarcoma: Rhabdomyosarcoma of the bladder, prostate and vaginal tissues (figs. 255-257) was previously considered to be a death sentence on diagnosis. However, modern cytotoxic therapy, even without radical tumour excision, is now producing an 80% 2-year survival.

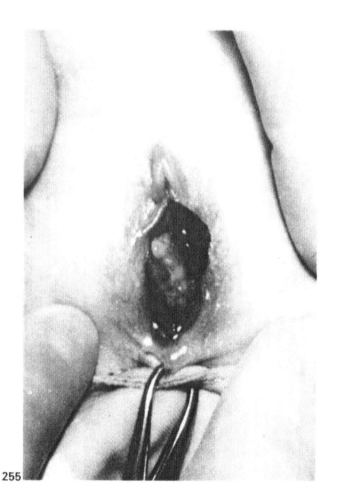

255

Rhabdomyosarcoma

255 Sarcoma botyroides, with tumour emerging from the urethra.

256 Bladder rhabdomyosarcoma, showing filling defects of tumour masses in a micturating cysto-urethrogram.

257 Prostatic rhabdomyosarcoma, producing urethral obstruction.

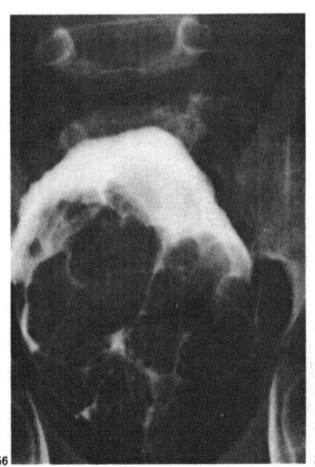

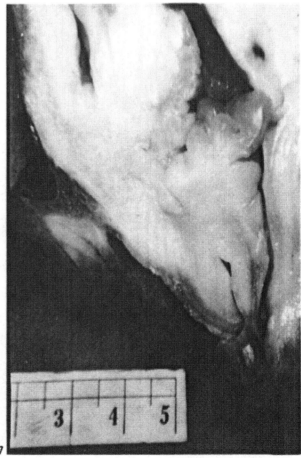

256   257

Other Neoplasms: Other types of genitourinary neoplasm in children are rare, and include:

1) Adenocarcinoma of the kidney — with a poorer prognosis than a Wilm's tumour
2) Retroperitoneal pelvic tumours (sarcoma) — with a very poor prognosis
3) Ovarian and uterine malignancy — also with a poor prognosis.

Neuropathic Bladder

This may be classified as:

Upper Motor Neurone Bladder: Resulting from spinal trauma, neoplasm and infection and uncommon in children.

Lower Motor Neurone Bladder: This is the usual form encountered in children, with the common lesion being spina bifida with myelomeningocele (figs. 258-261). Less commonly other forms of spinal dysplasia (spina bifida occulta, diastematomyelia, sacral agenesis (chapter IX fig. 166)) may also produce a lower motor neurone type of bladder dysfunction.

The treatment of these patients is discussed in detail in the chapter on The Neurogenic Bladder (chapter XI). Irrespective of chemotherapy, sphincterotomy, penile appliances, intermittent catheterisation by the parents, electronic or hydrometric prostheses, the results are poor and it is rare for urinary control to be achieved. Upper tract damage is usually progressive in most children and they eventually require urinary diversion (chapter VIII).

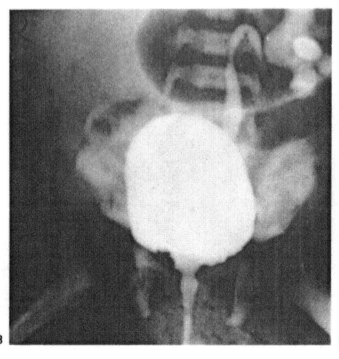
258

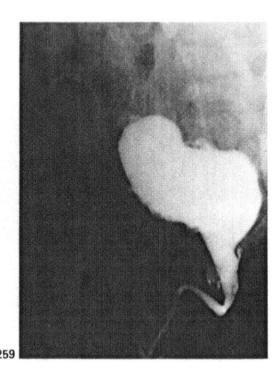
259

Neuropathic bladder in spina bifida with myelodysplasia: I.
This is an example of the most common type with a patulous open urethra and continuous incontinence. The urethra is open in all phases of the radiographs.
258 A neonate. The bladder is quite smooth at this stage. Ureteric reflux is present in about 20% of patients.

259 In an older child the bladder is beginning to become sacculated.

Neuropathic bladder in spina bifida with myelodysplasia: II.
The less common type (about one-third of the patients) with an obstructive sphincter mechanism. Note that the obstruction is not at the bladder neck, which is open throughout, but in the distal half of the posterior urethra. The patients are incontinent but dribbling is less frequent and the bladder is palpable.

260 Arrow points to the closed distal posterior urethra. Manual expression produces a weak flow.

261 In early life the bladder is often quite smooth and reflux is common.

262 Unrelieved obstruction produces gross bladder sacculation and deterioration of the upper tract, often with reflux.

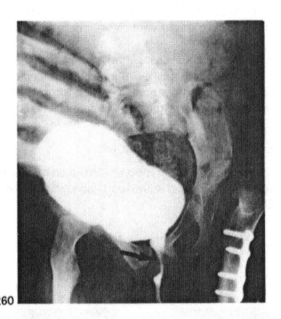

260

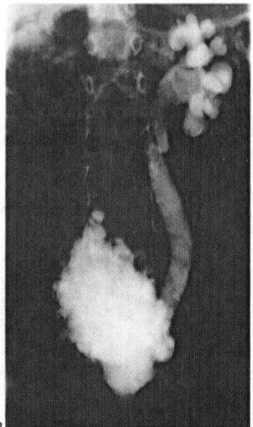

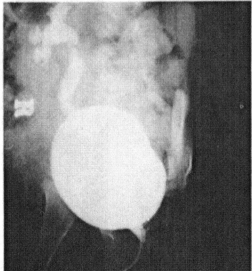

261

262

*Lesions of the
External Genitalia*

*Lesions in Male
Children*

Hypospadias. In hypospadia the urethra terminates proximal to its normal site on the ventral surface of the penis (p. 20). The most common site of the orifice (75%) is at or near the coronal groove (fig. 263), less commonly, more distally on the glans, or proximally on the shaft, peno-scrotal junction, or perineum (figs. 264-265). There may be an associated chordee deformity (ventral angulation) and a deficiency of the ventral prepuce.

Clinical aspects: This is a very common anomaly (1 in 300 newborn males) and the following considerations should be borne in mind:

1) The degree of chordee must be assessed separately from the site of the orifice as it may be quite significant, even with distal hypospadias (or even no hypospadias): it may necessitate a major reconstruction, belied by the seemingly innocent site of the orifice.
2) Non-palpable gonads may suggest an intersex state (see later).
3) Patients present with misdirection of the urinary stream. (In adults there may be inadequate penetration in sexual intercourse and, in severe cases, inadequate insemination of the vagina. Cosmetic embarrassment is common if the chordee is severe.) The condition does not affect urinary control.
4) There is a slight familial factor but direct chromosomal aberrations are rare.
5) Urological investigations for associated abnormalities are not necessary in the common subglandular type, but there is a slightly increased incidence of other anomalies in severe hypospadias, and an intravenous pyelogram and micturating cysto-urethrogram are essential investigations in these children.

Treatment: The objectives of treatment are:

1) To produce a straight penis on erection and a terminal orifice on the tip of the glans, from which to void in the long axis of the penis in the standing position (fig. 266).

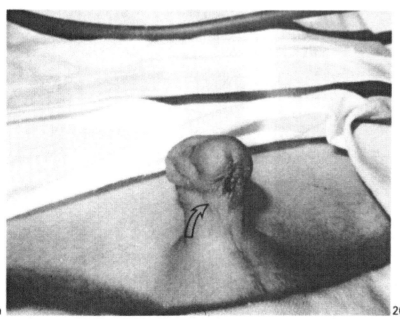

263a

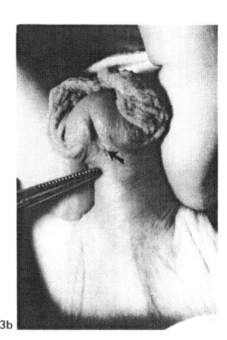

263b

Hypospadias

263a,b Subglandular or distal penile hypospadias — the most common site of the orifice. Note the site of the orifice in the coronal groove and the associated stenosis (b). There is often a blind pit at the site where the orifice should normally be. The prepuce is typically deficient on the ventral surface and 'hooded' on the dorsal surface. The penile raphe (a) is often eccentric (arrow). Chordee may or may not be present (marked in a, minimal in b).

264 Peno-scrotal hypospadias (orifice of urethra shown by arrow) and severe chordee deformity.

265 Perineal hypospadias and severe chordee.

266 Result of hypospadias repair by author's technique. Straight stream from the glans, no chordee, and appearance of a normal circumcised boy. Arrow indicates site of original hypospadiac orifice.

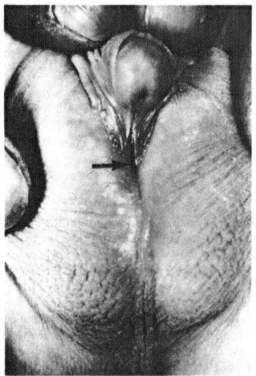

264

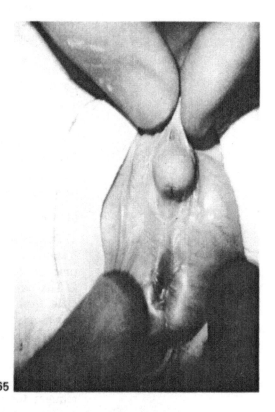

265

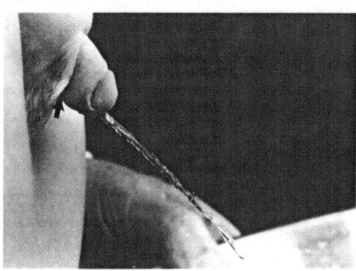

266

2) To make possible insemination well into the vagina.
3) To achieve a good cosmetic appearance.
4) To achieve a urethra free of fistula, stricture, sacculation or meatal stenosis.

There is controversy about whether these objectives can best be achieved by a one-stage or a multi-staged procedure. More than 150 variations in operative technique have been described.

For distal glandular orifices (i.e. on the distal half of the glans) only meatotomy and/or circumcision is required and is carried out between 2 and 3 years of age. For all other types, including proximal glandular and coronal orifices, a full reconstruction is necessary, and is carried out at 3.5 years of age, whether a 1 or a 2-stage technique is used. The author prefers a 2-stage procedure (Holder and Ashcraft, in press) but irrespective of the technique used the chordee must be corrected initially and then the urethra reconstructed.

Complications of the prepuce: These conditions which are commonly encountered in adult practice include:

1) Balanoposthitis which, if severe and recurrent, is treated by circumcision.
2) Phimosis, which usually requires circumcision if it is severe and persists beyond the age of 3 years.
3) Paraphimosis, which often requires circumcision if it recurs or cannot be manually reduced.
4) An adherent, non-retractile prepuce which may also require circumcision.

In children there are certain features which should be noted:

1) The prepuce is normally adherent to the glans into the second year of life. It should not be forcibly retracted before this time, as to do so may split the prepuce with the subsequent scarring, resulting in phimosis.
2) The parents should begin to retract the prepuce, in the uncircumcised child, from about the third year of life, and teach the child to continue to do this regularly for normal hygiene.
3) The case for 'routine' neonatal circumcision, under the current conditions offered for such procedures (non-aseptic conditions in the nursery), cannot be sustained in view of the unacceptably high incidence of complications.
4) Apart from religious reasons and the surgical indictions listed above, a request for circumcision on hygienic grounds is, in the opinion of this author, not unreasonable. However, certain features are insisted upon:

   a) The operation is never done in the first year of life (in view of the risks of anaesthesia, ammoniacal dermatitis, and a still adherent prepuce)
   b) Availability of expert general anaesthesia, and
   c) Full aseptic theatre conditions
   d) A technique that avoids haemorrhage, uses neat suturing and an adequately planned skin exicision
   e) Postoperative dressing of soft paraffin and soft wool to avoid meatal ulceration.

The complications of circumcision may be:

   1) Local and general infection, especially in the neonate
   2) Haemorrhage
   3) Too little or too much skin excision
   4 Meatal stenosis
   5) Urethral fistula.

Meatal Stenosis

Apart from hypospadias a narrow terminal urethral meatus is rarely congenital, but may result from a poorly executed circumcision operation. The usually accepted explanation is ammonaiacal dermatitis, with ulceration in the diaper area, including the tip of the exposed glans. Ulceration is followed by cicatricial scarring of the orifice. Although this mechanism undoubtedly occurs the author's contention is that the usual cause is an inadequate dressing technique in the immediate post-circumcision period. If a dry dressing is applied, or a tight diaper is pressed hard up against the exposed delicate epithelium of the glans, a tip abrasion occurs, followed by scarring. Observations in neonatal nurseries, in the days after 'routine' circumcision, will often reveal an ulcerated tip, which is either not noticed or ignored in the general swelling of the penis. Meatal erosion also occurs more commonly following circumcision with mechanical bells and cups, again from pressure necrosis. The 'bone forceps' technique of circumcision can inadvertently nip off the tip of the glans and is easily recognised later by a flattened tip to the glans with central stenosis. The stenosis is usually eccentric, with the scar encroaching from ventrum to dorsum. The stream is jet-like and often flows tangentially at an angle from the long axis of the penis.

Apart from misdirection of the stream stenosis itself is of little consequence. Rarely should one ever be concerned about back pressure effects and it does not cause wetting, despite the hopes some hold of a quick cure of enuresis.

The real problem of stenosis is that it is the precursor of *meatal ulceration*. Why an ulcer forms is not clear; eddy currents with statis in the dilated fossa navicularis are postulated but this is unconvincing. The fact is that a meatal ulcer is invariably associated with meatal stenosis. A meatal ulcer reveals itself by painful micturition and/or a drop of blood at the end of the stream. The fear of voiding may precipitate acute retention.

Although some temporary relief is obtained with analgesic ointment the cure of meatal ulcer necessitates a meatotomy. Once the meatus is of adequate size further ulcers do not appear. Dilatation of the meatus is not an alternative to meatotomy — it is painful and distressing to the child, of temporary benefit only and the orifice invariably narrows down again. The meatotomy should be very generous and suture of the urethral mucosa to the glandular epithelium with fine catgut (6/0) is essential to prevent a recurrence of the stenosis.

Undescended Testes

A distinction must be made between an undescended testis and a retractile testis, as the latter is a normal variant for which no treatment is required (chapter I section 2.5). More than half the testes seen in consultant practice are retractile, mistakenly referred as 'undescended'. The confusion rests upon an inadequate technique of examination.

Examination: The patient must be lying down with the legs wide apart. The examining hand is laid flat on the abdomen (not the scrotum) and several firm movements of massage down along the inguinal canal region are made. A finger, or thumb, then occludes the external ring and only then is the scrotum grasped, in a claw-like action, with the fingers and thumb of the other hand, pushing upwards until the testis is grasped and manipulated into the scrotum. If the testis can be confidently placed in the scrotum, and it lies there briefly, it is retractile. If it cannot be brought into the scrotum its degree of lateral mobility in the superficial inguinal pouch is assessed. An impalpable testis means it is either in the abdomen, in the canal, or absent altogether.

Some classifications attempt to define 'ectopic' sites from those 'arrested in the line of normal descent'. Although some sites are clearly ectopic (e.g. a perineal testis) the distinction is often difficult and is of little help in treatment or prognosis. The amount of mobility of the testis, indicating the adequacy or not of the cord length and hence the ease or difficulty of attempted orchidopexy, and the size of the testis, indicating the eventual functional result, are the important clinical considerations.

Complications: The traditional list of complications of undescended testes has been exaggerated:

1) Trauma: very few undescended testes become traumatised.
2) Inguinal hernia: this is not a complication but is commonly associated with undescended testes.
3) Torsion: more torsions occur in descended than in undescended testes (p. 70, 80).
4) Neoplasm: The risk of malignancy is very low. Operative correction does not avoid the risk of malignancy even if it exists.
5) Cosmetic embarrassment: adolescent boys are usually embarrassed by the persistence of an undescended testis.
6) Infertility: there is good evidence that the testis not in the scrotum during puberty is retarded in spermatogenic development. Histological studies show delayed development of the tubules from at least the age of 5 years (see chapter XVIII). The chance to faciliate fertility, the prevention of cosmetic embarrassment and the correction of an associated hernia constitute the main reaons for surgical intervention.

Treatment: There is little place for *hormone* therapy. It is ineffective and animal studies have shown that it may retard spermatogenesis.

Surgical treatment comprises orchidopexy, with or without herniotomy, and is performed at 4 to 5 years of age. If there is a clinical hernia present this may precipitate an operation at an earlier age. If the testis is less than half normal in size it may be better to excise it, unless both testes are small, on the grounds of very poor function and its potentiality for malignant change. A testicular prosthesis is available if required.

Painful inguino-scrotal masses: A series of lesions producing pain and swelling of the inguino-scrotal area constitute a very common clinical entity in children and adults and are discussed in further detail on page 80. In some the diagnosis is obvious but where doubt exists a sound rule is, *A unilateral painful scrotum in children is torsion of the testis until proved otherwise by open operation whereas bilateral swollen painful testes are most likely to be mumps epididymo-orchitis, and can be safely observed provided there is progressive clinical improvement.*

Lesions in Female Children

Labial adhesions: This very common condition (fig. 267) causes much confusion and is often interpreted as an absent vagina, which is a very rare anomaly. The labia minora are simply fused by the sticky adhesion of mucous. The labia of infants can be separated by the fingers on the examination couch, without anaesthesia, except in older children, in whom there may be actual skin union. The mother is asked to thoroughly wash the area daily and to apply a little soft paraffin to the labia with the finger, for some months, to prevent recurrence.

Imperforate hymen: This is a rare condition (fig. 268). It may be noticed in infancy as a mucocolpos abdominal mass, or at the menarche with recur-

267 Labial adhesions. The inner labia are fused across the vestibule, obscuring the site of the fourchette.

268 Imperforate hymen. A neonate with bulging hymen from a vagina distended with mucus (mucocolpos).

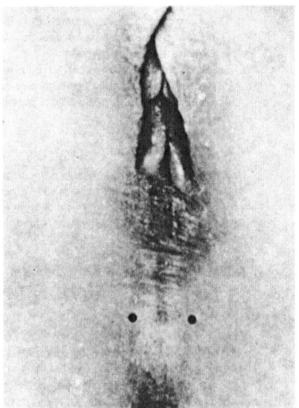

267

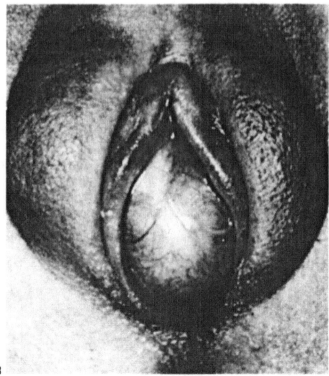

268

rent abdominal pain and amenorrhoea. Treatment consists of excision of the membrane.

Vaginal Discharge

Some mucous discharge is common in children and often causes parents considerable anxiety; although the vast majority of discharges are harmless (see page 82) the causes may include:

1) A hormonal discharge occurring in the early weeks after birth from the effects of maternal hormones. It ceases spontaneously
2) Obesity and poor hygiene
3) Infection. Specific infection is rare, and swab cultures are rarely necessary. They only confuse and usually lead to over-treatment
4) Foreign body. Suggested by a profuse offensive or bloodstained discharge
5) Associated vulvitis
6) Worm infestation.

Hormone creams and excessive topical antibiotics are not indicated in the treatment of children and may readily produce a chemical dermatitis, which causes the discharge to persist. Simple irrigation by the mother using an antiseptic lotion in a rubber infant 'ear syringe', is all that is necessary in the majority of children.

A bloodstained or very purulent discharge calls for examintion under anaesthesia, both to look for a foreign body and to check for a serious malignancy.

Lesions Common to Both Sexes

Epispadias. This lesion is much less common than hypospadias and is especially rare in females. It usually consists of a dorsal defect extending up to the bladder neck (fig. 269). Unlike patients with hypospadias these patients are incontinent. Bladder neck and urethral reconstruction occasionally restores continence but most patients eventually require permanent urinary diversion.

Ectopia Vesicae (extrophy of the bladder). This is one of the most serious of the congenital anomalies of childhood (figs. 270-271). The unfused bladder is open to the exterior with an associated epispadias whilst the sphincter mechanisms are splayed open. The treatment is staged as follows:

1) A sacro-iliac osteotomy, performed at 3 to 6 months of age, closes the separated pubic symphysis.
2) Closure of the bladder and urethra is performed 1 week after the osteotomy.
3) If continent, completion of the epispadiac repair and penile lengthening; in the female, vulval reconstruction.
4) If incontinent, a repeat attempt at bladder neck repair, or permanent urinary diversion, followed by penile lengthening or vulval reconstruction.

Most patients eventually require permanent urinary diversion.

269 Epispadias. The urethra is an open groove on the dorsal surface of the penis. The urethral defect extends to the bladder neck and the boy is incontinent — the most serious aspect of epispadias.

Ectopia vesicae (exstrophy of the bladder).
270 Female. The bladder is visible on the surface of the abdomen and the mucosal surface of the bladder is exposed. Clitoris and labia are unfused and the urethra opens between them.

271 Male. The penis is short and an epispadiac urethra is continuous with the bladder.

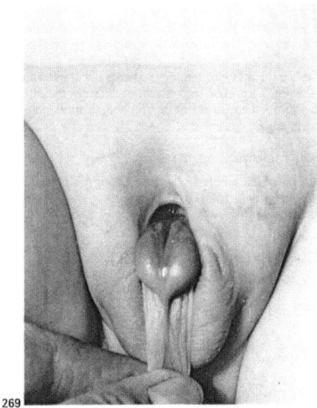

269

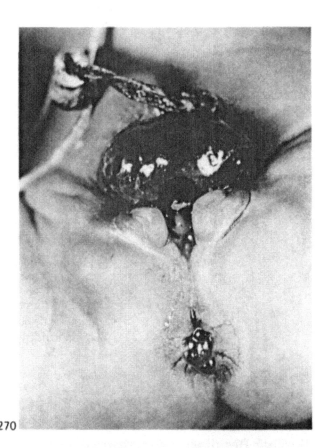

270

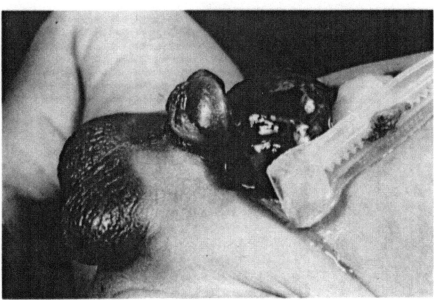

271

Intersex States

This difficult area is beyond the scope of this chapter, but the practitioner should recognise certain principles:

1) When ambiguous genitalia are noticed specialist referral to determine the sex of rearing is urgent, in order to avoid the vast problems of a misappropriate choice necessitating later conversion.

2) In deciding on the sex of rearing the size and adequacy of the phallus is critical, irrespective of any other consideration. If the phallus is small and inadequate for erection the sex of rearing should be female, as no amount of surgery can correct this; if the phallus is adequate the sex of rearing can be in either direction and will be determined by other tests.

3) The adreno-genital syndrome (p. 46) must be excluded. These patients are normal females capable of normal sexual fulfillment and fertility. A delay in diagnosis may result in death from electrolyte loss or lead to later stunted growth.

4) Apart from the hormonally induced types intersex patients are sterile and the type of gonad is irrelevant. Castration and hormone therapy may be necessary, to correspond with the chosen sex of rearing and, in some conditions, because the gonads are pre-malignant.

Investigations: Initially these comprise:

   1) Clinical findings, with particular emphasis on the size of the phallus
   2) A buccal smear and a karyotype analysis
   3) Hormone and electrolyte serum levels.

Later investigations comprise:

   1) Urogenital sinugram and vagino-hysterosalpingogram
   2) Urethrograms and cysto-urethroscopy
   3) Long bone x-ray
   4) A laparotomy and gonadal biopsy.

Reference

Stephens, F.; Douglas, W.J. and Hewstone, A.S.: True, false and sham urinary tract infection in children. Medical Journal of Australia 2: 840 (1966).

Further Reading

Stephens, F.D.; Whitaker, R.J. and Hewstone, A.S.: True, false and sham urinary tract infection in children. Medical Journal of Australia 2: 840 (1966).

Holder, T.M. and Ashcraft, K.W.: Surgery of Infants and Children (Saunders, Philadelphia in press).

Kakalis, P.P.; King, L.R. and Belman, A.B.: Clinical Paediatric Urology (Saunders, Philadelphia 1976).

Stephens, F.D.: in Webster (Ed) Congenital Malformations of the Rectum, Anus and Genito-urinary Tracts (Livingstone, Edinburgh 1963).

Whitehead, E.D. and Leiter, E.: Current Operative Urology (Harper and Row, Hagerstone in press).

Williams, D.I.; Barratt, T.B.; Eckstein, H.B.; Kohlinsky, S.M.; Newns, G.H.; Polani, P.E. and Singer, J.D.: Urology in Childhood (Springer-Verlag, Berlin 1974).

Chapter XV

Adult Urinary Incontinence

Urinary incontinence offers an important diagnostic and therapeutic challenge to the urologist. Precise diagnosis is an essential requirement for successful therapy and usually requires the use of specialised urodynamic equipment. The difficult therapeutic problem of severe male sphincter deficiency incontinence has recently been greatly helped by the development of artificial sphincter prostheses, while Zacharin's abdominoperineal urethral suspension operation has greatly improved the results of selected cases of female stress incontinence operations.

Urinary incontinence is a condition which is socially disabling and at times therapeutically frustrating. As such we need our utmost efforts to diagnose it accurately and treat it appropriately. Adult eneuresis is rare and is only briefly discussed in this chapter.

Classification

The following classification is based on symptom presentation (p. 77):

1) Stress incontinence: this implies temporary loss of urinary control which accompanies raised intra-abdominal pressure. The loss of control may be quickly reversed when the patient notices the urine leak.
2) Urgency incontinence: this implies urgency of micturition with loss of urinary control when the patient has been unable to reach a toilet in time.
3) Overflow incontinence (retention with overflow): this implies mechanical overflow incontinence which may occur with a grossly distended bladder (see chapters X and XI).

Incontinence may be partial or complete.

Aetiology

Sphincter Incompetence

Examples of sphincter incompetence include:

a) Congenital bladder outlet sphincter deficiency, which is a common cause of stress incontinence in the female.
b) Neurogenic incontinence (see chapters IV, XI and XVI).
c) Traumatic sphincteric damage resulting from a severe pelvic fracture with an associated posterior urethral disruption (see chapter XIII), or post-prostatectomy external sphincter trauma (p. 250).

Detrusor Malfunction

1) Poor contractile function of the bladder detrusor, arising from mechanical, fibrotic, or neurological abnormalities, may result in inefficient emptying of the bladder and resultant incontinence.
2) Hyperactive function may arise from infection, inflammatory bladder disease (tuberculosis, irradiation cystitis) or idiopathically, to such a degree that a resultant urgency incontinence occurs (Nordling et al., 1979).
Severe anxiety may also produce urgency incontinence. Detrusor overaction in the erect position may be an associated factor in stress incontinence (Arnold, 1974).

Other Abnormalities

Other congenital or acquired anatomical abnormalities which may result in incontinence include:

Congenital Abnormalities

a) A short female urethra, which reduces urethral resistance and restricts sphincter efficiency
b) Ectopic insertion of a ureter, which may pass to the vagina or the urethra below the sphincteric mechanism
c) Ectopia vesicae
d) Neurogenic deficiencies (e.g. spina bifida)
e) Weak posterior pubo-urethral ligaments (Zacharin, 1972).

These abnormalities are discussed in chapter I.

Acquired Abnormalities

a) Damaged posterior pubo-urethral ligaments
b) A shortened female urethra as a result of surgical operations such as a urethral diverticulum excision
c) Vescio-vaginal fistulae, a complication which may result from an infiltrating neoplasm of the cervix or bladder and rarely, hysterectomy. Birth delivery forceps or pressure necrosis resulting from obstructed labour may also be responsible (p. 310)
d) Uretero-vaginal fistulae are a very rare complication of pelvic surgery (p. 294).

The mechanism of enuresis is not known.

Investigation of the Incontinent Patient

A full history and a thorough general examination, with particular reference to the genitourinary system, is needed as well as chemical and microscopic examination of the urine (chapter III).

Special Investigations

The following investigations, which are described fully elsewhere, may be indicated:

a) Tuberculosis cultures
b) An intravenous pyelogram which may display anatomical and functional abnormalities
c) A micturating cysto-urethrogram demonstrates the vesico-urethral angle, which should be about 90°, the length of the urethra and any associated vesico-ureteric reflux
d) A urodynamic evaluation is essential to both the diagnosis and treatment of many patients with urinary incontinence, particularly those with known or suspected partial or complete nerve or muscle causes (Farrar et al., 1975)
e) An assessment panendoscopy may reveal bladder or urethral abnormalities.

Treatment of Adult Incontinence

Medical Treatment

Weight Loss and Smoking. Moderate or gross obesity is common and overweight females suffering from mild to moderate stress incontinence of urine may be made continent by disciplined dietary weight loss. Such weight loss is also an important prerequisite to successful surgical treatment. Cigarette smoking causes coughing and raised intra-abdominal pressure and should be discontinued both for this and general health reasons.

Perineal Muscle Exercises. Increased muscular development of the levator ani muscle (p. 60) increases urethral resistance. The patient is told to vigorously interrupt the urinary flow during voiding and to voluntarily refrain from voiding while increasing the intra-abdominal pressure (e.g. while coughing).

Drug Treatment. *Enuresis:* Enuresis is rare in adults; imipramine therapy is successful in 25% of patients and improves a further 25%.

Imipramine has a complex action on the voiding mechanism. There is a central stimulatory effect and a peripheral sympathomimetic effect. A nocturnal dose of 10 to 25mg is given, for enuresis but it may be 2 months before a beneficial effect is seen. Adult stress incontinence may be alleviated by a dose of 10 to 25mg 3 times a day. Imipramine overdosage is a serious problem and parents must be warned to keep the tablets away from children. Overdose side effects include tremulousness, weakness, drowsiness, insomnia, blurred vision, dry mouth and postural hypotension.

Incontinence due to infection: Appropriate chemotherapy should be used to treat specific infections according to the organism and its drug sensitivity pattern (see chapter V).

Incontinence due to sphincter incompetence: Sympathetically innervated smooth muscle is found throughout the bladder neck and sphincter regions (p. 54). Stimulation of the adrenergic receptors at the bladder neck by giving ephedrine, which acts by liberating noradrenaline from its storage sites and also by increasing the action of endogenous amines, causes contraction of the bladder outlet and increases the urethral resistance. A dose of 15mg 3 times a day, is usually effective. Side effects include insomnia, tremulousness, palpitations and urinary retention (Stewart et al., 1976).

Incontinence due to detrusor malfunction: Various autonomic agents are helpful depending on the mechanism of incontinence.

Poor contractile function: Detrusor inactivity may result in overflow incontinence in the presence of a full bladder. This may be improved by using cholinergic drugs, such as bethanecol, which increase detrusor tone, or α-adrenergic blocking agents such as phenoxybenzamine, which reduce the tone of the bladder outlet (p. 56). Bethanecol is a potent, orally active, synthetic cholinergic agent. It acts on the post-ganglionic neurones and on the effector muscle cells. It causes contraction of both the detrusor and urethral smooth muscle components and beneficial bladder emptying depends upon a dominant detrusor muscle effect. A dose of 5mg 4 times a day is given at first and increased, if necessary, to 10mg 4 times a day. Side effects include abdominal cramps, urinary urgency, nausea, faintness, sweating and excessive salivation. Phenoxybenzamine is given in a dose of 5mg 3 times a day initially, which may be increased to 10mg 3 times a day if side effects such as postural hypotension, palpitations, blurred vision, dry mouth or nasal stuffiness permit. If the patient has a moderate bladder residual urine phenoxybenzamine may aggravate the problems of incontinence — in such situations it may be used in combination with bethanecol. Phenoxybenzamine is contraindicated in patients with cardiac failure and cerebrovascular disease (Krane and Olson, 1973).

Detrusor hyperactivity: Anticholinergic drugs such as propantheline, emepronium and flavoxate inhibit detrusor contractions and reduce intravesical pressure. Propantheline is given in doses of 15mg 3 times a day initially. The dose can be increased to 30mg 4 times a day. A slow-release preparation can be used to produce a smoother dose-time curve. Possible side effects include blurred vision, dry mouth, constipation, urinary retention and drowsiness. Unfortunately toxic and therapeutic dose levels are similar and side effects are common at therapeutically effective doses. Should such side effects occur, ephedrine may be given with propantheline.

Females
Surgical Treatment

Sphincter
Incompetence

Surgery for Sphincter Incompetence and to Increase Urethral Resistance

Stress incontinence: This is the most common form of female incontinence treated surgically but the results depend upon careful patient selection as previously indicated. The causative factors in female stress incontinence which may need to be overcome surgically include:

1) Vaginal prolapse, which results in loss of the normal urethrovesical angle
2) Congenital or acquired sphincter incompetence and/or posterior pubo-urethral ligamentous damage
3) Congential or acquired shortness of the urethra.

Specific operations for *female stress incontinence* of urine are:

Vaginal prolapse repair: Plication of the peri-urethral tissues at the vesico-urethral angle results in increased mechanical bladder outlet resistance and more effective sphincter action. The urethra is not elongated in this procedure. Careful patient selection results in a 90% success rate.

Correction of an abnormal urethro-vesical angle: abdominal extra-peritoneal *urethro-cystopexy operations* involve suturing the para-urethral tissues to the symphysis pubis and the bladder to the posterior rectus sheath (Marshall et al., 1949; Marshall and Begaul, 1968). Urethral sling operations, using a strip of rectus sheath (Millin, 1947) or synthetic materials, passing behind the urethra and attached anteriorly to the posterior rectus sheath have also been effective, provided that they are broad enough to overcome postoperative urethral kinking.

Stress
Incontinence

Synchronous combined abdominoperineal urethral suspension operation: Zacharin and Gleadell (1963) first reported this operation for female patients with stress incontinence of urine due to weak or damaged posterior pubo-urethral ligaments. The procedure requires a synchronous combined extra-peritoneal abdominal and perineal approach. Two 3-inch strips of rectus abdominus sheath are cut and sutured to the para-urethral posterior pubo-urethral ligaments on both sides. A special grasping instrument is used to pull the aponeurotic bands into position. The results, in carefully selected patients, are very good, with a 5-year cure rate of 72%.

Increased Urethral
Resistance

Elongation of the urethra: Procedures to elongate the urethra in the female may be performed, either at the vaginal or the bladder end, and can be useful in difficult cases of sphincter deficiency. Lapides (1961) has achieved considerable success with this method in selected patients.

Males
Surgical Treatment

Specific operations for *male stress incontinence* of urine are as follows:

Synthetic prosthesis implantation: The most difficult cases of incontinence to treat are those resulting from traumatic sphincter damage, non-surgical or surgical. The recently developed prostheses (Scott et al., 1976; Rosen, 1976; Das and Kaufman, 1977) now appear to offer a better means of treating these unfortunate patients than an indwelling bladder catheter or permanent urinary diversion.

Electronic implants: These have recently been used to treat male sphincter incompetence (Glen, 1974) but their precise positioning requires considerable expertise.

Surgery for Detrusor Malfunction. Correction of mechanical (prostatectomy for chronic retention of urine) or neurological (spinal neoplasm) causes may be possible, and very small capacity bladders may be enlarged by operations such as ileocystoplasty or colocystoplasty (p. 156).

Surgery for Congenital or Acquired Anatomical Abnormalities. This includes excision of an ectopic ureter, attempted ectopia vesicae reconstruction (p. 354), traumatised ureteric repair or vesico-vaginal fistula correction (p. 310).

References

Arnold, E.P.: Cystometry-postural effects in incontinent women. Urologia Internationalis 29: 185 (1974).

Das, S. and Kaufman, J.J.: The use of a silicone gel prosthesis in the treatment of post-prostatectomy incontinence. British Journal of Surgery 64: 600 (1977).

Farrar, D.J.; Whiteseide, C.G.; Osborne, J.L. and Turner-Warwick, R.T.: A urodynamic analysis of micturition symptoms in the female. Surgery, Gynecology and Obstetrics 141: 875 (1975).

Glen, E.S.: Electrical stimulation controls incontinence. 16th Congress of the Society Internationale d'Urologie 2: 343 (1974).

Krane, R.J. and Olson, C.A.: Phenoxybenzamine in neurogenic bladder dysfunction. I. A theory of micturition; II. Clinical considerations. Journal of Urology 110: 650 (1973).

Marshall, V.F. and Begaul, R.M.: Experience with suprapubic vesico-urethral suspension after previous failures to correct stress incontinence in women. Journal of Urology 100: 647 (1968).

Marshall, V.F.; Marchetti, A.A. and Krantz, K.E.: The correction of stress incontinence by simple vesico-urethral suspension. Surgery, Gynecology and Obstetrics 88: 509 (1949).

Millin, T.: Discussion on stress incontinence in micturition. Proceedings of the Royal Society of Medicine 40: 364 (1947).

Nordling, J.; Meyhoff, H.H.; Andersen, J.T. and Walter, S.: Urinary incontinence in the female. The value of detrusor reflux activation procedures. British Journal of Urology 51: 110 (1979).

Rosen, M.: A simple artificial implantable sphincter. British Journal of Urology 48: 675 (1976).

Scott, F.B.; Bradley, W.E. and Timm, C.W.: Treatment of urinary incontinence by implantable prosthesis urinary sphincter. Journal of Urology 112: 75 (1976).

Stewart, B.H.; Banowsky, H.W. and Montague, D.K.: Stress incontinence: conservative therapy with sympathomimetic drugs. Journal of Urology 115: 558 (1976).

Zacharin, R.F. and Gleadell, L.W.: Abdominoperineal urethral suspension. American Journal of Obstetrics and Gynecology 86: 981 (1963).

Further Reading

Lapides, J.: Stress incontinence. Journal of Urology 85: 291 (1961).

Westmore, D.D.: Urinary incontinence, which drugs to use. Current Therapeutics 4: 33 (1979).

Zacharin, R.F.: Stress incontinence in the female (Harper and Row, New York 1972).

Chapter XVI

Renal Failure

Renal failure may result from solitary or combined impairment of the kidney's blood supply, parenchymal tissue or calyceal-pelvi-ureteric conducting mechanism. The result may be acute or chronic potentially reversible, or irreversible failure, hence the importance of prophylaxis, early diagnosis and adequate treatment.

Aetiology

Although some types of obstruction, glomerulonephritis, incompatible blood transfusion, poisons and the crush syndrome will cause *acute renal failure* the most common cause is an inadequate pre-renal blood supply. Causes include:

1) Severe bleeding
2) Renal artery trauma or disease (atherosclerosis, fibrosis, aneurysm, embolus)
3) Acute or chronic heart failure
4) Sudden fluid and electrolyte loss (vomiting diarrhoea burns)
5) Septicaemic shock (Eremin and Marshall, 1969)
6) Aortic aneurysm
7) Acute pancreatitis
8) Renal vein thrombosis
9) Incompatible blood transfusion
10) Pre-eclampsia
11) Heavy metal poisoning (mercury, lead)
12) Chemical poisoning (phenol, carbon tetrachloride)
13) Traumatic crush syndrome (myoglobin release and resultant tubular necrosis).

Progressive post-renal obstruction and parenchymal damage are the most common causes of *chronic renal failure*. The damage may arise from:

1) Post-renal urinary obstruction (chapters X, XI and XII)
2) Severe vesico-ureteric reflux (p. 134, p. 334)
3) Infection (chapter V)
4) Glomerulonephritis (see later)
5) Benign or malignant hypertension (chapter XVII)
6) Staghorn calculi, gross medullary sponge kidneys or the rare tubular acidosis
7) Analgesic nephropathy and other causes of papillary necrosis (p. 274)
8) Collagen diseases (polyarteritis nodosa, systemic lupus erythematoses)
9) Diabetes mellitus (papillary necrosis)
10) Hyperuricaemia
11) Nephrocalcinosis (chapter IX)
12) Polycystic disease (chapter I)
13) Irradiation
14) Paroxysmal haemoglobinuria, porphyria, amyloidosis, sickle cell anaemia (papillary necrosis)

15) Balkan nephropathy [unknown but presumed dietary aetiology causes glomerulonephritis, papillary necrosis and, occasionally, renal calyceal and pelvic neoplasms (p. 172)].

Acute Renal Failure

In acute renal failure the kidney is pale and swollen with usually an ischaemic cortex and a congested medulla.

Surgical Pathology

An inadequate blood supply produces hypotension and vasoconstriction. When the glomerular filtration rate is less than 5ml per minute and the urine production less than 20ml per hour renal failure will occur. Arteriovenous anastomoses may shunt blood away from the already hypotensive renal cortex and this may produce infarction, or so-termed renal cortical necrosis (Trueta et al., 1947). The tubules become blocked with desquamated dying cells and may also infarct and rupture.

Renal parenchymal damage may also result from tubular obstruction due to post-renal causes such as calculi, papillary necrosis impaction, or to intra-tubular collections of haemoglobin, uric acid crystals or myoglobin, and from direct tubular cell destruction resulting from infection, glomerulo-nephritis, heavy metal or chemical poisoning.

Clinical Features

The aetiology of the acute renal failure may dominate the clinical presentation as occurs with severe haemorrhagic blood loss, Gram-negative septicaemia and acute coronary infarction; alternatively the patient may present with a symptomatic or asymptomatic undiagnosed oliguria or anuria.

Diagnosis of Acute Renal Failure

A full history, including a knowledge of all drug therapy, with particular empahsis on known nephrotoxic agents or any possibility of ingested poison, and a thorough general examination with particular emphasis on the detection of a distended bladder or large kidneys, often enables a diagnosis to be made. However, it is essential that post-renal obstructive causes be excluded and this usually necessitates a cysto-urethroscopy and bilateral pyelo-ureterograms.

Occasionally there is doubt as to whether the patient is oliguric or in renal failure. A diuretic trial in conjunction with the above findings usually clarifies the situation but *should only be attempted after all fluid deficits have been replaced*. Intravenous 20% mannitol (1ml/kg bodyweight) or 120mg of intravenous frusemide should produce a rapid urinary flow rate unless renal failure is present. A second dose of mannitol should not be given unless these has been an adequate initial response but frusemide can be safely repeated, 2-hourly, to a maximum dose of 1 gram, even in the absence of any response (Cantarovich et al., 1971).

Generalised arterial (malignant hypertension) or local renal artery or vein occlusion (aneurysm, embolus, thrombus) and glomerular disease (glomerulonephritis) should be excluded and this may require a renal biopsy, arteriogram and/or a venogram.

Management of
Acute Renal Failure

Prophylaxis. Careful preoperative, operative and postoperative monitoring of both the central venous pressure and the arterial pressure and the prompt administration of intravenous fluids or blood will prevent many cases of acute renal failure, particularly in those high risk patients undergoing major cardiovascular or excisional surgery, or being treated for burns or the crush syndrome (Eremin and Marshall, 1969).

Established Acute Renal Failure Management. Patients with renal failure should be managed in specialised centres with expert staff and dialysis facilities (Mahoney, 1977).

The primary cause must be urgently treated, if this is possible, and the patient kept alive for the next 2 to 6 weeks while awaiting renal recovery. Severe acute renal failure requires either intraperitoneal dialysis or haemodialysis, using an artificial kidney machine, as these means provide the only accurate way of controlling the large metabolic nitrogenous protein tissue breakdown and associated dangerous intracellular potassium release, resulting from severe trauma or septicaemia. Haemodialysis provides the more rapid means of controlling these metabolic changes and is the only method possible in the presence of peritonitis.

The patient's fluid intake is restricted to about 1,000ml per day, sufficient to replace the usual adult breathing and sweating losses. As there is often massive body protein breakdown, dietary protein intake is replaced by 1,000 calories per day of carbohydrate so as not to contribute to further nitrogenous accumulation (Giovanetti and Maggiore, 1964). Electrolytes and the serum potassium in particular, are carefully monitored and maintained within normal limits.

Renal Recovery: Provided that the patient can be kept alive during this critical period the returning glomerular filtration and associated phagocytic action clears the recoverable tubules and urine passes down the collecting ducts. The recovering distal tubule is initially unable to retain salt and water and this usually results in a massive diuresis with resulting fluid and electrolyte imbalance which must be carefully monitored and controlled. The degree of recovery is dependent upon the severity of the renal failure and the adequacy of management.

Chronic Renal Failure

Chronic renal failure may result from:

1) Fibrosis resulting from acute renal failure.
2) Specific known or unknown renal parenchymal or obstructive diseases. Urinary tract obstruction, glomerulonephritis, pyelonephritis, or any of the other diseases or agents listed previously may cause chronic renal failure but it is not always possible to determine, at the contracted, scarred end-stage, precisely which mechanism has been responsible (Hodson, 1965; Sherwood, 1973).

Common Causes of
Chronic Renal Failure

The following causes of chronic renal failure are discussed elsewhere:

Urinary Tract Obstruction. (See chapters X and XII.)

Vesico-ureteric Reflux. (See chapter V and figure 272).

Pyelonephritis. (See chapter V.)

Analgesic Nephropathy. [See p. 274 (Kincaid-Smith, 1969).]

272 Renal Failure. A small scarred kidney may result from congenital or acquired causes. The destruction of this right kidney resulted from vesico-ureteric reflux. Note the hypertrophied left kidney which has been able to maintain normal renal function.

The most common cause of acute renal failure results from a sudden gross reduction in blood supply whilst the most common causes of chronic renal failure are obstruction, vesico-ureteric reflux, infection and glomerulonephritis.

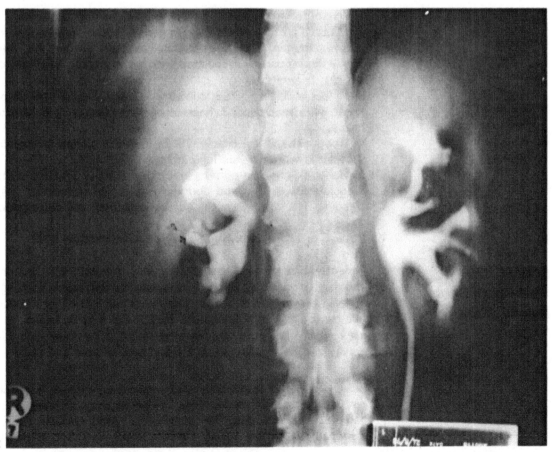

272

Glomerulonephritis: Glomerulonephritis is an uncommon disease but a common cause of chronic renal failure (Kincaid-Smith et al., 1973). Its aetiology is unknown and it is classified according to the histological changes occurring within the kidney. Such changes are either focal or more general and range from:

1) Minimal basement membrane lesions, where electron microscopy studies reveal that the foot processes (p. 37) of Bowman's cells have been damaged and are no longer separate. This is manifested clinically by selective *proteinuria* (albumin, being smaller than globulin, is filtered through the glomerulus and appears in the urine).
2) More severe lesions, where the basement membrane becomes swollen and compresses the capillary. This is termed *membranous glomerulonephritis* and results in filtration of both albumin and globulin.
3) The most severe form of glomerulonephritis involves damage to the capillary endothelium in addition to the basement membrane. The capillary endothelium swells and both red and white cells pass through into Bowman's capsule. Groups of these cells, together with protein molecules and sloughed capsular cells, are termed crescents and the appearance is described as *proliferative glomerulonephritis.*

In severe cases fibrosis occurs around the glomeruli and vessels. The severity of the histological appearance usually enables an accurate diagnosis and prognosis and in particular may assist treatment; however, renal biopsies are not free from complications and may result in severe bleeding, even when performed by experts.

Clinical presentation: The clinical presentation of glomerulonephritis (Bright, 1836) varies greatly:

1) Asymptomatic proteinuria and/or microscopic haematuria.
2) Massive proteinuria resulting in general tissue oedema due to the loss of plasma albumin. This presentation has been termed the 'nephrotic syndrome' and is usually associated with hypertension, renal failure and, occasionally, haematuria.
3) A febrile illness, often following a streptococcal sore throat, of rapid onset, with macroscopic haematuria hypertension and occasionally renal failure.
4) Goodpasture's syndrome (1919), in which severe glomerulonephritis is associated with a severe lung infection.
5) Henoch-Schonlein purpura in which the presentation described above is associated with joint and abdominal pain and occasional gastrointestinal bleeding. The disease usually occurs in children and has a good prognosis.

Benign or Malignant Hypertension. (See chapter XVII).

Some Clinical Features of Chronic Renal Failure

Patients with chronic renal failure may present with tiredness, nausea, anorexia or vomiting, hypertension, muscle and nerve wasting, bone pain and, if the renal failure is associated with salt and water retention, congestive cardiac failure. A pericardial friction rub may be heard, polycystic kidneys may be palpable, and the urine found to be dilute with a low specific gravity and to contain red, white and tubular cells and casts (p. 86).

Bone x-rays may reveal several changes. Less calcium is absorbed by the gut in patients with chronic renal failure, resulting in rickets in children and osteomalacia in adults. The parathyroid gland releases parathormone in response to the low serum calcium levels, resulting in possible osteitis fibrosa cystica. Because of the high serum phosphate levels and the bone demineralisation, calcium phosphate crystalisation may occur in many tissues, including bone, and this apparent paradox may result in adjacent areas of bone demineralisation and bone deposition, to which the term osteodystrophy is applied.

Diagnosis

The serum creatinine, urea and potassium levels are raised while the serum bicarbonate is low. A normocytic, normochromic anaemia occurs (p. 45).

A straight abdominal and pelvic x-ray is an essential investigation, particularly to assess the renal size and to detect the presence of any radio-opaque obstructing calculi; the injection phase of the intravenous pyelogram is often of little diagnostic value as the kidney is unable to concentrate the medium if the blood urea is greater than 200mmol/per litre (Kelsey Fry and Cattell, 1971). Urinary tract obstruction should always be excluded however and this usually requires cysto-urethroscopy and bilateral pyelo-ureterograms. A renal biopsy may be indicated.

Treatment of Chronic Renal Failure

Diet and General Medical Management: The protein requirement depends upon the renal function. Reduction of the daily protein intake to 20g may maintain a patient in reasonable health if his creatinine clearance is at least 3ml per minute but the diet is unpleasant and poorly tolerated (Giovanetti and Maggiore, 1964).

In salt-losing renal failure added dietary salt is required and oral sodium bicarbonate may be needed for the associated acidosis. Potassium levels can be reduced by oral or rectal ion-exchange resins.

The anaemia of chronic renal failure is not adequately treatable as the loss of renal erythropoietin inactivates the bone marrow production. Short term packed red cell transfusions may be necessary if the haemoglobin falls below 6g per 100ml.

Congestive cardiac failure, nausea, hypertension and bone pain may all require specific treatment.

Failed Dietary and Medical Management: When the creatinine clearance rate falls below 3ml per minute then dietary manipulation and drug therapy are insufficient to maintain life. A doctor/family/community decision must be made as to whether chronic renal dialysis and/or renal transplantation should be undertaken or whether the patient should no longer be treated.

Renal Dialysis

Haemodialysis: A forearm arteriovenous shunt is created, resulting in large varicose forearm veins. Blood is taken, at arterial pressure, from one of these veins heparinised and allowed to flow across a semi-permeable membrane within the dialysis machine. The membrane separates the patient's blood from a saline mixture and allows water, salt, potassium, urea, creatinine, phosphate and calcium osmotic interchanges to occur so that the blood, returned to the patient's venous system, has been cleared of excess metabolites and fluid and essential constituents, such as calcium, replaced. The procedure is usually performed twice a week either within hospital or the patient's home, depending upon the family and community facilities and attitudes (Brescia et al., 1966; Robinson, 1971).

Peritoneal dialysis: A silastic catheter is inserted into the peritoneal cavity, using a careful aseptic technique, and the peritoneal lining cells utilised as

the 'semi-permeable membrane'. A measured volume of appropriately prepared saline mixture is introduced through the catheter and then removed
after the osmotic exchanges have achieved the same results as haemodialysis (Rae and Pendray, 1973).

Peritoneal dialysis is cheap and relatively simple to perform but it is unsuitable for severe acute renal failure as the osmotic exchanges are much slower
than those achieved with haemodialysis. Intermittent peritoneal dialysis is
being increasingly used in the treatment of end-stage renal failure. Both the
introduction of closed systems of dialysate delivery, and permanent indwelling peritoneal catheters, have reduced the previously high incidence of
peritonitis, which is still the major complication of the procedure.

Renal Transplanation

If a suitably tissue-matched cadaver or living kidney and ureter is available
then it may be removed and anastomosed to the recipient's iliac vascular
system and bladder (fig. 273) utilising an anti-reflux ureteric tunnel implantation technique (Brown, 1968). The surgical operation is usually not
difficult but the subsequent control of the recipient's immunological defence response to the donor kidney determines whether or not the operation will be successful (Ewing et al., 1967). Transplants between identical
twins do not result in such immunological host defence problems. At present about 70% of all cadaver grafts survive for at least 12 months (Calne,
1976).

Renal transplantation requires a competent team of medical and para-
medical personnel including nephrologists, dialysis technicians, experienced
nursing staff, immunologist, bacteriologist, haematologist and a urologist,
as well as adequate facilities and a constant supply of kidneys.

A successful renal transplant provides a better quality of life than long term
intermittent dialysis. Unsuccessful renal transplantation requires dialysis
treatment until such time as a suitable second kidney is available although
such secondary cadaver grafts have a poorer prognosis than the primary
operation (Brown, 1969).

273 Renal homotransplantation. Renal homotransplantation. Here the donor artery has been anastomosed to the internal iliac artery and the vein to the common iliac vein. The ureter enters the bladder through a long submucosal anti-reflux tunnel, thus protecting the kidney facilitating postoperative retrograde pyelo-ureterogram studies.

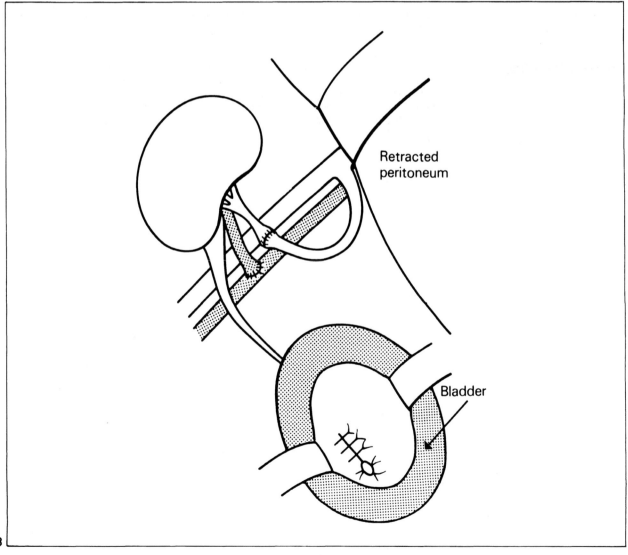

273

References

Brescia, M.J.; Cimino, J.E.; Appel, K. and Hurwich, B.H.: Chronic haemodialysis using venepuncture and a surgically created arteriovenous fistula. New England Journal of Medicine 275: 1089 (1966).

Bright, R.: Cases and observations illustrative of renal disease accompanied with the secretion of albuminuric urine. Guy's Hospital Report 1: 396 (1836).

Brown, R.B.: Urological complications of renal homotransplantation. British Journal of Urology 4: 492 (1968).

Brown, R.B.: The fate of double-header cadaveric renal allografts. British Journal of Urology 5: 386 (1969).

Cantarovich, F.; Locatelli, A,; Fernandez, J.C.; Perez, L. and Cristhot, J.: Frusemide in high doses in the treatment of acute renal failure. Postgraduate Medical Journal (Suppl.) 13: 13-18 (1971).

Eremin, J. and Marshall, V.C.: The diagnosis and management of refractory shock. Medical Journal of Australia 1: 778 (1969).

Ewing, M.R.; Brown, R.B.; Marshall, V.C.; Johnson, M. and McLeish, D.G.: Cadaveric renal transplantation. Lancet 2: 59 (1967).

Giovanetti, S. and Maggoire, Q.: A low nitrogen diet with proteins of high biological value for severe chronic uraemia. Lancet 1: 1000 (1964).

Goodpasture, E.W.: The significance of certain pulmonary lesions in relation to the aetiology of influenza. American Journal of Medical Science 158: 863 (1919).

Hodson, C.J.: Natural history of chronic pyelonephritic scarring. British Medical Journal 2: 191 (1965).

Kelsey Fry, I. and Cattell, W.R.: Radiology in the diagnosis of renal failure. British Medical Bulletin 27: 148 (1971).

Kincaid-Smith, P.: Analgesic nephropathy: a common form of renal disease in Australia. Medical Journal of Australia 2: 1131 (1969).

Mahoney, J.F.: Treatment of acute renal failure. Current Therapeutics 4: 73 (1977).

Robinson, B.H.B.: Intermittent dialysis in the home. British Medical Bulletin 27: 173 (1971).

Rae, A.I. and Pendray, M.: Advantages of peritoneal dialysis in chronic renal failure. Journal of the American Medical Association 225: 937 (1973).

Sherwood, R.: Ureteric reflux 1973: chronic pyelonephritis versus reflux nephropathy. British Journal of Radiology 46: 653 (1973).

Further Reading

Calne, R.V.: Renal transplantation; in Blandy (Ed) Urology p.488-520 (Blackwell, Oxford 1976).

Kincaid-Smith, P.; Mathew, T.H. and Lovell Becker, E.: Glomerulonephritis: Morphology, Natural History and Treatment (Wiley, New York 1973).

Trueta, J.; Barclay, A.E.; Daniel, P.M. Franklin, K.J. and Pritchard, M.M.L.: Studies of the Renal Circulation (Blackwell, Oxford 1947).

Chapter XVII

Renal Hypertension and Vascular Disorders

Renal parenchymal or vascular disease may result in primary renal hypertension, or non-renal hypertension may so damage the vessels in the kidney that secondary renal hypertension develops (fig. 274). Identification of the cause of renal hypertension is important as occasionally the condition is curable.

Primary Renal Hypertension

Mechanism

Partial occlusion of the renal artery reduces the afferent arteriole pressure and stimulates the release of renin from the juxtaglomerular cells (p. 37). Renin converts a liver protein angiotensinogen into angiotensin I which splits into a smaller protein, angiotensin II, which both vasoconstricts peripheral blood vessels, producing hypertension, and also stimulates the adrenal cortex to produce aldosterone, which acts on the renal tubules and results in increased sodium and water retention and further hypertension.

274 The causes of renal hypertension and related vascular disorders.

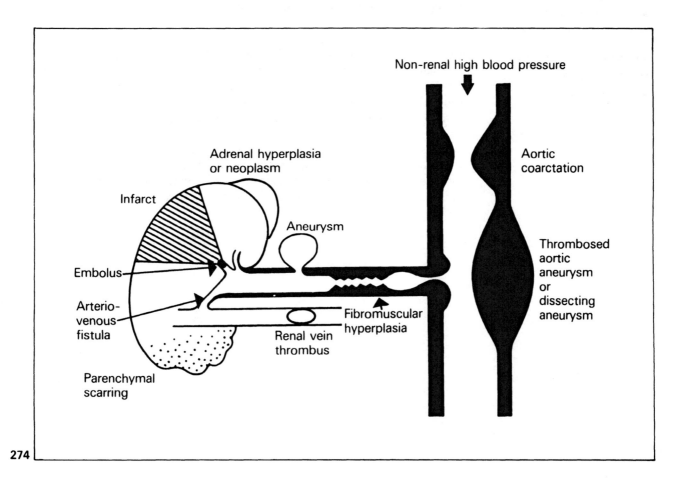

Renin release is inhibited by excess aldosterone and stimulated by both a low afferent arteriole pressure and low serum sodium levels.

Diagnosis

If the history and physical examination reveal hypertension then an intravenous pyelogram is an essential special investigation (DeCamp and Birchall, 1958).

Intravenous Pyelogram Findings: Hypertensive kidneys usually have a partial or total delay in excretion due to the vascular or parenchymal abnormality responsible for the excessive renin release. The intravenous pyelogram is diagnostic in 80% of unilateral and 60% of bilateral primary hypertensive kidneys (fig. 275).

Other Investigative Procedures: A selective renal angiogram which displays the complete arterial pattern of the kidney may reveal the cause of the hypertension. Renal angiography catheterisation (p. 96) enables the direct collection of blood for renal vein renin estimation at the same time (Kaufman et al., 1970). Direct renal vein renin level measurements are more diagnostic of renal hypertension than measurements of peripheral venous renin levels.

Renal scan studies (for suspected infarction) and renal venograms (for a suspected venous thrombosis) may also be indicated (see below).

Parenchymal Causes of Primary Renal Hypertension

Primary renal hypertension may result from parenchymal damge caused by pyelonephritis, glomerulonephritis, obstruction, neoplasm or cystic changes, all of which are discussed fully elsewhere.

Vascular Causes of Primary Renal Hypertension

Renal Artery Stenosis. *Fibromuscular hyperplasia:* Hypertrophy and associated degeneration of the main renal artery or its branches may result in renal hypertension and is easily diagnosed by selective renal angiography. The narrowed segment may require partial excision and vein patch grafting or a by-pass operation using venous, arteriole or synthetic tubes.

Atherosclerosis: Atheromatous plaques may occlude the origin of the renal artery and, provided that the diagnosis is made before irreversible renal damage has occurred, may be correctable by either open excision of the plaque or by-passing the area as indicated in figure 276.

275 **Renal hypertensive kidneys** usually have a relative delay in excretion as illustrated here on the right side.

276 **Reconstruction of the renal artery.**

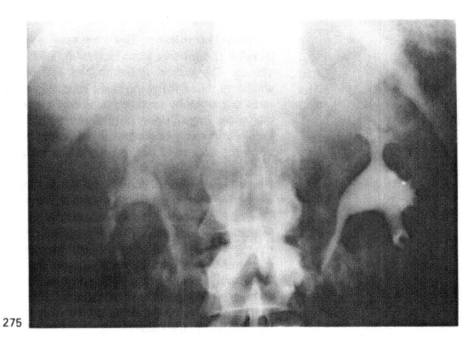

275

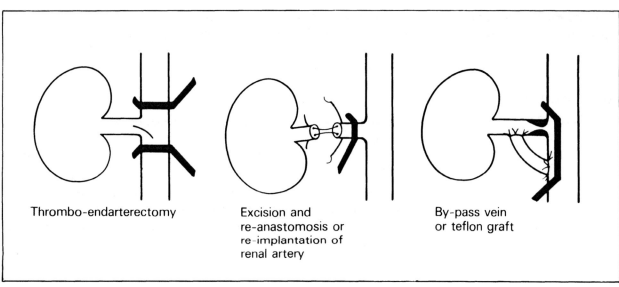

276

Thrombo-endarterectomy

Excision and
re-anastomosis or
re-implantation of
renal artery

By-pass vein
or teflon graft

Renal Artery Embolus: As indicated on page 40 the renal arteries are end-arteries and complete occlusion of the main renal artery will result in infarction of the kidney. Complete occlusion of a main branch will result in infarction of the wedge-shaped area it supplies (fig. 277). Emboli may result from heart valve disease, detachment or dissection of atheromatous arterial plaques, open heart surgery or trauma. Depending upon the degree of infarction, the patient experiences:

1) Sudden severe loin pain and haematuria with the development of hypertension
2) Slowly developing hypertension
3) Neither pain, haematuria nor hypertension.

Renal infarction may be diagnosed by intravenous pyelogram and/or renal scan studies which reveal a partial or completely non-functioning kidney with an early swollen and a later shrunken appearance. Selective renal angiography confirms the diagnosis (Lang et al., 1968; Abel and Kennedy, 1978). Partial or total nephrectomy is required to remove infarcted and hypertension-producing ischaemic tissue.

Venous Thrombosis: The main renal vein, or one of its tributaries, may develop thrombosis from unknown, inflammatory, infective or neoplastic causes. The clinical presentations and special investigative findings are similar to those following renal infarction with the exception that selective renal angiography reveals no arterial blockage; a venogram confirms the diagnosis. Urgent open surgical removal of the thrombus from the vessel is required in most cases but a nephrectomy may be necessary depending upon the degree of occlusion and the resultant renal damage.

Renal Artery Aneurysm: Saccular, fusiform or arteriovenous aneurysms may arise from congenital, traumatic, neoplastic or inflammatory causes. They are diagnosed by the occasional auscultation of a loin bruit or by selective angiography. They are sometimes calcified which may confuse the diagnosis with that of a renal calculus. Aneurysms are often multiple and rarely cause primary renal hypertension unless they are associated with renal artery stenosis (fig. 278). Large solitary aneurysms are best removed as they may rupture and aneurysms shown to cause renal hypertension must also be removed although the operation is difficult and may necessitate removing the kidney.

Treatment of Primary Renal Hypertension

As has been stated the cause of renal hypertension should be treated surgically if possible. Renovascular hypertension is difficult to control with antihypertensive drugs and patient compliance with long term drug regimens is also a problem.

Secondary Renal Hypertension

Secondary renal hypertension may result from:

1) Essential hypertension which usually responds to hypotensive drug therapy
2) Malignant hypertension which is difficult to control with drug therapy
3) Adrenal neoplasms.

Conn's tumour: Conn et al. (1964) first described an aldosterone-producing adrenal cortex neoplasm which results in hypertension and, in view of the loss of potassium and associated sodium retention, muscle weakness. Surgical excision cures the condition.

277 A renal artery embolus has completely occluded the main right renal artery.

278 Renal artery aneurysms. Even multiple renal artery aneurysms, without renal artery stenosis, rarely produce renal hypertension.

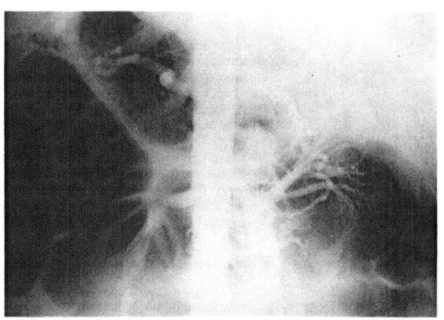

277

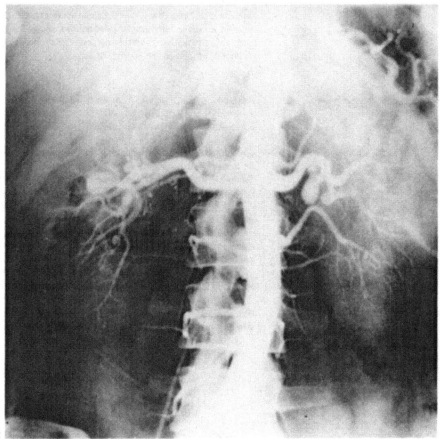

278

Phaeochromocytoma: The secretion by this tumour of excessive amounts of noradrenaline and adrenaline can produce hypertension (Hill and Smith, 1960) and the diagnosis is made by measuring the 24-hour break-down product of one of these catecholamines (vanillyl mandelic acid, VMA) in the urine (p. 89). The neoplasm is removed by surgical excision, controlling the hypertension which results from handling the neoplasm with ganglion blocking drugs throughout the procedure.

Cushing's disease: The over-production of cortisol also produces hypertension and the diagnosis is made by measuring the urinary 17-hydroxy-corticosteroid levels. An adrenal neoplasm does not respond to pituitary control while adrenal hyperplasia does and this enables an accurate distinction to be made before surgery is undertaken. An adrenal neoplasm is removed by excision while adrenal hyperplasia is treated by subtotal resection of both glands.

Although in *severe coarctation of the aorta* renin release results in hypertension, the aortic stenosis protects those parts of the body distal to the narrowing. The results of resecting the narrowed area, or replacing it with a graft, are excellent provided the condition is diagnosed at an early age.

References

Abel, B.J. and Kennedy, J.H.: Severe hypertension following traumatic renal infarction. British Journal of Urology 50: 54 (1978).

Conn, J.W.; Knopf, R.F. and Nesbit, R.M.: Clinical characteristics of primary aldosteronism from analysis of 145 cases. American Journal of Surgery 107: 159 (1964).

DeCamp, P.T. and Birchall, R.: Recognition and treatment of renal artery stenosis associated with hypertension. Surgery 43: 124 (1958).

Hill, F. deM. and Smith, D.R.: Phaeochromocytoma. A report of 12 cases. California Medicine 92: 125 (1960).

Kaufman, J.J.; Lupu, A.N.; Franklin, S. and Maxwell, M.H.: Diagnostic and predictive value of renal vein renin activity in renovascular hypertension. Journal of Urology 103: 702 (1970).

Lang, E.K.; Mertz, J.H.I. and Nournse, M.: Renal arteriography in the assessment of renal infarction. Journal of Urology 99: 506 (1968).

Further Reading

Alexander, F. and Grimason, P.: Aldosterone production and juxta-glomerular granule. British Journal of Experimental Pathology 48: 540 (1967).

Butler, A.M.: Chronic pyelonephritis and arterial hypertension. Journal of Clinical Investigation 16: 889 (1937).

Cushing, H.: The basophil adenomas of the pituitary body and their clinical manifestations (pituitary basophilism). Bulletin of Johns Hopkins Hospital 50: 137 (1932).

Glenn, J.F. Adrenal surgery; in Urologic Surgery p.1-30 (Charper and Row, New York 1975).

Goldblatt, H.; Lynch, H.; Hanzall, R.F. and Summerville, W.W.: The production of persistent hypertension in dogs. American Journal of Pathology 9: 942 (1933).

Harrison, E.G. and McCormack, L.V.: Pathological classification of renal artery disease in renovascular hypertension. Mayo Clinic Proceedings 46: 161 (1971).

Kaufamn, J.J.: Surgical treatment of reno-vascular hypertension. Journal of Urology 94: 211 (1965).

Kirkendahl, W.M.; Kiechty, R.D. and Culp, D.A.: Diagnosis and treatment of patients with phaeochromocytoma. Archives of Internal Medicine 115: 529 (1965).

Moore, H.L.; Katz, R.; McIntosh, R.; Smith, F.; Michael, A. and Vernier, R. D.: Unilateral renal vein thrombosis and the nephrotic syndrome. Pediatrics 50: 598 (1972).

Poutasse, E.F.: Renal artery aneurysms. Journal of Urology 113: 443 (1975).

Ward, J.N. and Dias, R.: Iatrogenic renal artery thrombosis. Journal of Urology 118: 13 (1977).

Chapter XVIII

Male Infertility

Males are responsible for at least 40% of all infertile marriages. An infertile male who presents with a varicocele, a potentially correctable mechanical obstruction, or non-obstructive moderately impaired spermatogenesis has a good chance of improving his fertility with modern surgical or medical treatment. Most other infertile men, who have more severely impaired spermatogenesis or uncorrectable mechanical obstructions, are not usually sufficiently improved by any form of treatment.

Aetiology

Idiopathic Infertility: This is the most common cause and results from unknown defects in spermatogenesis.

Infective Causes of Infertility: Rarely, mumps and Coxsackie viruses produce such a severe orchitis that gross ischaemia of the testis results. A testicular gumma is extremely rare.

Undescended, Abnormal or Traumatised Testes: The testis may be:

1) Congenitally hypoplastic
2) Still undescended
3) Ischaemically damaged during attempts to place it in the scrotum or as a result of other surgical or non-surgical trauma.

These causes of infertility are discussed in more detail in chapters I and XIV.

Varicocele: A varicocele decreases the motility of the sperm (p. 72) and usually results in the formation of many tapered types.

Obstruction to the Flow of Semen: This can vary from obstruction of the efferent ductules of the testis, which is not surgically correctable, to simple strictures of the vas deferens which may be. Urethral strictures and phimosis, if severe, will inhibit the flow of the thicker semen to a greater degree than urine.

Incompetent Bladder Neck: Congenital or acquired incompetence of the bladder neck (p. 250) may result in retrograde ejaculation and subsequent infertility.

Drugs: Cyclophosphamide and sulphasalazine, used to treat ulcerative colitis, are only 2 of many drugs which are known to inhibit spermatogenesis. If possible a choice of drug therapy which does not produce infertility should be made.

Hyperthermia: Raising the temperature of the scrotum by living in hot climates or wearing warm, tight, underwear may inhibit spermatogenesis and reduce sperm motility.

Severe General Illness: All serious illnesses inhibit spermatogenesis and usually cause a partial impotence and this is particularly evident in Cushing's syndrome, paraplegia and diabetes mellitus.

Chromosomal Abnormalities: The genotype XXY results in Klinefelter's syndrome (see later).

Gonadotrophin Deficiency: This is uncommon but may result from abnormalities of the pituitary gland or hypothalamic areas.

Investigation

The couple should be interviewed together. An adequate history includes details concerning the wife's fertility, general health and attitude towards pregnancy and adoption.

History Taking

The patient's past and present history of pubertal development, fertility, mumps, venereal disease, genitalia, abdominal or pelvic trauma, tuberculosis, occupations, type of underclothes and exposure to irradiation must be known, together with the details concerning any previous investigations or treatment. Details concerning libido, erection, penetration, orgasm and frequency of intercourse should be noted. The patient's sense of smell and vision should be questioned in view of a possible pituitary or hypothalamic disorder.

Physical Examination

In addition to a full general examination, including a chemical and microscopic examination of the urine, particular attention is given to the aspects discussed below.

The Body Appearance. *Klinefelter's syndrome:* Mental retardation, a 'straight across' hairline, gynaecomastia, small soft testes, a female distribution of pubic hair and long limbs are characteristic of the syndrome. A chromosomal karyotype will reveal the XXY genotype.

Cushing's syndrome: A moon face, cervical hump, hirsutism, obesity and purple abdominal striae are common findings, together with the high excretion levels of free urinary cortisol (normally less than 330mmol/day).

The External Genitalia and the Prostate Gland: The genitalia and prostate gland are examined to assess the size, shape and position of the testes and appendages and to detect the presence of abnormalities such as prostatitis, phimosis, hypospadias, epispadias, Peyronie's disease or evidence of previous trauma to this area or to the abdomen or pelvis.

Olfactory and Optic Function: These senses should be tested to detect a possible pituitary or hypothalamic lesion.

Special Investigations

Semen Analysis: At least 2 specimens should be examined by an expert with a continuing interest and involvement in the problem of male infertility. The specimen is obtained by masturbation or coitus interruptus, after sexual abstinence for 1 week, and ejaculated into a sterile plastic container. Semen coagulates within 25 minutes but liquifies after the next 25 minutes. The specimen should be examined as soon as is possible after ejaculation. The following characteristics of the specimen are noted.

Volume: The normal volume is between 1 and 5ml. As previously indicated the semen volume is derived mostly from the seminal vesicles and a low volume indicates possible disease (e.g. tuberculosis) in this area.

Sperm Count: The normal value is 20 to 200 million per ml. The presence of one sperm in a semen analysis count can, medico-legally, be taken as evidence of fertility, but few patients with a sperm count of less than 5 million per ml are helped by any form of therapy.

Sperm Morphology: Although 85% of the sperm in a normal semen ejaculation are normal 15% exhibit large heads, double heads, taper forms or some other abnormality. The lower the sperm count the greater the percentage of such abnormal forms.

Sperm Motility: If the specimen is examined within the first hour following ejaculation then 70% of the sperm should be motile. A varicocele inhibits motility.

Fructose Estimation: A low or absent fructose level indicates a deficiency of seminal vesicle volume and/or function.

Review of Evidence

On the evidence provided by the history, physical examination and semen analysis the patient can be put into one of 5 infertile groups:

Group 1	Azoospermic or severely oligospermic (less than 2 million sperms per ml) with very small testes
Group 2	Azoospermic or severely oligospermic Klinefelter's or Cushing syndrome patients
Group 3	Azoospermic with normal or moderately small testes
Group 4	Oligospermic with normal or moderately small testes
Group 5	Normal findings.

Group 1 usually does not justify any further investigation or treatment and the couple should be told that, because of microscopic changes within the male testes, the husband is not capable of fertilisation but that he is otherwise healthy.

In Group 2 the spermatogenesis of Klinefelter's syndrome is usually so impaired that no treatment is of value. Primary Cushing's syndrome-induced oligospermia can usually be helped by surgical excision of the abnormal adrenal tissue (p. 374).

Groups, 3, 4 and 5 require further investigation.

Further Investigations   **Testicular Biopsy:** This is more kindly performed under general anaesthesia and the bilateral specimens placed in Bouin's fluid, which enables a more accurate histological study to be than does formalin preservation.

The biopsy may show:

1. *Normal spermatogenesis and normal Leydig cells with or without tubular blockage (20% of patients)*
This is suggestive of an obstructive cause (fig. 279); a vaso-seminal-vesiculogram (vasography) may indicate the site of obstruction but will not indicate occlusion of the efferent ductules. If the vas deferens, seminal vesicles and ejaculatory duct are unobstructed then a vaso-epididymostomy by-pass operation may overcome an obstruction in the body or tail of the epididymis, provided that the efferent ductules are normal, but the results of joining one large tube (the vas deferens) to a number of smaller tubes (the head of the epididymis) are poor. By contrast, the results of excising a simple obstruction in the vas deferens and rejoining the two healthy vas ends, using an operating microscope, are excellent.

2. *Poor spermatogenesis with normal Leydig cells (25% of patients)*
This is termed germinal cell arrest (fig. 279). If there are reduced levels of follicle stimulating hormone (see later) then spermatogenesis may be improved by giving human gonadotrophins (2000-5000 units of human chorionic gonadotrophin 3 times per week or 60-80 units of human follicle-stimulating hormone [human menopausal gonadotrophin] in combination). Clomiphene citrate (50mg per day for 3 months) may also assist spermatogenesis.

3. *Sloughed germinal epithelium with normal Leydig cells (45% of patients)*
This is the most common biopsy finding in infertile men (fig. 279). The tubules are filled with sloughed epithelia. Some spermatogenesis may be achieved by giving androgens (1.5mg of methyl testosterone per day for 3 months). This therapy suppresses normal spermatogenesis by inhibiting pituitary gonadotrophin secretion. Cessation of the testosterone may result in a 'rebound' rise of sperm production. Mesterolone (25mg 4 times a day) is an androgen which does not inhibit pituitary function and may also be of value, as may clomiphene citrate, thyroid extract or cortisone.

4. *Germinal cell aplasia or,*

5. *A fibrosed, atrophic testis with little, if any, functioning tissue*
There is no treatment available for these patients and many of them do not require a testicular biopsy in order to make this diagnosis. The aetiology of germinal cell aplasia is unknown but a fibrosed atrophied testis often results from trauma or infection (mumps).

279 Normal and abnormal spermatogenesis.

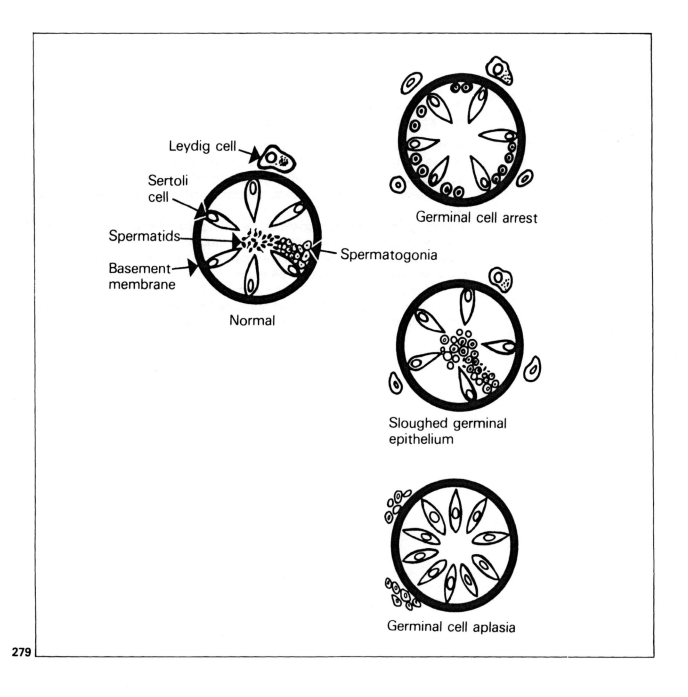

Leydig cell

Sertoli cell

Spermatids

Basement membrane

Spermatogonia

Normal

Germinal cell arrest

Sloughed germinal epithelium

Germinal cell aplasia

Table I. Serum hormonal levels in male infertility and the likely response to treatment

Hormone	Level	Response potential
Follicle-stimulating hormone	Normal	May respond to androgen or clomiphene citrate
Luteinising hormone	Normal	
Testosterone	Normal	
Follicle-stimulating hormone	High	Usually nil
Luteinising hormone	Normal	
Testosterone	Normal	
Follicle-stimulating hormone	High	Nil
Luteinising hormone	High	
Testosterone	Low	
Follicle-stimulating hormone	Low	Nil
Luteinising hormone	Low	
Testosterone	Low	

Further Review of Evidence

The testicular biopsy results, taken in conjunction with the previous findings, allow the identification of 3 groups of patients:

1) An obstructed group: The testicular biopsy investigation and the associated vasography, when indicated, may have suggested a potentially correctable obstruction and an attempted surgical correction may follow.
2) Germinal aplasia and testicular fibrosis: there is no treatment for this group.
3) Oligospermia with poor spermatogenesis ± sloughing: As indicated this is the largest group and may benefit from drug or other therapy and advice. Before beginning drug therapy an estimation of the patient's gonadotrophin and testosterone levels should be made; normal male values are shown in chapter III tables II and III. The levels should be estimated on at least two separate occasions. Estimation of hormone levels can be of help with both the prognosis and the choice of treatment (table I).

Other Considerations in the Management of Male Infertility

Undescended Testes: These should be brought down into the scrotum before the age of 5 years (p. 349).

Severe Orchitis: This may require several tissue tension-relieving incisions through the tunica albuginea in order to prevent gross ischaemia (p. 71)

Varicocele Ligation: As indicated earlier a varicocele may decrease the motility of the sperm as well as altering their morphology. Ligation of the varicocele (p. 72) results in an improved semen analysis in 60% of patients (Rodriguez-Rigou et al., 1978).

Urethral Stricture and Phimosis Surgery: This may aid the urethral transmission and release of the semen. See chapters X (p. 254) and XIV (p. 348).

Reducing Scrotal Temperature: An improvement in spermatogenesis may follow the move from a warm to a cooler climate and/or from wearing cooler, looser, underclothing.

Surgical Reconstruction of an Incompetent Bladder Neck: The results of such attempted surgery are extremely disappointing.

Emotional and Psychological Considerations: As the majority of cases of male infertility come from the group of patients who have more severely impaired spermatogenesis or uncorrectable mechanical obstructions, and are not usually significantly improved by any form of therapy, their investigation and suggested treatment must always acknowledge this fact. At no stage should over-investigation or over-optimistic estimates of likely results of treatment be given to the couple. Their personal relationships are more important than an unhelpful and expensive academic pursuit of the precise aetiological factor, explained in such a way that the couple become convinced that the male partner is abnormal.

Reference

Rodriguez-Rigou, L.J; Smith, K.D. and Steinberger, E.: Relationship of varicocele to sperm output and fertility of male partners in infertile couples. Journal of Urology 120: 691 (1978).

Further Reading

Amelar, R.D.: Infertility in Men (Davis, Philadelphia 1966).
Jenkins, I.L. and Blacklock, N.J.: Experience with vasovasostomy: operative technique. British Journal of Urology 51: 43 (1979).
Mancini, R.E. and Martini, L.: Male Fertility and Sterility (Academic Press, New York 1974).
Silber, S.J.; Galle, J. and Friend, D.: Microscopic vasovasostomy and spermatogenesis. Journal of Urology 117: 299 (1977).

Chapter XIX

Venereal and Non-venereal Diseases and Discharges

The word 'venery' is derived from two sources, the Latin *venari*, 'to hunt' and from Venus, and meaning the pursuit of sexual pleasure.

Venereal disease is increasing. A careful clinical and laboratory assessment must be performed so that the causative agent can be determined. The recent emergence of penicillinase-producing *Neisseria gonorrhoea* emphasises the importance of accurate diagnosis and adequate therapy. Males commonly present with a discharge or ulceration but 60% of women with gonorrhoea display no obvious symptoms and 50% of all patients with syphilis are also asymptomatic or have minimal symptoms initially.

The identity of recent sexual contacts must be established so that they too may be examined to exclude the presence of infection. It is often necessary to treat the sexual contacts even if proof of infection cannot be found. Multiple and recurrent infections are not unusual.

Public health education, pre and post sexual hygiene, contraceptive vaginal foam, prophylactic chemotherapy and the use of condoms are important factors in the prevention of venereal disease.

Clinical Presentation

Patients may present with:

1) *Urethritis, vaginitis, pharyngitis and proctitis*
The most common symptoms of sexually transmitted disease are those of urethritis and vaginitis although these symptoms are not always due to sexually contracted disease. The discharge may be associated with irritation, dysuria (p. 154), pruritis and dyspareunia.
2) *Ulcers and nodules of the genitalia, oral cavity or rectum*
Although rare, syphilis is the most important exlcusion diagnosis because of its serious systemic effects. Not all ulcers or nodules of the genitalia, oral cavity or rectum are caused by venereal disease and malignancy must always be considered as a possible diagnosis.

Infective and Inflammatory Discharges

Gonorrhoea

Table I lists the causes of infective and inflammatory urethral and vaginal discharges.

Neisseria gonorrhoea is transmitted by sexual contact. This may produce urethral, vaginal, cervical, rectal or pharyngeal infection and is followed by a prolific, yellow, purulent discharge 4 to 10 days later. Further extension of the disease, either locally (prostatitis, epididymitis) or generally (arthritis, meningitis, endocarditis), is now rare because of early diagnosis and treatment.

Diagnosis: The urethral discharge is examined unstained in normal saline to detect trichomonal infection (p. 83). Gram and methylene blue stains are then prepared to detect *N. gonorrhoea*, recognised by its characteristic Gram-negative, intracellular, kidney-shaped, diplococci appearance.

Table I. The causes of infective and inflammatory urethral and vaginal discharges

Patient group	Cause of discharge
Male and female (common)	Gonorrhoea Nonspecific urethritis
Female (common)	Trichomoniasis Candidiasis *Haemophilus (corynebacterium) vaginalis* Senile vaginitis Chemical vaginitis Foreign body vaginitis
Both sexes (less common)	β-haemolytic streptococci[1] *Chlamydia trachomatis,* *Treponema mycoplasma*[2] Cytomegalovirus[1,3]

1 May infect newborn.
2 May cause nonspecific urethritis.
3 May cause systemic disease e.g. mononucleosis, pneumonia.

Culture with a chocolate blood agar medium, in an atmosphere of 10% CO_2, may be necessary in cases where the diagnosis is doubtful. Swabs and scrapings of urethral, vaginal, cervical, pharyngeal and rectal mucosal lesions are similarly examined. This should establish the diagnosis although it may be difficult in asymptomatic adult females and children, where a precautionary swab of the endocervical region and the vulva should be taken in all suspected contacts. The identification of penicillinase-producing *N. gonorrhoea* calls for specialised laboratory experience.

Complications of Gonorrhoea. *Epididymitis:* This is the most common complication and occurs in 2% of patients.

Para-urethral duct inflammation, abscess formation and prostatitis: These are all now uncommon complications because of earlier diagnosis and treatment.

Chronic gonorrhoea: In our society this is uncommon in males but commonly occurs in women patients, producing salpingitis and often sterility. Although gonorrhoea in females may cause dysuria and a vaginal discharge it is often asymptomatic.

Urethral stricture: Gonococcal strictures occur 2 months or more after infection and are usually situated in the anterior urethra. They are now rare.

Treatment. *Prophylaxis:* Benzathine penicillin (2.4 million units intramuscularly) and the use of a condom will prevent infection. Routine antenatal screening for both gonorrhoea and syphilis is essential (see later).

Established infections: N. gonorrhoea is very sensitive to most antibiotics and combined therapy, using 1.5 million units of intramuscular penicillin daily for 3 days, with probenecid, 2.5g, 30 minutes before each injection, is usually curative although penicillinase-producing *N. gonorrhoeae* have been detected in increasing numbers since 1976. At present there are two identifiable strains of penicillinase-producing organism, one in Southeast Asia and one in West Africa, both areas where the incidence of gonorrhoea has always been high. The Vietnam war, greatly increased international tourist air travel, increased promiscuity and homosexuality, poor quality control of antibiotic prescribing and inadequate therapy (Editorial, 1977) have combined to favour both the development and spread of these penicillin-resistant strains.

Spectinomycin cures 95% of penicillinase-producing *N. gonorrhoea* infections but because of its high cost its beneficial effects are denied many patients; however kanamycin and chloramphenicol are far less expensive drugs which are almost as effective.

Most treated patients continue to have a progressively diminishing non-infective clear white urethral discharge for some months. Proof of cure is essential and is established by examining this discharge, or the affected area, for the absence of gonococci 7 days after cessation of drug treatment. If the combined penicillin-probenecid therapy suggested above has failed to achieve a cure then the presence of penicillinase-producing organisms must be suspected and urethral or endocervical smears forwarded to an appropriate laboratory for accurate diagnosis.

In recent years there has been a trend away from prescribing penicillin by injection for established gonorrhoeal infections. This has the double disadvantage that alternative oral antibiotics may not be taken correctly and that associated unrecognised syphilis may persist (see later).

Nonspecific Uethritis

This is an increasingly common cause of urethral discharge and may exist in conjunction with a gonorrhoeal infection. In our community it now accounts for approximately 60% of cases of urethral discharge in male patients. The discharge may be accompanied by dysuria and a varying degree of urethral discomfort.

Aetiology: Although the cause is difficult to detect in most cases, *Chlamydia trachomatis* (the so-called TRIC agent which also causes trachoma) is the causative organism in at least 40% of patients , with *Treponema mycoplasma* as an occasional finding.

Diagnosis: Cell culture techniques may be employed to detect the *C. trachomatis* organism but the diagnosis is often assumed after the exclusion of other infections such as gonorrhoea and trichomoniasis.

Treatment: Tetracycline, 500mg 6-hourly, for 2 weeks, is administered to the patient and the sexual partner or partners. Tetracyclines should never be given during the first 4 months of pregnancy; erythromycin is equally effective and does not stain fetal teeth.

Complications. *Epididymitis:* As with gonorrhoea approximately 2% of patients with nonspecific urethritis develop an associated epididymitis.

Stricture: Hancock (1959) has estimated that 4% of patients with non-specific urethritis develop a urethral stricture.

Reiter's disease: Approximately 2% of patients will develop associated polyarthritis and iritis (Catterall and Nicol, 1976).

Trichomoniasis

This is a common infestation and patients present with vaginitis, urethritis and, occasionally, prostatitis, The parasite can be acquired by direct contact with infected objects and does not necessarily result from sexual intercourse. The incubation period is approximately 1 week.

Diagnosis: The pear-shaped organism with its 4 flagella is easily identified by taking a sample of the vaginal discharge, mixing it with normal saline, and then, using a coverslip, examining the preparation under a microscope. In males the parasite is best demonstrated by swab scraping a specimen from just inside the external urinary meatus. There is considerable evidence to suggest that the parasite is present in all men whose female partners are infected (Catterall and Nicol, 1976).

Treatment: Metronidazole 200mg, 3 times a day for 1 week, is given to both the patient and the sexual partner or partners. The topical organic mercurial, hydrargaphen, 2 pessaries at night for 2 weeks, is used for those few patients who do not respond to metronidazole therapy.

Candidiasis

Infection with the yeast-like *Candida albicans* is common and although pruritis, with a 'cheesey' discharge, is common there may be no symptoms. Candidal infection is often associated with diabetes mellitus, pregnancy, chemotherapy or chronic illnesses and the use of antibiotics which may suppress the growth of other organisms which normally prevent *C. albicans* from becoming invasive. The infection is also thought to be more common among women taking oral contraceptives but this has not always been demonstrable (Goldacre et al., 1979).

In males candidal infection results in a balanitis with a reddening and irritation of the glans penis, particularly after sexual intercourse.

Diagnosis: The fungal spores or hyphae are detected either in a saline preparation of the vaginal discharge or in a scraping of the glans or prepuce. Diagnostic difficulty may require a Gram stain film or culture of the fungus in Sabouraud's medium.

Treatment: As indicated, known causes should be corrected. One nystatin vaginal pessary is inserted morning and evening for 3 weeks and the pathological examination is then repeated. Sexual intercourse should not take place during this treatment period.

Resistant organisms are uncommon but usually respond to alternate day painting of the vagina with 0.5% gentian violet for 2 weeks. If there are recurrent infections a careful search for the source, including the patient's intestinal tract, external genitalia, fingers and sexual partner, should be made. Intestinal infections are treated with nystatin oral tablets and skin infections with nystatin cream or powder.

Haemophilus Vaginitis

Haemophilus vaginitis is not transmitted by sexual contact but produces a malodorous grey discharge which may be confused with venereal disease. The vaginal squamous cells, covered with *Haemophilis vaginalis* organisms, are easily identified from a saline preparation of the discharge. The organism commonly inhabits the vagina and treatment is only required if there is excessive contamination.

Treatment: Ampicillin, 500mg 4 times a day for 7 days and in resistant cases 1 neomycin suppository, inserted high into the vagina each evening before retiring, for 10 days, usually resolves the infection. Topical triple sulphonamide cream is of value in ampicillin-resistant cases.

Senile Vaginitis

The occasional highly purulent but non-infective discharge of an atrophic vaginal mucosa may also be confused with venereal disease.

Treatment: Dienoestrol cream (two applicators-full per day) administered intra-vaginally for 2 weeks, with a variable maintenance dose, is usually effective. The vulval and introital pruritis is treated with topical applications of the cream.

Chemical Vaginitis

Chemical lubricant aids for sexual intercourse, vaginal douches, medicated soaps and antiseptic solutions, particularly when used excessively, may result in a non-infected discharge.

Treatment: The cause should be identified and eliminated; temporary relief of the discomfort may be gained from the use of 1% hydrocortisone cream and sedation.

Foreign Body Vaginitis

The occasional presence of a foreign body causing vaginitis (p. 352) emphasises the necessity for a thorough physical examination of all patients, of all ages presenting with a vaginal discharge.

Summary

1) A full history and a thorough general examination is necessary, particularly in relationship to previous genitourinary pathology and the possible source of the present infection.
2) Gonorrhoeal discharges are yellow in colour while those from other causes, or partly treated gonorrhoea, are greyish white.
3) A saline specimen of the discharge should be examined microscopically and Trichomonas, Candida and/or *Haemophilis vaginalis* infection confirmed or excluded. A second discharge specimen is Gram stained and cultured and this should enable the identification of *Neisseria gonorrhoea.* Nonspecific urethritis and senile vaginitis are usually diagnosed by exclusion, although cell cultures may detect *Chlamydia trachomatis.*
4) The medical management of venereal and non-venereal discharges involves:

a) educating the public about the spread, morbidity and mortality of venereal disease
b) accurately detecting and adequately treating the causative agent
c) treating all sexual contacts
d) mature handling of the often delicate personal and matrimonial situation.

Ulcers and Nodules of the Genitalia

Many venereal diseases cause genital ulceration or nodules (table II); apart from syphilis and herpes, other causes are rare in most non-tropical developed countries, although they have become more common with increasing international travel.

Syphilis

Treponema pallidum causes syphilis, with an incubation period of between 2 and 4 weeks. The early infective lesion begins as a red papule which usually ulcerates. The ulcer is painless and, if small and transient, may not concern the victim sufficiently for him, or her, to seek medical advice. The inguinal lymph nodes become rubbery but not tender. The secondary manifestations of the disease develop approximately 2 months after the original infection and consist of dull red skin lesions and macula and ulcerated mucosal lesions, together with fever, falling hair, lymphadenopathy and general malaise. Rarely, jaundice may occur. The mucosal lesions, in particular, are highly infectious.

Diagnosis: The detection of *T. pallidum* by dark-field microscopic examination of scrapings from the ulcers or from an endocervical swab is usually diagnostic if an adequate specimen is taken. Serological tests for syphilis are usually negative when the ulcer first appears but rapidly become positive.

Reagin or non-treponemal tests: The Wassermann reaction has now been replaced by the Venereal Diseases Reference Laboratory test (VDRL).

Specific or treponemal tests: The VDRL test is usually diagnostic but, when the diagnosis is not clear, other specific tests are necessary. These include, the treponemal pallidum haemagglutination test (TPHA); the fluorescent treponemal antibody-absorbed test (FTA-ABS) and the treponemal pallidum immobilisation test (TPI).

Treatment. *Prophylaxis:* Benzathine penicillin 2.4 million units intramuscularly, and the use of a condom.

Table II. Some features of ulcerative venereal diseases commoner in tropical countries

Feature	Chancroid	Lymphogran-uloma venereum	Granuloma inguinale	Balano-posthitis
Causative agent	*Haemophilus ducreyi* (Ducrey's bacillus)	Chlamydia bacterium	*Calymmato-bacterium granulomatis*	*Borrelia refringens*
Incubation period	2-9 days	2-20 days	2-3 months	2-7 days
Genital appearance	Macule-papule, then the formation of an ulcer	Papule or macule	Superficial ulcer	Single or multiple ulcerations which fuse and spread
Pain	Very painful	None	Little	Very painful
Inguinal involvement	Usually enlarged and tender	Becomes matted 4 weeks after infection and then suppurates with multiple sinuses	Nil	Slight tender enlargement
Diagnosis	Skin test, stained smear, culture or biopsy	Frei test and complement fixation test	Stained organisms in scrapings from ulcer or biopsy	Spirochetes and fusiform bacilli on dark-field examination or stained smear

Treatment Tetracycline, 500mg 6-hourly for 2 weeks (all conditions)

Established infection: Procaine penicillin 600,000 units, intramuscularly, daily for 8 days.

Herpes Genitalis

Herpes simplex virus type I commonly infects the face, particularly the lips but may also infect the genitalia. Herpes simplex virus type II *(Herpes genitalis)* invasion results from sexual intercourse and infects the genitalia but oral sexual intercourse can result in transfer of the infection. The incidence of herpes genitalis is increasing at a rapid rate. The incubation period of the virus is unknown. Multiple superficial vesicles form on the prepuce, glans, cervix, vagina or vulva and rapidly coalesce to form superficial ulcers, which usually heal spontaneously with minimal discomfort. The inguinal lymph nodes are not involved and the condition tends to become recurrent.

Diagnosis: Active herpes lesions are highly contagious and every care should be taken to avoid contracting the serious complications of herpetic conjunctivitis and opthalmia during diagnostic examination. Cell culture of the virus is diagnostic but it is essential that syphilis and other ulcerative-nodular lesions of the genitalia be excluded.

Treatment. *Prophylaxis:* There is no cure for recurrent herpes and in modern society the importance of sexual hygiene, contraceptive vaginal foam and a prophylactic condom must be stressed.

Established infections: Reassurance and local analgesic ointment can be of help. The patient should be told that the condition commonly recurs and that sexual partners should be informed and prophylactic precautions taken. Idoxuridine painted on the lesion at frequent intervals at the prodromal stage (Platts, 1980) can help, but has not been shown to prevent recurrence. Jose and Minty (1980) reported improvement in recurrence rates of genital herpes in patients taking oral levamisole. Other new anti-herpes drugs, such as acyclovir, are being tested clinically.

Differential Diagnosis: Any ulcer or nodule on the genitalia should suggest the possibility of syphilis or a carcinoma. Herpes is not uncommon; occasionally scabies forms genital papules, but there is always a history of nocturnal pruritis and the mite is generally easily identified by its characteristic burrows beneath the skin. Scabies is treated by twice daily showering and the daily application of gamma benzene hexachloride cream.

Table II sets out the characteristic features of chancroid, lymphogranuloma venereum and granuloma inguinale, which because of the increase in air travel, are now occasionally seen outside endemic areas. Balanoposthitis (erosive balanitis) occasionally occurs in elderly, debilitated males.

Pregnancy and Sexually Transmitted Diseases

Sexually transmitted diseases can persist or occur during pregnancy and routine antenatal screening is mandatory. Any patient with such a history or suspicion should be carefully examined throughout the pregnancy and specifically tested for infection in the last month. This particularly applies to syphilis, gonorrhoea, haemophilis vaginitis, β-haemolytic stretpcoccal and cytomegalovirus infections.

References

Editorial: Control of penicillinase producing gonococci. British Medical Journal 1: 1618 (1977).

Deture, F.A.; Drylic, D.M.; Kaufman, H.E. and Centifanto, Y.M.: Herpes virus type II: Study of semen in male subjects with recurrent infections. Journal of Urology 120: 499 (1978).

Goldacre, M.J.; Watt, B.; London, N.; Milne, L.J.R.; London, J.D.O. and Vessey, M.P.: Vaginal microbial flora in normal young women. British Medical Journal, 1: 1450-1453 (1979).

Hancock, J.A.H.: Relationship between relapsing non-gonococcal urethritis in the male and urethral stricture. Urologia Internationalis 9: 258 (1959).

Jose, D.G. and Minty, C.C.J.: Levamisole in patients with recurrent herpes infection. Medical Journal of Australia 2: 390 (1980).

Oriel, J.D.; Reve, P.; Powis, A.P.; Miller, A. and Nicol, C.S.: Chlamydial infection. Isolation of chlamydia from patients with nonspecific genital infections. British Journal of Venereal Diseases 48: 429 (1972).

Platts, W.M.: Sexually transmissible diseases; in Avery (Ed) Drug Treatment, p. 1169 (Adis Press, Sydney 1980).

Segura, J.W.; Smith, T.F.; Weed, L.S. and Pellersen, G.R.: Chlamydia and non-specific urethritis. Journal of Urology 117: 720 (1977).

Further Reading

Catterall, R.D. and Nichol, C.S. Sexually Transmitted Diseases (Academic Press, New York, 1976).

Schofield, C.B.S.: Sexually Transmitted Diseases (Churchill-Livingstone, Edinburgh 1972).

Symposium on Venereal Diseases, Medical Clinics of North America 56: 1057 (1972).

Chapter XX

Impotence and Ejaculation Problems

These problems are common. Impotence and premature ejaculation generally result from psychological difficulties and require expert counselling.

The development of modern penile prostheses has greatly assisted many impotent patients but a careful assessment of both the patient and the prosthesis is necessary before proceeding with such surgery.

Impotence

Impotence implies failure either to achieve penile erection or to maintain an erection during or after vaginal penetration.

This definition is independent of the female response which may vary from full orgasm in the presence of male impotence to indifference in the presence of full erection, penetration and ejaculation. Although commonly occurring together, a distinction should be made between decreased libido due to low secretion of testosterone, and psychological, drug-induced, neurogenic, vascular, hormonal and other causes (fig. 280) inhibiting or preventing penile erection or ejaculation; only thus can specific therapy be offered.

The mechanism of penile erection and maintenance is discussed on page 66. Mental, visual, penile, touch, auditory and olfactory efferent stimuli may result in parasympathetic S2,3,4 cholinergic dilatation of the 3 corpora arteries. Ejaculation is dependent upon a normally functioning T12-L2 sympathetic nervous system (Hotchkiss, 1970) and is reinforced by the adrenal release of adrenaline and noradrenaline.

The external emission of semen depends on the presence of anatomically normal pathways and S2,3,4 contraction of the bulbocavernosus and ischiocavernosus muscles and the pelvic floor.

An orgasm represents the pleasurable consequences of the total sensations occurring at the climax of ejaculation and emission.

Impotence may be partial or total and may have lasted for a lifetime or several months. The incidence is difficult to assess but independent questioning in the author's practice indicates that 1 in 500 males between the ages of 20 and 60 years experience some periods of at least partial mostly psychological impotence lasting 1 month or more.

Investigation

Patients presenting with impotence require a detailed past and present medical and social history taking, with emphasis placed on previous and present sexual difficulties and interests, venereal disease, drug therapy, and any serious medical or surgical past or present history such as diabetes mellitus or undescended testis operations. Penile shaft fracture is discussed on page 68.

In the physical examination special attention is given to the nervous system, testicular size, androgenic characteristics, alcohol-related symptoms and a urine chemical examination to detect the presence of sugar.

If an androgen deficiency is suspected the serum prolactin (normal — less than 10mg/ml), serum follicle stimulating hormone, luteinising hormone and testosterone levels are measured to accurately determine the site and severity of the condition (see chapter III table II).

Noctural penile tumescence can be measured in those patients who deny that it occurs by the use of mercury-filled strain gauges which record changes in penile circumference. The normal 30-year-old male has 3 mocturnal erections each night with partial tumescence occurring in up to 30% of his total sleeping time. Nocturnal penile tumescence tracings in those patients with organic impotence show reduced or absent tumescence with smaller than normal penile circumference changes while those patients with psychological impotence have normal tracings. Such findings often clarify the aetiology and assist in the management (Moss, 1979).

Aetiology and Management

Psychological Causes: The vast majority of patients presenting with impotence have a psychological cause resulting from past or present personal relationships, or sexual or work stress situations. Almost all of these patients experience early morning erections and some are able to have sexual intercourse with other partners.

Psychological counselling: Expert psychological counselling of both partners is often successful in identifying and allowing discussion of the cause (Haslam, 1978). This approach is not likely to be successful if the female partner will not cooperate. In recent years surrogate therapy has been popularised but, although it may achieve erection, penetration and ejaculation, it has very little to offer in terms of establishing a better personal relationship for the particular couple.

Penile implant prostheses: Many impotent patients have now been treated with a permanent or removable silastic penile prosthesis (Pearman, 1972; Scott et al., 1973) and such aids have been developed to include sophisticated 'blow-up' permanently implanted prostheses. It is essential that a careful assessment of both the patient and the prosthesis is made before proceeding with such surgery.

Drug therapy: Patients are always receptive to the idea that impotence may respond to drug treatment but, other than by increasing libido and providing some psychological benefit, it is rarely of value.

Some response may be achieved by androgen replacement therapy (weekly injections of testosterone enanthate, 250mg), if the serum testosterone has been shown to be lower than 10mmol per litre. However, this form of treatment is not free from side effects including jaundice, liver neoplasm, polycythaemia and raised serum cholesterol. Drug replacement therapy is also occasionally of value in those few cases of impotence resulting from disordered hormonal activity (see later).

Drug-induced and Organic Causes: Alcholism is a common cause of impotence as it:

1) Diminishes awareness and libido
2) Inhibits nerve pathways
3) Causes permanent liver and brain damage.

Alcohol-induced impotence may persist for several months after drinking has ceased.

Antihypertensives and antidepresasnts are among the drugs which commonly contribute to or cause impotence. These are listed in figure 280, and as will be seen, many of them act at more than one site.

Neurological and vascular disorders, severe illnesses, and endocrine disorders such as hyperprolactinaemia, hypogonadism, hypothyroidism and hyperthyroidism may also cause partial or complete impotence. Liver disease may raise the serum oestrogen levels and thereby decrease the libido. Radical pelvic surgery, pelvic trauma and congenital or acquired genital abnormalities may result in erection or ejaculatory difficulites or both.

Indentification of an organic cause of impotence, or a change of prescription when it is drug-induced may lead to recovery but often this is not possible and supportive functional therapy is subsituted.

Prognosis

As previously discussed the prognosis depends on the aetiology.

Complete impotence since puberty, whatever the cause, rarely responds to any therapy but partial psychological impotence, due to emotional stress, responds well. Organic impotence due to severe neurological or vascular causes rarely responds to therapy but alcoholic or other drug-induced partial impotence responds well when the causative agent is withdrawn.

Ejaculation Problems

Premature Ejaculation

This condition, often associated with a highly excitable, anxious, personality responds well to psychological counselling with associated advice concerning sexual technique (Clarke and Clarke, 1979).

Failure to Ejaculate

This may be due to congenital or acquired failure of the bladder outlet to occlude during orgasm, to disordered sympathetic ganglia (e.g. the use of ganglion-blocking drugs), or to a congenital or acquired stenosis of the ejaculatory ducts. If semen enters the bladder it can be recovered and, once concentrated, used for artificial insemination.

Haemospermia

This is a not uncommon problem and usually greatly concerns the patient but, in the presence of a normal physical examination, including a detailed examination of a prostatic gland massage specimen (chapter V; page 159), the condition can be assumed to be due to rupture of a seminal vesicle, prostatic or posterior urethral blood vessel and does not require further investigation. Abnormal physical examination findings, such as infection, or sterile inflammatory or neoplastic cells, necessitate further investigation to exclude prostatitis, tuberculosis, rarely bilharziasis or, extremely rarely, neoplasm in this area.

280 Erection and ejaculation. Mechanisms of penile erection and ejaculation and some of the factors responsible for abnormal function.

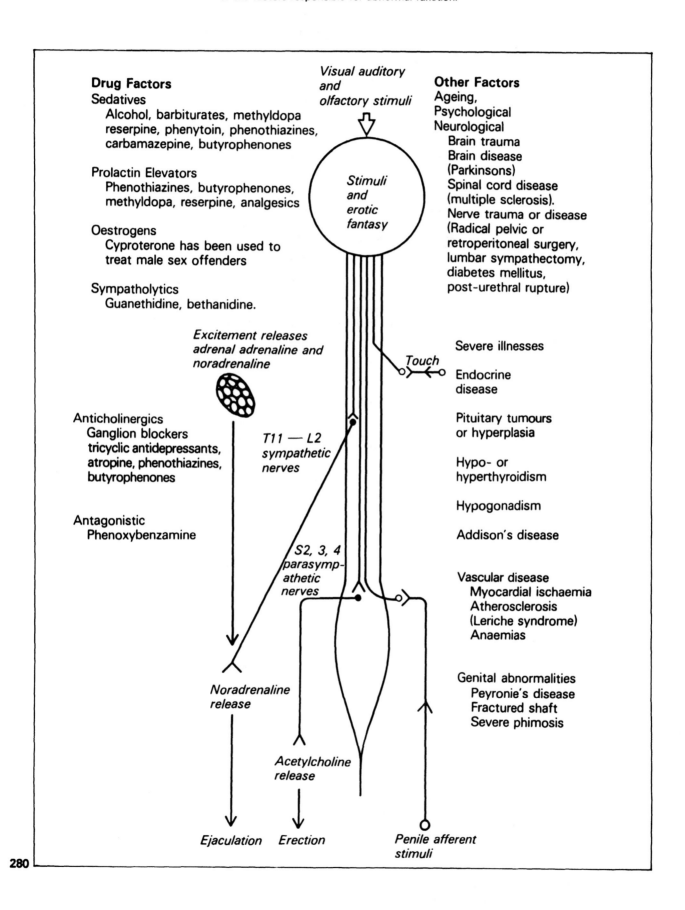

Drug Factors
Sedatives
    Alcohol, barbiturates, methyldopa
    reserpine, phenytoin, phenothiazines,
    carbamazepine, butyrophenones

Prolactin Elevators
    Phenothiazines, butyrophenones,
    methyldopa, reserpine, analgesics

Oestrogens
    Cyproterone has been used to
    treat male sex offenders

Sympatholytics
    Guanethidine, bethanidine.

*Excitement releases
adrenal adrenaline and
noradrenaline*

Anticholinergics
    Ganglion blockers
    tricyclic antidepressants,
    atropine, phenothiazines,
    butyrophenones

Antagonistic
    Phenoxybenzamine

*Visual auditory
and
olfactory stimuli*

*Stimuli
and
erotic
fantasy*

Touch

*T11 — L2
sympathetic
nerves*

*S2, 3, 4
parasymp-
athetic
nerves*

*Noradrenaline
release*

*Acetylcholine
release*

Ejaculation   *Erection*   *Penile afferent
stimuli*

Other Factors
Ageing,
Psychological
Neurological
    Brain trauma
    Brain disease
    (Parkinsons)
    Spinal cord disease
    (multiple sclerosis).
    Nerve trauma or disease
    (Radical pelvic or
    retroperitoneal surgery,
    lumbar sympathectomy,
    diabetes mellitus,
    post-urethral rupture)

Severe illnesses

Endocrine
disease

Pituitary tumours
or hyperplasia

Hypo- or
hyperthyroidism

Hypogonadism

Addison's disease

Vascular disease
    Myocardial ischaemia
    Atherosclerosis
    (Leriche syndrome)
    Anaemias

Genital abnormalities
    Peyronie's disease
    Fractured shaft
    Severe phimosis

280

Semenorrhoea

This occurs uncommonly after straining defaecation, when it is assumed that pressure on the seminal vesicles and ampulla of the vas deferns has released semen. In the presence of a normal physical examination no treatment other than reassurance is required. Occasionally patients notice a slight mucous discharge from the external meatus which is not related to any previous urethritis. This discharge does not contain sperm and possibly originates from Cowper's glands. Reassurance and regular sexual intercourse usually resolves the problem.

References

Hotchkiss, R.S.: Physiology of the male genital system as related to reproduction; in Campbell and Harrison (Eds) Urology, p.161 (Saunders, Philadelphia 1970).

Moss, D.: Nocturnal penile tumescence (NPT) monitoring in penile surgery. British Journal of Urology 51: 423 (1979).

Pearman, R.O.: Insertion of a silastic penile prosthesis for the treatment of organic sexual impotence. Journal of Urology 107: 802 (1972).

Scott, F.B.; Bradley, W.E. and Timm, G.W.: Management of erectile impotence. Use of inflatable prostheses. Urology 2: 80 (1973).

Further Reading

Clarke, M. and Clarke, D.: Sexual Joy in Marriage (Adis Press, Sydney 1979).

Haslam, M.T.: Sexual Disorders: A Practical Guide to Diagnosis and Treatment for The Non-specialist (Pitman, Melbourne 1978).

Masters, W.H. and Johnson, V.E.: Human Sexual Inadquacy (Little, Brown and Co., Boston 1970).

Subject Index

Lightning Source UK Ltd.
Milton Keynes UK
UKOW01f1616070914

238136UK00002B/4/P